THE REFLEXOLOGY

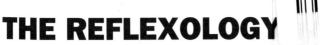

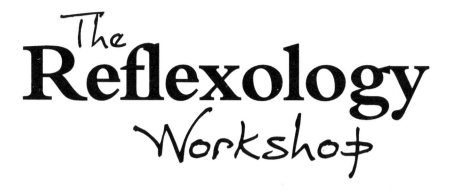

Jenny Hope-Spencer

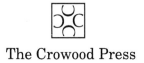

The Crowood Press

First published in 1999 by
The Crowood Press Ltd
Ramsbury, Marlborough
Wiltshire SN8 2HR

British Library Cataloguing-in-Publication Data
A catalogue record for this book is available from the British Library.

ISBN 1 86126 203 5

This book is written for the student in training in reflexology and those interested in learning more about the therapy. It is recommended that advice is sought from a professionally trained reflexologist and/or doctor before embarking on self-treatment, or before receiving treatment from an untrained practitioner. The author takes no responsibility for adverse effects experienced as a result of treatments received, or self-treatment administered, under any circumstances.

Acknowledgement
The list of the effects of excess sugar on health on page 205 is reproduced from *Lick the Sugar Habit* by Nancy Appleton © 1996. Published by Avery Publishing Group, Inc., Garden City Park, New York, 1-800-548-5757. Used by permission.

Typefaces used: Galliard and Franklin Gothic.

Typeset and designed by
D & N Publishing
Membury Business Park, Lambourn Woodlands
Hungerford, Berkshire.

Printed and bound in Great Britain by
WBC Book Manufacturers Ltd, Mid Glamorgan.

Contents

Acknowledgements

This book has been a joy and a trial to write. A joy because it has been half-written for six years and I have been itching to write it but never found the time, and a trial because of the complexity of knowing what to write in a first volume and what can wait until the next!

However, it is done and I would like to give grateful thanks to the following people: Hazel Goodwin, chairman of the Association of Reflexologists for her unstinting support and encouragement over the years I have known her; Jennifer Harrison, for writing the Foreword to this book and for her patience and support in reading one edited version after another; Jan de Planta, for her support, encouragement, undying energy in propping me up throughout writing, making suggestions, corrections and collating of material; Gail Maxted, for her dedication, energy, patience and enthusiasm in typing the anatomy and physiology; Jenny Gribble for general typing; Jane and Wim Vandeveld, who gave up their holiday, Wim for providing food and sustenance, and Jane for helping me type and edit my material; my students in training who offered to wait for further training until the book was finished; Tony Reynolds from East Dorset Drug and Alcohol Advisory Service for information on drug and alcohol misuse and to Jenny Chambers of the Birmingham Women's Hospital Obstetric Cholestasis Support Group; my friends who have not heard or seen me for months because of the pressure they knew I was under; special thanks to David Price-Goodfellow and his team at D & N Publishing for their patience, thoughtfulness, and technical expertise in designing the book, and most importantly in managing to retain a sense of humour; and last, but by no means least, the publishers for their patience and support whilst preparing the final manuscript.

To all of them, I say 'Thank you' and I hope that readers find the content encouraging, stimulating and thought-provoking with a therapy that has, to my thinking, been undervalued as a major contributor to healthcare in this country for far too long. Most importantly, I hope it can be enjoyed and used to advantage by students in training, those thinking of training, those who are thinking of having treatment or those who simply have an interest in reflexology.

Foreword

It is with feelings of pride and excitement that I have agreed to write this Foreword. For many years the nursing profession has declared an interest in patient-centred treatment and the concept of holistic care for patients and clients. With the writing of this book comes an opportunity to implement and develop these theories. Nurses have long taken the view that they know best how to care for patients and clients, indeed by the nature of their work they have a duty to provide that care. In this provision, nurses have become increasingly attracted to complementary medicine as they explore a philosophy of care that centres around the whole, unique person and not just elements of their illness or disease. This book though is not just for the benefit of health professionals, it will allow others an insight into the world of anatomy and physiology and the art of reflexology. Nurses and others, by studying this book, will gain the information required to develop this practice and to truly promote the concept of prevention and therapy.

Men and women do not live in isolation from the environment and they need to develop strategies to coexist with nature.

This book began as a result of Jenny's contribution to the art of reflexology over the last few years. She became aware of the need to inform others of the background and developments in complementary medicine. Jenny brings a depth and commitment to the work that is rarely found in writers these days. As a nurse I find this book takes me back to primary knowledge that is helpful, informative, directed and useful, as well as providing me with new knowledge on the history and development of medicine and reflexology. In this way, it is also particularly helpful for students studying reflexology for the first time or for those developing an interest from other health-care fields. If carefully read and understood, this book will enable the student to develop a breadth of knowledge that will allow them to develop their practice with integrity and commitment.

The author has drawn on her own considerable knowledge as well as historical data, and has linked theory with experience. In this way she brings complementary medicine to life for the reader. Jenny neither avoids nor oversimplifies the anatomical element of reflexology, but explores it in a way that all can understand. She thus provides a map to the primary sources of knowledge readers may wish or need in order to develop their practice. Practitioners without academic preparation can, with careful reading, improve their understanding of the key issues that will underpin the decisions in their practice. The reader is introduced to a number of historical orientations and perspectives, and Jenny demonstrates how the cultural beliefs and health practices that vary from Western medical models can be utilized in the care of the whole. Each approach is introduced with a brief historical background.

This book goes a long way to bridging the gap between the student and the practitioner, conventional and complementary believer. It will help the reader negotiate a pathway through relevant theory in a way that respects priorities and the individualistic approach to caring.

I commend this book to lay people and nurses alike in their journey along a path that will challenge, inform and develop their practice in complementary medicine and the art of caring for the whole unique being that is human.

Jennifer Harrison, SRN, DMS

There is a light that shines beyond all things on earth, beyond us all,
beyond the heavens, beyond the highest, the very highest heavens.
This is the Light that shines in our heart.

The Upanishads, Chandogya Upanishad

Introduction

I have been asked many times over the years how I came to learn reflexology. It is not so strange a story, given that when we are meant to do something, it repeatedly jumps in front of us, or taps us on the shoulder! So it was with me. In 1979 a friend wrote a letter telling me that a training school had come to England from America and would I be interested to learn and teach for them. My personal life at that time did not allow me to investigate the possibility and I dutifully ignored it. However, wherever I went about in my locality, I encountered leaflets and people who slowly enlightened me about reflexology.

In 1981 I had my first reflexology treatment. It seemed that I wasn't going to be allowed to escape this word 'reflexology'! I was amazed at the reaction – I felt ill for two days after the treatment, which showed just how much I had needed it! At about the same time, I had a friend who encouraged me to train in reflexology – he said that I would be a 'natural' as I had always enjoyed massaging feet. My mother also used to tell me repeatedly that I had 'needle' fingers when I learnt to play the piano as a child, and I began to understand how my fingers could have other helpful possibilities. As a result, I became encouraged to investigate this strange idea for myself.

Neither I, nor those close to me, had any idea where reflexology would lead me. Whenever I have considered stopping my practice, someone inevitably telephones to ask for my help with a problem and, knowing that I will probably be able to help them, I continue in the work. It seems that once you begin the 'healing pathway' you cannot step off – so be prepared if you are contemplating training in this wonderful therapy!

This was the beginning of my journey into the world of complementary medicine and associated doctrines. Over the years, I have become fascinated with the concept of the human being as an energy in motion and the interconnectedness of life and events, which has led my continuing education into training in counselling and psychotherapy. I had recognized that our emotions (emotion meaning energy-in-motion) have a direct effect upon the physical health and the emotional, mental and spiritual counterparts of the self. By helping the patient look at the reasons why they may be feeling the way they do, release of tension can be obtained from areas of the body where they are held. This, as I see it, is the way forward within holistic health-care, getting to the cause before the cause gets to the body!

WHO THIS BOOK IS WRITTEN FOR

The aim of this book is to raise awareness of how people can help themselves with a more clinical approach to reflexology, through integrating medical knowledge in the sciences of anatomy and physiology and integrated biology.

The layperson who is thinking of going to a reflexologist but is unsure of what the therapy is about, or the prospective student who may be contemplating training, or those who are already practitioners who are interested in gaining another perspective on reflexology will, hopefully, gain insight into aspects on the theory and practice of reflexology.

There are many books available on the subject of reflexology, all of which give different information and different methods of working the feet. There is no 'right' or 'wrong' way of working with reflexology – all methods will assist those seeking help. What is important is that different perspectives of the therapy are available so that the individual can compare and decide on what method of reflexology they want to receive or train in.

The Theory and Practice explained in this book has its roots in Eunice Ingham's research and methods. This amazing lady spent a good part of her life researching the practice and theory behind the therapy and has given us a valuable tool to offer others on the road to health and well-being.

THE PSYCHOLOGY OF HEALTH

Health problems can be symbolic of unconscious emotional perceptions and memories that can be 'held' as energy blocks in different parts of the body. Our culture has, for two hundred years, separated the mind, spirit and emotions from the physical body with the result that we fail to see our bodies as an integrated part of our being. Mental attitudes, feeling and emotions are a part of the whole human being, not separate entities that need to be dealt with in a compartmentalized way. As we lock these unexpressed feelings into our bodies, the key to their release is important to find before pathological disturbance sets onto the energy field,

creating specific health disorders. Through reflexology, counselling and energy-based therapies, the individual can find out why they may have created a particular problem through holding tension in an area of their body to such an extent that blood fails to reach nerve endings, with the result that the particular part eventually becomes diseased.

Reflexology, and other forms of body-work contribute to the individual reclaiming their 'wholeness' by: releasing physical tensions, so that blood flow reaches peripheral nerves and helps to keep parts of the body well supplied with oxygen and nutrients; creating contact with the world and others in feeling alive; bringing colour and humour into their lives and the lives of others; and engendering spontaneity and finding inner peace. There is insufficient space in this book to delve into the fascinating subject of the psychology behind health disorders; theories will be put forward in a further book.

THE PLACE OF REFLEXOLOGY IN SOCIETY TODAY

Reflexology has been an original method of healing and helping without the use of surgery or medication for over 5,000 years. It has its roots in Eastern philosophy, where the non-separatist understanding of life as a matrix, or interconnected web of life, has used the healing arts as the route to the wholeness of the individual.

The Western need for scientific validation as proof of effectiveness has meant that we have denied the realization that true health depends on the balance of all parts of the human psyche, not just the physical. In the East, things just *are the way they are*, without the need for validation or proof. Health-related philosophies have therefore gained a liberation that we in the West are searching to achieve in our hi-tech culture, but which a lot of time elude us because of our craving to validate and 'prove' theories of what it means to enjoy good health.

Over the last twenty years training standards and methods of practice have developed and become more sophisticated in the requirements for professional practice of reflexology. A growing understanding of the human being as an energetic, multi-layered being whose life and vitality depend on contributory life-style factors, perceptions of life-events, emotional response, mental attitudes and spiritual awareness has led to and encouraged investigation from health-care professionals and the individual into the new territory of how to keep a healthy body, mind and spirit. This growing understanding has flourished and has developed reflexology, and holistic health-care philosophies generally, into more clinical methods of practice. With increasing interest, individuals are discovering how they can aid their health disorders, feel happier and more alive, enjoy increased energy levels and calmness by the simple application of the hands working systematically over feet and hands.

More knowledge has been gained about reflexology as more people work and research with the therapy. Over the years, I have 'discovered' reflexes that add further to the general knowledge already available.

COMPLEMENTARY OR ALTERNATIVE MEDICINE?

The definition of the word 'alternative' means to be that which can be replaced. The definition of the word 'complementary' is that which completes.

In the early days of 'alternative medicine', many people had the notion that practitioners of these therapies wished to assume an 'instead of' approach to health, where the practitioner wished to take over the role of the GP or health-professional. However, practitioners wish to work *alongside* conventional medicine and we are, therefore, in essence, *complementary* to our medical friends. This word carries an important message to the public and the medical profession as there still remains some confusion of the role of complementary medicine within health-care.

Complementary practitioners wish to work with the conditions that patients present and to have a collaborative relationship with the medical profession in the care and outcomes of treatment for their patients. The people who come to holistic practitioners for help have usually tried every medical approach and are desperate to help themselves and their health problems.

Very often, practitioners refer their patients to their GP or other health-care professional and liaise with them for the best route forward for the patient. Increasingly, medical professionals are referring their patients to selected complementary practitioners for help where they recognize that conventional medication can be of no assistance. It is, therefore, every holistic health-care professional's duty to develop their knowledge to the best of their ability to gain credibility with the medical profession so that confidence in referring their patients for reflexology or other treatments is established.

The advances in medical technology and knowledge have been enormous in the last fifty years and the results in the increase in quality of health and life are manifold. Longevity has doubled over the last century, giving the last phase of life more enjoyment and quality than ever before. In enhancing this gift of a healthier life, preventative medicine has a role to play in raising the individual's awareness as to how they can remain healthier, for longer.

THE MESSAGE OF 'FLOWER-POWER'

The flower-power days of 1960s and 1970s may have carried considerable negativity with them but they may also have reflected the essence of the mood at that time, where to relax, accept and just be, heralded a new way of thinking about the individual's purpose for being alive and an expanded awareness of how we affect our health through our thoughts, feelings and emotions. Try just sitting and staring into space, or meditate – be with yourself, listen to your thoughts, feelings and body – what do they tell you? Every cell in your body has a memory and knows exactly what it has to do, every minute of your life – it has intelligence all of its own and will obey whatever messages you give it! Make sure those messages are nurturing, by telling your body and reinforcing your spirit with a desire to work for its welfare so that they will work for you into a healthy old age.

BECOMING A REFLEXOLOGIST

Becoming a complementary therapist requires the attributes of caring, patience, calmness and a genuine concern for others, as well as the self-motivation to become a self-employed person. Learning to detach from others' concerns is equally important and training in basic counselling skills is a good route to developing this attribute.

Reliability, good professional skills, an enthusiastic, positive and confident manner, and a thorough understanding of the theory and practice of reflexology will enable the newly qualified practitioner to establish a clientele in time. The most important ingredient in the profession of a complementary practitioner is to enjoy helping others. Without enjoyment in a working career, whatever it may be, generates a sense of purposelessness and a half-hearted approach that leads eventually to health-related problems for the person involved.

Very often, students are sceptical about the benefits of reflexology whilst in training, but soon realize through case studies and experience the benefits and efficacy of this wonderful and greatly undervalued healing science.

THE WAY FORWARD

Reflexology has enormous possibilities as an integrated therapy with conventional medicine – let us encourage this path by giving reverence, respect and responsibility to the ancient healers and philosophers whose knowledge has given us, what we call today, 'reflexology'.

The foundations of all complementary therapies are concerned with the senses, sensing, feelings and emotions and the building of relationships. The practitioner and client travel a personal and, sometimes, intimate journey through new realms of self-understanding, where a new perception of our personalized world creates personal growth for both concerned.

As we enter the twenty-first century, the world of new physics opens up awe-inspiring possibilities with the concept of human life. Our bodies are a living intelligence and wish to work for us as healthily and for as long as they can. Despite the abuse we inflict on them, they lovingly do what we wish them to do and, nurtured and cared for, they continue to serve us.

The time is coming when we will understand that we can no longer live as isolated beings on our planet and in the universe. Our bodies are our personal energy fields, which interact and have a direct effect internally on our bodies and externally on our environment and with those with whom we come into contact. Health problems will be seen as a reflection of a 'sick' spirit that needs healing from a fragmented way of being, and health-care services offering complementary therapies as a vital route back to wholeness will be available alongside conventional medicine.

The journey for those involved in the work, whether practitioner, student or patient, leads into exciting unknown territory where expectations, realizations and ideas evolve and flourish.

The human spirit remains forever an enigma and reflexology attracts those who wish to care for others and where the person who seeks help and healing embarks with the practitioner on a never-ending journey of self-discovery.

Learn, experience and enjoy the wonderful art of reflexology!

Section 1

Science, Philosophy and Concepts of Health and Healing

We are too much accustomed to attribute a single cause to that which is the product of several, and the majority of our controversies come from that.

Attributed to: Baron Justus von Liebeg (1803–73), German chemist

This section of the book is concerned with the history of reflexology, cultures and concepts of healing throughout the ages, new physics and energy concepts, 'stress' and its meaning, and some methods of study for the beginner student.

CHAPTER 1
History

WHEN DID REFLEXOLOGY BEGIN?

As early as 5,000 years ago, the science of reflexology was known in India. Buddhism and Hinduism are two of the oldest religions in the world and reflect the worship of many divinities, or gods, through art and sculpture. The three most important gods are: Brahma, the creator of the universe; Vishnu, its preserver; and Shiva, its destroyer. The feet are thought to symbolize the unity of the universe and the Ultimate One, with all of the elements of the universe represented by the signs on the soles of the feet.

If we study the Sanskrit symbols contained on the feet of Vishnu, although the true significance of them has been lost over time, they appear to correspond with the anatomical reflexes on the feet (*see* the Hindu Foot Chart in the colour section).

REFLEXOLOGY THROUGH THE AGES

The dominance of Buddhist and Hindu philosophy in India led to the migration of Buddhism to Japan, Korea, China, Tibet and Vietnam, where we can trace foot massage and other healing systems and their movement to China.

Chinese Medicine and Reflexology

Within Chinese traditional medicine, reflexology is a sub-division that stems from thousands of years of philosophy and theory of health and disease. A doctor called Sima Qian wrote during the second-century BC that there was a doctor named Yu Fu (Yu means healing and Fu means foot, together they form 'foot healing') who did not work with herbs or acupuncture but only massage and who stated that, 'the illness responded to every stroke of his'. In the oldest classic of the theory of Chinese traditional medicine, six important energy channels in the human body were defined as running to and from the foot, connecting sensitive points over the skin and internal organs. A total of 600 points comprise the body, with 66 points located in the feet. Although China had its own system of healing and traditional foot massage techniques, the Indian foot massage techniques were also introduced to China along with Buddhism. The Chinese method of reflexology, called 'Rwo Shur' is practised with the knuckles, short sticks and an extremely hard pressure.

The Chinese tradition refers to human energy as 'vital-forces', 'Chi' or 'Prana' – where there is no movement, there can be no life. For the body to be healthy, the natural flow of energy running throughout must be fluid and harmonious. The martial arts exemplify this tradition with movement containing concentrated Chi in each posture and muscle tension.

Egyptian Medicine and Reflexology

We have historical evidence that the Egyptians worked with herbs, astrology, sacrificial offerings and an advanced understanding of energy flow, and we now know a lot about their way of life. Mystery surrounds the Egyptian pyramids, and research today reveals that the Egyptian dependence on the placement of the stars and planets in our solar system were of major significance within their culture and the healing sciences. The oldest documentation that could be interpreted as the practice of reflexology was brought back to Europe in 1979 by Dr Gwendoline Raines; it consists of an Egyptian papyrus scene dating from 2500BC and depicts treating the hands and feet of patients by medical practitioners. Egyptian medicine was held in great esteem and tombs of important physicians depicted healing sciences. At Saqqara, there is the tomb of the physician, Ankhmahor, who was an influential official, second only to the King. A wall painting depicting the possible practice of reflexology was discovered as belonging to the 6th Dynasty, about 2330BC. The hieroglyphics behind the patient and practitioner are translated as the patient's plea, 'Don't hurt me'; the practitioner replies, 'I shall act so you praise me' (*see* colour section).

Interestingly, Egyptian physicians sometimes had professions other than medicine, with some being metaphysicians, astrologers, engineers, master builders, scribes and architects. At death, the physician was entitled to have his professions depicted by paintings around the walls of his tomb, which held religious significance as well as a biography of the person's life. In Ankhmahor's tomb, carvings into stone depict embalming, dentistry, childbirth, pharmacology, circumcision and reflexology. These paintings and carvings provided a gateway for the soul when returning to the earth from the afterlife, so that by the carvings and paintings the same body would be found and re-inhabited.

Not only can we produce evidence of the Egyptians working with the feet and hands, we also know that Egyptians from Upper Egypt were practitioners who travelled to Lower Egypt to treat the sick. Study of the pictograph reveals that the patient on the left of the picture has his right hand on his right knee and his left hand under his armpit, with the other patient in reverse. If we interpret the picture to represent a relationship between the problem the patient has and where the practitioner touches, it would appear that the patient works with the practitioner in working with associated pressure points.

Zone Therapy

In the sixteenth century, a book on the subject of 'zone therapy' was written. Until recently it was thought that the concept of reflexology was largely unknown by Western civilization but we now know that zone therapy was understood and practised. Zone therapy is thought to relieve stress and pain with the application of pressure to zonal points on the body and through this pressure a reflex action occurs within the same zone.

Germany's Discovery of Reflex Actions

In the eighteenth century, a German physiologist called Johann August Unzer published a work in which he was the first to use the word 'reflex' with reference to motor reactions (muscular movement stimulated by nerves) in the body. In 1833 Marshall Hall, an English physiologist, introduced 'reflex action' when he demonstrated the difference between *unconscious reflex actions*, such as coughing, sneezing, vomiting, blinking, etc., governed by a part of the brain called the medulla oblongata, and *conscious reflex actions* governed by the spinal cord and decision making.

By the mid-nineteenth century, the scientific study of the behaviour of animals and human beings began and indications show that reflexology may have developed in the 1890s with Sir Henry Head of London and his neurological studies. He worked with the Nobel prize winner, Sir Charles Sherrington towards understanding the effect of the environment on humans and their reaction to it.

Reflexzonenmassage

In the early 1900s, massage techniques were developed in Germany, called 'reflexzonenmassage'. This was the first time the benefits of massage techniques were credited to reflex actions. Dr Alfons Cornelius was the first to apply massage to reflex zones, even though he was unaware of the work of Sir Henry Head at about the same period of time. An important consequence of Dr Cornelius' work was that he established that pressure points worked within nerve pathways, following the anatomy of the body, although there were some exceptions to this anatomical concept.

Like Sir Henry Head, Dr Cornelius chartered different classifications of pain according to intensity. He found pressure points in the skin, over the surface of the body and in the deeper musculature. He also found that different intensities of pain responded to different pressures, which stimulated the healing process, and further, that there are two types of painful sensation. As a result of his research, Dr Cornelius established the important conclusion that *all* conditions reveal themselves as sensitive pressure points, which indicates imbalances in the body, long before they manifest as the neurological problems of pain.

Connective Tissue Massage

Another major contributor to understanding the body as an integrated neurological energy field was made by Elisabeth Dicke who was a physical therapist. Her development of connective tissue massage, based on the concept of reflex zone massage, applied massage techniques to connective tissue within the segmental zones established by Sir Henry Head. Dicke's discovery that pathological changes can also take place in the subcutaneous tissue within the connective tissue layer is currently used not only for the treatment of diseases of the circulatory system and other pathological conditions with excellent results, but also for diagnosis.

Sir Charles Sherrington (1861–1952) investigated and proved that stimuli are produced within the organism by movement in its own tissue, especially by a reflex action, and subsequently called this the 'proprioceptive system', where the sensory end-organs in the body provide information about the position of the body and movements that occur mainly in the muscles, joints, tendons, joint capsules and the bony labyrinth of the inner ear. In 1906, Sherrington published his paper on the reflex action of the nervous system, called *The Integrative Action of the Nervous System*.

Sherrington explained how the nerves coordinate and dominate body functions and he demonstrated a process by which the brain, spinal cord and reflex pathways control activities in the body. Thus, through this reflex action the entire body can create a spatial map of where it is in time and space. Sherrington's work greatly influenced modern physiology. In 1932, he received the Nobel prize.

Russian Tests with Reflexology

The Russians have also pursued the study of reflexology, with the use of physiological and psychological scientific tests to find the effects of reflexology on patients with a range of ailments. It is viewed today as being an effective complement to allopathic medicine.

The Native American Indians and Reflexology

The biggest influence on the practice of reflexology has come from America, where the practice of massaging the reflex zones comes from ancient folk medicine used by Native American Indians, probably passed down by the Incas who refined the Asian Indian techniques. There are no scripted accounts of Inca healing systems and this remains a speculative concept. The North American Indians alluded to the human spirit as being interconnected with the universe, with this energy channelling through the physical body by the feet being planted on the earth. Hence the expression 'plantar', which corresponds to the sole of the foot in contact with the earth. Again, there are no recorded accounts of working with the reflexes but there are living descendants within certain tribes who confirm various methods of practice of working with the feet, dependent on the needs of the individual at the time of treatment.

THE REDISCOVERY OF REFLEXOLOGY

More recently, in 1942, Dr William Fitzgerald conducted studies with zone therapy. Dr Fitzgerald received his medical degree from the University of Vermont in 1895 and practised in Boston City Hospital for two-and-a-half years before travelling to London where he spent a further two years at the Central London Nose and Throat Hospital. In light of historical evidence, Dr Fitzgerald was not the first to work the reflexes and zones of the body as previously thought, but 'rediscovered' the science after becoming aware of the work whilst in Vienna. As Dr Fitzgerald gives no written account of how he became acquainted with the theory of zone therapy, speculation predisposes that he could easily have heard of Dr Cornelius' 1902 treatise, *Pressure Points, Their Origin and Significance*, whilst he was in Vienna. However, through the knowledge he gained whilst in Europe and his own research, Fitzgerald theorized that the body can be divided into ten longitudinal zones, running from head to toe. We can compare this concept with the Chinese theory of acupuncture, where the body was divided into longitudinal meridians by the period of approximately 2500BC.

Although there are no direct connections between Eastern and Western energy therapy, definite links can be made as, for example, Dr Fitzgerald confirming Sir Henry Head's theory that stimulation of the skin causes a reflex action to occur by working anywhere in a zone where everything within that zone has a response. There does not appear to be any written evidence or illustrations supporting Dr Fitzgerald's zone theory although Dr George Starr White hints that records were kept.

Dr Joe Shelby and his wife Elizabeth were staunch supporters of Dr Fitzgerald's work and Dr Riley used the teachings of Dr Fitzgerald extensively in his practice for many years and probably used the therapy more than any other method of healing, making detailed drawings and diagrams of reflex points located on the feet. He also added his discovery of eight horizontal divisions that also control the body, and researched reflexes and zones included in the ear, known now as 'auriculotherapy'. Although these reflexes were limited, he was the first exponent to extend zonal therapy within Chinese traditional medicine. More recently, Dr Paul Nogier found that working the reflexes of the ears is effective with problems associated with the muscular system.

Dr Riley developed the 'hooking' technique commonly used when working the reflex points on the feet and hands when he dispensed with Dr Fitzgerald's idea of using spring clothes-pegs and rubber bands and other bizarre gadgets to work the reflexes.

The sensation of the therapist's thumbs and fingers against the patient's skin is necessary if sensitivity to pain and 'blocked' energy channels are to be found accurately. The therapist's intuition plays a key role in interpreting the map of the body on the feet and hands with various methods of assessing the psychological, emotional and mental balance of the person as a whole. This cannot be done if an instrument is used as an intermediary to the sensation of touch.

THE WORK OF EUNICE INGHAM

During the 1930s pioneering work was done by Eunice Ingham (1879–1974) who worked with Dr Riley as his therapist in St Petersburg, Florida. Ingham's basic philosophy was to help people to help themselves if their doctor was not interested in using reflexology. From this perspective, her work was profound as it encouraged people to take more responsibility for their health and to become more autonomous in personal decision-making about health issues. By separating the reflexes in the feet and hands from zone therapy, she called her work 'compression massage' but later changed the word to 'reflexology'.

In her life, Eunice Ingham contributed two major theories to the practice of reflexology. The first was that she realized that anyone could learn reflexology to help their ailments and those of family and friends, and over the years she was asked to talk at conventions to share her techniques and knowledge. Her second contribution was that she found an alternating pressure, rather than having a numbing effect, stimulated healing. In her early days, she padded and taped the tender reflexes with cotton so that as the patient walked about the reflexes would continue to be stimulated. Although patients improved, she realized that over-stimulation of reflexes brought about the same reactions as the condition.

Since the worldwide popularity of reflexology, largely brought about by Eunice Ingham, divergent methods and applications of the therapy have developed, all of which have a role to play in helping people to help themselves when more allopathic (conventional) medicine fails to aid recovery.

CHAPTER 2
Cultures and Concepts

STAYING ALIVE

For thousands of years civilizations have known that survival depended on maintaining a healthy body. Different cultures developed individual philosophies, concepts and applications to rectify physical and temperamental disorders, with nature and the elements viewed as being all-powerful. Through the worship and sacrificial offerings to appease the gods and deities as beneficent spirits, the elements would send appropriate weather conditions for crops to flourish and ensure abundant food, necessary in the preservation of the self and society.

Even as we draw near to the beginning of the twenty-first century, animal sacrifice is still seen in some cultures as an omnipotent force for protection, survival and safety of the individual and the society in which he or she lives. This interconnectedness with nature as an unseen power and energy flow between themselves and the natural world has sustained an understanding that people respond to plants and herbs to cure their ailments. Different areas of the body were also viewed as an unseen energy field, responding to stimulation by varying interventions. The understanding that, as human beings, we are a thread of the ecological web of the planet, and where, for example, tribal traditions in Africa and Australia still practise ancient healing rites to cleanse the body, these remind us of our ancient heritage.

The Ayurvedic Tradition

The Ayurveda healing tradition has been in use for over 4,000 years and has its roots in the Indian system of Brahman, the source of life. In a similar way to the Taoist tradition of Yin and Yang, the three Gunas act as expansion and contraction of energy movement, which set up polarities within every aspect of our lives. The elements of water, fire, air, earth, wood and metal are seen as a fundamental part of healing and if one or more of the elements appears to be out of balance, disharmony and disease result. Imbalances within the elements can be restored with foods grown either in, on or above the ground, together with the preparation of herbs.

Tibetan Medicine

Today, Tibetan medicine uses herbs and prayer to activate and release the healing potential within the herbs gathered in the scree slopes of the Himalayas by the Amchi (Tibetan doctor). Combined with an energetic understanding of the individual taken from the personal astrological birth chart, the Amchi prescribes and prepares the herbs that remedy imbalances within the body. This, again, gives consideration to the fact that we as human beings are composed of the same elements that surround us in our external environment, and with the use of herbs, which have had prayers chanted over them by

Buddhist lamas and monks, the healing properties held within them cure and re-balance the person back to health.

The Aboriginal Tradition and Shamanism

The Aboriginal culture is one of healing with herbs and shamanic healing (a role which tends to be passed down through families), where a man or woman is able to deliberately alter their state of consciousness, when they make contact with the spirit world on behalf of members in their community. The initiate in to the shamanistic magical career goes through the process of circumcision and subincision, with the disciplines of shamanhood extending beyond the rites of manhood. The shaman is especially gifted in three ways: productive magic, which is concerned with fertility rites, rain-making and love-making; protective magic, concerned with healing or counteracting accident or misfortune; and destructive magic, concerned with bringing sickness, death and injury. Aboriginal dream-time places emphasis on the contents of dreams as symbols with, for example, the unborn child's specialness represented by food, a place or a creature, which will be significant to the child in life. The dream might be seen as a bridge across which those living in time can wander in the world of eternity and where specialness of being in the world is 'chosen' because of its relationship to a sacred place and where the child will probably dream about it. Interestingly, in the West we believe in the symbolism of dreams – it was Sigmund Freud, the grandfather of psychoanalysis at the turn of the century who described dreams as the 'royal road to the unconscious'. The difference between the two systems of dream symbolism is that the Aborigines believe that the eternal spirits move in our direction. Man is therefore seen as more than a physical being, with the unseen world of spirits, of which he is one, interrelating in many different areas of life.

BIOLOGICAL AND SPIRITUAL CONSCIOUSNESS

One of the most powerful and influential images in Greek mythological concepts of the psyche is found in Plato's philosophy, the *Phaedrus*, where the soul is pictured as a charioteer driving two horses, one representing bodily passions and the other the higher emotions. This metaphor encompasses two approaches to consciousness – the biological and spiritual – which have been pursued without being reconciled throughout Western philosophy and science. It is this conflict which has created the 'mind/body' existential division within the individual and society.

Greek Medicine and Mythology

We can trace the root of traditional Western medicine and healing to Greek Hippocratic science, which has existed since pre-Hellenic times. To the Greeks, healing was a spiritual phenomenon and was linked to many deities, the most prominent one being Hygeia (meaning 'health'), who was a manifestation of the Cretan goddess, Athena, and whose symbols were mistletoe, used as all-healing, and the snake. As social order and religion became changed by invaders from other cultures, the myths of the goddess became distorted into a new culture. In this particular myth, Hygeia was made to be the daughter of the healing god, Asclepias, who became the dominant god and who was worshipped in temples all over Greece. As the name Asclepias had its origin in mistletoe and snakes, mythology continued to play a dominant role in Western healing traditions, with the coiled serpent around the Asclepian staff becoming the symbol of Western medicine.

The word 'physician' means 'natural knowledge' and in the Asclepiad traditions, the

Greek physicians, Hippocrates (460–375BC) and Galen (200–130BC) studied medicine in Alexandria. Out of the Asclepiad traditions, where medical Guilds were set up to promote empirical knowledge as a form of medicine, Hippocrates represented the culmination of Greek medicine. These ancient healing arts are as relevant today as they were in Ancient Greece and are centred around prevention and therapy. The Hippocratic Corpus are voluminous writings attributed to Hippocrates but were probably written by several authors at different times. These writings represent the knowledge taught in the Asclepian guilds with the core of the Hippocratic teachings describing illness as natural phenomena and not due to evil spirits, demons or supernatural forces, as had previously been thought. With studied scientific and therapeutic procedures appropriated to the wise management of a person's life, health disorders were recognized as natural phenomena that could be controlled in a preventative way, as well as the use of diagnosis and therapy. Although medicine today honours and reveres Hippocrates, successors of the tradition barely touch on the depth of philosophical thought and breadth of vision encompassed in the Hippocratic writings.

One of the most significant books of the Hippocratic Corpus, *Airs, Waters and Places*, represents and describes what we would now call a treatise on human ecology, where the well-being of the individual is influenced by environmental factors – the quality of the air, water and food, general living habits and the area lived in. Sudden changes in these factors and the appearance of disease is emphasized. To the physician, understanding the significance of these factors is the essential basis for medical practice and the importance of balance within environmental influences, personality, temperament and ways of life. These components are described in terms of 'humours' and 'passions' that need to be in balance for physical health to be present.

The forces inherent in living organisms, which Hippocrates called 'nature's healing power', gave recognition to the importance of creating favourable conditions for the healing process to take place. As the original meaning of the word 'therapy' comes from the Greek *therapeuin* (to attend), the therapist's role was viewed as assisting and attending to the natural healing process. In addition, the Hippocratic writings contain a strict code of medical ethics, known as the Hippocratic Oath, which has remained a prerequisite of ethical practice to this day for those in medical practice.

Personality and the Humours

In the second century BC, the eminent Greek physician Galen outlined a theory of personality that was comprised of three domains, each of which comprise the human psyche: the cognitive, or intellectual; the conative, or intentional; and the affective, or emotional. Each domain was viewed as important for human functioning with the conative and affective domains forming the driving force of human behaviour, and the cognitive domain guiding and directing how these energies were used.

In the Middle Ages, the explanation of human personality was derived from the concept of the 'humours' where the personality was shaped by physiological factors. The idea behind this theory was that the body contained different humours, or fluids, and that different personality types arose from one of the four fluids being in excess in the body. Those who had a greater preponderance of blood were thought to be cheerful, lively and energetic – the *sanguine* temperament; those with a greater proportion of phlegm were consider to be placid and calm – the *phlegmatic* temperament; those with a high proportion of black bile were thought to be gloomy and depressive – the *melancholic* temperament; and those with yellow bile were thought to be irascible and hot-tempered – the *choleric* temperament. We can see how influential this theory still is today with the source of the word 'humour' meaning mood. Interestingly, the word sanguine comes from the French *sang*, meaning 'blood' and 'ruddy'. This led to the belief that people with high fever had too much blood and thus blood-letting with leeches came into being.

EASTERN AND WESTERN PHILOSOPHIES

What then, has caused our Western culture to move away from such a profound understanding of the 'web' of interrelated life into such a separatist existence, where humans have striven to control nature, seeing it as something to be subjected to human mastery?

Eastern philosophy and tradition refers to the understanding that nothing can exist in isolation and everything animately and inanimately manifested is seen as interrelated. In Zen Buddhism, everything manifested in the universe is viewed as an illusion with things accepted as they appear to be and in a state of constant change and '*being-ness*', without the need for validation or proof. Human life is considered to be a combination of mental, emotional, psychological and spiritual currents of energy that form the physical body with energy centres, called 'chakras' (a Hindu word used to define each of the seven major energy centres running from the tail of the spine to above the crown, and minor chakras found over the body). Chakras are directly related to life issues and must spin and rotate at the correct speed and in the correct direction for physical harmony to be in place. These traditions refer to the energy of the human being, where the description that we are a combination of energies that converge with the physical body to form the 'whole' person are given specific terms and language.

The main themes of health, healing and practice were developed by the Chinese in a very different cultural context to the Greeks. As in the Greek culture, there was the same emphasis on environmental influences, nature's inherent healing power and the interdependence of mind and body, which was an important root in healing practice. The difference between the two cultures was that classical Chinese medicine had its roots in the shamanistic traditions and was moulded by two philosophical schools of the Classical period: Taoism and Confucianism.

Unlike the early Greek scholars, the Chinese were not interested in the *cause* of a health problem but in the synchronistic *patterning* of things and events. For example, the healthy individual and the healthy society represent integral parts of a great patterned order, with an imbalance in either individual or society resulting in illness.

The Chinese developed acupuncture based on the theory that energy travels through the body by lines called 'meridians'. When health disorders occur, treatment is effected by the insertion of needles into the skin's surface to redirect energy into the correct path, thereby balancing the body to wholeness.

The Taoist ('Tao' meaning neutral essence of all life) has its tradition rooted in the concept of negative and positive energy polarities, called 'Yin' and 'Yang'. These energies flow around the body with *Yin* representing the negative, feminine, receptive, passive force and *Yang* the positive, masculine, outgoing force. For us to be in physical, emotional, mental and spiritual harmony, both poles of expression must be in balance. When there is an excess of Yin, there is an insufficient functioning of the parasympathetic nervous system and when

Yang is present in excess, excessive organ activity, stimulated by the sympathetic nervous system, is present. Imbalance within either polarity results in illness. The human being is seen as a microcosm of the universe, with the social and natural being in dynamic balance, with all components swinging between the two archetypal poles.

From these concepts we can see that health, from early Western and Eastern perspectives, was based on philosophies where the tangible is obscured by a belief that energy movement and spiritual atonement act as predominating factors in creating a balanced and harmonious physical, emotional, mental and spiritual state of well-being.

The Use of Herbs

In Eastern cultures, herbs are used as an interrelated 'whole' in the pure state and working with the individual on energetic levels enhances their properties and healing powers. In the West, herbs lose their intrinsic energy and powerful essence as chemicals partially destroy them or replace them artificially. Drugs are largely used to suppress energetic symptoms and imbalances in health and, whilst they have a role to play, we need to begin to look deeper for the origins of disease, where we treat the whole person, rather than a set of symptoms. Fewer side-effects from medication would present themselves if drugs were administered on an individual holistic diagnosis. In this way, the same illness, one-drug syndrome would largely disappear and negate the need for additional medication to suppress the side-effects of the first.

Cultural Integration

Western science and philosophy have created a materialistic outlook where something or someone outside of ourselves will make us better, happier, or will do it for us – usually the doctor! Responsibility for ourselves, our happiness, our health and our spiritual welfare is a personal process and one which the partner, doctor or clergyman may be able to assist with but who cannot solve our problems for us. Responsibility for others extends to helping them to become 'response-able', where they do what they can for themselves and feel supported by those around them.

Both East and West health-value systems have within them valuable offerings with which to build a new concept of what is needed for human beings to create a healthy body, mind and spirit. Slowly, Eastern philosophies and Western scientific thought are moving closer together with the advent of the New Physics – this new understanding of health and life will educate and imbue modern-day society with concepts which in the past have been referred to as either mystical, or just plain cranky!

Through understanding the ancient healing sciences and applying them to twentieth- and twenty-first-century society, people will be helped to become more responsible for their health and contribute, ultimately, towards a healthier society. To a large extent, the responsibility for health and well-being lies with the individual, in learning how to listen to their body, thoughts, feelings and spirituality – to know *how* and *when* they can help themselves, when to seek help from a complementary therapist or when conventional medical intervention maybe the best solution for their problem.

SOME THEORETICAL CONCEPTS ON HOW REFLEXOLOGY WORKS

For many people, the time spent with a reflexologist will be the only opportunity they have to give time to themselves. The key to becoming a good practitioner is to develop the ability to form good relationships with those who come to you for help. Building a stable, trusting relationship with your clients may have a beneficial effect for them on all levels of their being. Reflexology not only encompasses the physical body but also the Subtle Bodies. It can aid in raising the client's self-esteem and improve self-image in caring about themselves, and increase feelings of self-worth as a result of the other two benefits. As a result, the person feels important and cared for.

We must not confuse reflexology with massage. The parts of the nervous system comprise many types of reflexes, which are found throughout the body and which perform functions in response to the external environment or emotional response. Sir Henry Head was responsible for discovering that through different parts of the nervous system, the skin can affect organs in the body and organs affect skin, and that the areas of sensitivity lay at a distance from the affected part. Both Sir Henry Head and Sir James MacKenzie proved that there is a connection between stimulation of the skin and internal organs through pressure, manipulation, stroking, heat, cold and electrotherapy. They found that therapeutic methods applied to the surface of a part of the body influence pathological conditions associated with an organ or part in a particular area. There are places on the body where large numbers of nerve cells are close to the skin's surface. These areas are found in the back of the hand and soles of the feet, the middle of the back, between the shoulder blades, and the cheeks. There are also a larger number of skin capillaries in the soles of the feet and palms of the hand.

The brain releases endorphins, which act as pain relievers. As the nervous system can only cope with a limited quantity of sensory information, the application of pressure with reflexology stimulates the brain to release more endorphins while at the same time producing an 'overload' for the nervous system, shutting down nerve pathways relaying pain signals to the brain. Endorphins are considerably more powerful analgesics than morphine.

During his lifetime, Dr Fitzgerald assessed four reasons why reflexology works.

- The first is that it is soothing because of magnetic fields interacting between therapist and client.
- The second is that by manipulation with the hand over sensitive areas, bruising is alleviated.
- The third reason is that applied pressure on sensitive parts of the foot inhibits, through the nervous system, knowledge of imbalances held in the body.
- The fourth reason is that applied pressure over bone or to zones corresponding to sensitivity relieves pain. Extended pressure may have an analgesic effect in the body, or in extreme cases can result in anaesthesia.

Dr Fitzgerald also believed that the control centres in the medulla of the brain stem are stimulated and maybe influenced by the pituitary gland and nerve pathways from it. As a result of inhibition to transmission of nerve impulses from the brain, through the zone worked on, pathological changes take place in the body with symptoms sometimes disappearing. It is thought that lymphatic relaxation is a result of pressure applied to the zones.

There are chemicals and hormones in every part of the body, which are relayed to a part of the brain called the hypothalamus. Nerves from the thymus gland and spleen are connected to the hypothalamus, which in turn affects the immune system (a part of the lymphatic system). From this, we can understand how complex the interaction of nerves, hormones, lymph fluid and blood are and how reflexology affects the entire body.

Dr J. S. Riley believed 'zone therapy' worked by inhibiting pain through manipulation, touch and pressure before nerve impulses reached the brain, with pressure the most important factor. This latter explanation has been my experience, that the more pressure applied within the client's pain threshold the greater the relief from symptoms in a shorter space of time.

Eunice Ingham's theory of how reflexology works involves stimulation of the sympathetic and parasympathetic parts of the autonomic nerve system, where adrenaline and other substances are involved in alleviating symptoms.

The healer, Robert St John, developed a theory that life before birth influences future health problems. He found that reflex zones in the spine corresponded to the nine months of pregnancy and he therefore centred his work around the spine, calling this method the metamorphic technique.

Dr Randolf Stone developed Polarity Therapy, which is based on the Eastern philosophy which describes the body as composed of energy pathways, called 'chi'. It is through these pathways, he believes, that reflexology works. Dr Stone's theory involves negative and positive poles of electrically charged energy, which stimulate reflex points and release energy blocks and restore balance. Central to this theory, reflex points are found covering the body.

Other theories explain the reflexes as different parts of the body, with the location and relationship of reflexes largely following an anatomical patterning which reflects that of the body. It is also thought that reflexes are closely related to acupuncture meridians. Acupuncture is based on the theory that there are twelve pairs of meridians, or energy pathways, which together form a single energy system through which health is maintained. These pathways are viewed as vehicles, which allow universal energy to flow through the body so that the universe and body remain in harmony with each other. As with reflexology, when a meridian of energy is blocked the harmony of the body becomes imbalanced. Acupuncturists use needles inserted into these pathways to release the blockages.

Reflexologists work on both acupuncture and acupressure points where nerve pathways follow meridian pathways. It is interesting to note that within the twelve meridians there is one major point for each pathway, with six of these points corresponding to the hands and feet.

The presence of lactic acid crystals, which may settle on the feet and hands, are thought to impede the flow of energy. By applying pressure to the reflexes, these deposits are crushed and eliminated by the body. It has also been suggested that there may be known and unknown connections between organs of the body and parts of the hands and feet, as reflexology directly affects different parts of the body through proprioceptive nerve receptors.

Many symptoms and health problems are stress related and one of the main benefits of reflexology is that the person's body has a chance to relax during treatment. Relaxation to nerves provides relief to imbalanced and sensitive parts of the body, whether consciously wished for, or unconsciously. From this, we can understand that it is not important whether or not the client believes in reflexology as the physical body will be affected anyway.

Research has shown that health problems have improved, as a result of a placebo effect, in the belief that reflexology will help. If a large proportion of clients feel benefitted by receiving reflexology, then this must necessarily be accepted as a theory for how it works.

27

Finally, the constitution of the individual may be more important than the symptoms of health problems and in this way we deal not only with the genetic make-up of the individual but with their attitude and approach to life problems. Positive results obtained from reflexology may be combined with energetic interaction between client and therapist, where a harmonious flow of energy is beneficial to both client and therapist.

Reflexology can be described as a science because it works directly on all systems of the body, especially the nervous, endocrine, circulatory and lymphatic systems. It becomes an art form in the skill of the practitioner and the interactive relationship between therapist and client.

CHAPTER 3
Physics

LIFE IS ENERGY

If we view reflexology as an energy-based science, based on flow of energy and the inter-relationship between therapist and patient, we can get a clearer understanding of how this and other energy-based therapies work if we consider the world of physics and how it will develop into the twenty-first century.

As we have already seen, Eastern perspectives of life and the universe revolve around a non-separatist idea of interconnectedness and interrelatedness. At the opposite end of the spectrum, Western scientific thought has sought to compartmentalize and separate human beings from their internal and material external environment over the last four-hundred years by the need for mathematical validation and experiment.

CARTESIAN THOUGHT

Mechanistic mechanical laws were theorized by the French mathematician, René Descartes (1596–1650). Descartes felt he had proved that the body and mind were independent of each other. The body was viewed as a complex mechanistic machine with the soul residing in the mind, where it interacted with the brain without being a part of it. Descartes' emphasis on rational explanation and thought in our culture is epitomized in his statement '*Cogito, ergo sum*' ('I think, therefore I am') and

encouraged the Western culture to separate the mind from the wholeness of an integrated organism. Thus, by using only our minds to rationalize we have forgotten how to think with our bodies; how to open our awareness to the knowledge of the body and respect it as an intelligent emissary for well-being.

NEWTONIAN PHYSICS

Descartes saw human beings as working parts of a clock, with each part treated separately; the body to be treated pathologically with health problems and the Church to deal with spiritual, mental and emotional problems. A little later, in the seventeenth and early-eighteenth century, Isaac Newton developed 'Newtonian Physics', which dealt with the principles of the laws of gravity, chemical reactions, thermodynamics and electromagnetism. This was a slight step forward but Newton's insistence on seeing physical life as solid, including the universe as disparate parts, narrowed human beings even further from the essence of the spiritual, emotional and mental counterparts of the self. However, mechanistic thought does describe the motion of the planets, fluids in continuous motion and mechanical machines. Our world as seen largely as unchanging and solid is a comforting thought, especially if we experience our bodies in a mechanical way. Our homes are still today Newtonian, except for electrical systems, with three-dimensional linear time enabling us to continue life in a structured, mechanical way. Newton's ideas continued into the nineteenth century, with the universe thought to be composed of building-blocks, called atoms.

ELECTROMAGNETIC FIELDS

In the early nineteenth century, Michael Faraday and James Clerk Maxwell discovered electromagnetic phenomena, which they described as 'field' theory. A field is a condition in space that has the potential (meaning, it may or may not happen) of producing a force. A charge creates disturbance or condition in space around it so that the other charge, when present, feels the force. The universe is filled with fields that create forces and that interact with each other. This theory has given us the scientific framework explaining how we can affect each other at a distance, other than sight or speech, through focused thought and feeling; we can, for example, 'sense' someone in the room – this is a field interaction. One-hundred years after physicists discovered electromagnetic fields of force, it is interesting that within the last fifteen to twenty years the concepts that describe personal interactions, other than by sight and speech are becoming recognized as existing!

SPACE AND TIME

By 1905, Albert Einstein had developed his Theory of Relativity and shattered the mechanistic view of life and the universe. Einstein's theory decreed that space is not three-dimensional and time is not a separate entity; both are intimately connected and create a fourth dimension, known as space/time. Thus, we can never talk about space without time for they describe everything we experience in life. What is more, there is no universal flow of time and, unlike Newton's idea of time, it is not viewed as linear but relative. For example, two observers will order events differently in time if they move at different speeds, relative to the observed events, which can even lead to two observers seeing two events in reverse time! For example, we may have an intuitive flash with a problem happening to someone we know who lives at a distance. Normally, we need to validate our intuitive sense mechanistically by using the telephone and if the psychic flash has not happened, we dismiss it. However, the law of probability within Einstein's theory would contend that the event could happen in the *future* as well as in the *past*. We need to listen to and become aware of our intuitive 'flashes' if we are to develop and integrate a more broadened understanding of 'reality'!

QUANTUM MECHANICS

In the 1920s, physics moved into the sub-atomic world. Max Plank discovered that heat left a radiator not as a constant emission but in 'energy packets'. This discovery began a field of physics known as quantum mechanics, where energy exists in indivisible units and our radiators, such as we have at home to provide heating, were designed on this theory. *Light waves* were also discovered as being particles, and when a small change in the experiment took place, the particles could be described as *waves*.

ORGONE ENERGY

A psychiatrist and colleague of Sigmund Freud, Wilhelm Reich, developed in the early part of this century, a theory called 'orgone'. From the 1930s into the 1950s, Reich experimented with energies using the latest electronic and medical instrumentation, and a high-powered telescope. He observed orgone pulsating in the sky, around all organic and inanimate objects and micro-organisms. Reich constructed a number of apparatuses for the study of the orgone field.

The *accumulator* was one, capable of concentrating orgone energy which he then used to charge objects. He observed that a vacuum discharge tube would conduct a current of electricity at a potential considerably lower than its normal discharge potential after being charged for a long period of time in an accumulator.

From this theory, Reich developed different *character structures*, where energy is held in lateral bands across the body. Eventually, methods by which we 'hold' emotions and feelings in our bodies construct a physical shape. These shapes give the therapist a clue to the type of defence and coping mechanisms used by the individual to survive in life. Dr Alexander Lowen was a student of Reich's who went on to develop exercises that allowed the person to let go of deeply held emotional pain and feelings. The release of these painfully held experiences help to transform the body shape.

INTERACTION AND COMMUNICATION

In 1964 we moved into the world of subatomic physics, where particles are connected in a way that transcends space and time; whatever happens to one particle affects other particles, with the result that there is an immediate effect where time is not needed to transmit them. Subatomic particles are sometimes *superluminal*, or faster than the speed of light, and from this theory we can see how we can be instantaneously conscious of interconnectedness with the world and each other. The enormity of this discovery is that we can affect the thoughts, feelings, actions and understanding of each other and the world by revolutionizing our personal interaction and communication.

CORE ENERGETICS

Dr John Pierrakos developed Reich's theories of character structure even further into core energetics, where, by diagnosis and treatment of psychological disorders based on visual and pendulum observations, inner healing took place as ego defences and personality were 'unblocked'. Once these energies are released, core energetics balances the subtle bodies and auric field, creating harmonious healing.

THE HOLOGRAM

Through understanding the interconnectedness of ourselves as a microcosm of the universe, operating on spiritual, mental and emotional levels simultaneously, which affect our personal well-being as well as those around us, we can begin to understand the deeper dimension of reality known as the hologram. Dr David Bohm believes that the hologram theory explains an implicate and explicate enfolded order. In his theory, physical laws cannot be discovered by a science that attempts to break the world into parts. The *implicate enfolded order* exists in an *unmanifested* state and is the foundation upon which all manifest reality exists; the *explicate enfolded order* is, therefore, one where all *manifested* phenomena exists and which is interconnected within a dynamical relationship. This unbroken 'wholeness' cannot be analysed into independent and separate parts. Some researchers believe that the deep structures of the brain are holographic, as well as the universe.

METAPHYSICS

Moving into the world of metaphysics, Rupert Sheldrake has developed a hypothesis called 'morphogenetic fields' (*morph* meaning form and *genesis* meaning to come into being). In his theory, not only are we regulated by energy and material factors but also by invisible organizing fields. These fields serve as a blueprint for behaviour and have no energy or mass. The effect of these fields is that they can reach across time and space barriers, normally applied to energy. Therefore, their effect is as strong at a distance as close-up. For example, whenever a member of a species learns new behaviour, the field for the whole species is changed, no matter how slight. If the behaviour is repeated long enough, its morphic resonance affects the entire species and can move across space/ time, where *past* events influence *current* and *future* events elsewhere, with physical laws outside of time determining how something is manifested.

SUPERLUMINAL CONNECTEDNESS

The theory of psychoenergetic systems, as understood by Jack Sarfatti, gives us a theory through which superluminal connectedness exists. He believes that there is a higher plane of reality above ours and that 'things' in that plane are connected through an even higher plane. By reaching this higher plane, we may be able to understand how interconnectedness works. The enormity of this discovery is that we can affect the thoughts, feelings, actions and understanding of each other and the world by revolutionizing our personal interaction and communication.

Eastern philosophy parallels scientific streams of thought with meditation. Zen Buddhist Masters give students a short sentence to concentrate on, called a 'koan', where meditation transcends the linear mind and allows connectedness of all things:

What is the sound of one hand clapping?

From this understanding we can begin to see a link with Eastern philosophy and Western science.

NEW PHYSICS

The world of new physics involves research into unifying Einstein's relativity theory ($E = mc^2$) and quantum mechanics into a new theory of subatomic particles. In the early 1960s, Geoffrey Chew and colleagues proposed a theory, which has resounding implications for the future of physics and our understanding of life. This new general philosophy of nature proposes that nature cannot be reduced to fundamental building-blocks, outside of ourselves or building-blocks of matter.

Traditional research in physics has always been concerned with finding fundamental particles of matter but Chew's 'bootstrap' philosophy abandons traditional methods of research and views the universe as a dynamic web of interrelated events. None of the properties of any part of this web are fundamental; they all follow from the properties of the other parts, with the overall consistency of their interrelation determining the structure of the web.

Because bootstrap physics does not accept any fundamental building-blocks of matter, it becomes a profound system of thought for Western minds and one which parallels Eastern Buddhist or Taoist philosophy. Methods of observation are essential in the framework and if properties of particles are closely related to methods of observation, then the basic structures of the material world are determined, ultimately, by the way we look at this world, meaning that patterns of matter are but reflections of patterns of mind.

It is interesting to think about the fact that maybe it is no coincidence that we have developed the 'world-wide web' of the Internet as a reflection of the growing consciousness that all nature is interrelated and that we are all part of this intricate and finely woven web of life.

As we near the year 2000, modern physics can be seen to have transcended the mechanistic Cartesian view of the universe, with a new holistic dynamical conception of the universe and one which, ultimately, will mean that science as we know it becomes extinct, as bootstrap and other similar theories provide understanding for different levels and aspects of reality.

If these theories are validated and expanded upon in the future, it has deeply profound and far-reaching implications for our understanding of life, human consciousness and the existence of the natural world. It will reverse the Western concept of looking *outwards* into the world to materially change things, where everything, including God, has been viewed as being external to the self with scant regard to the power of thought and action as an *internal* awareness.

The Eastern philosophies teach the importance of daily meditation and visualization, recognizing the power of thought, feeling and action as having an effect, on not only those we come into contact with, but with the whole world. Buddhist prayer flags waving in the wind send their prayers around the world – maybe soon, we will have Western scientific evidence that those prayers are powerful thought forms, which in the past have been categorized as mystical and part, only, of Eastern religious practices. The way we all create the world, will then, by thought, word and action be each person's ultimate responsibility.

REFLEXOLOGY AND NEW PHYSICS

From the history of exploration into health, healing and new physics, we can consider how energy-based therapies, such as reflexology, can find a place in medicine and society. We can view reflexology as a system of healing, operating on all levels of the human psyche and one that can shift consciousness into new ways of thinking about personal well-being and physical health. It can also integrate into conventional medicine, filling a void where there is little or no time to listen, touch (other than in formal medical examination), empathize, communicate, relate, encourage, show compassion, be kind, exchange ideas and beliefs, and believe in the patient's ability to heal their own soul and body. In short, allowing human contact from its highest aspirations, where the therapist or doctor is not seen as all-powerful but one who desires to assist in the patient's healing process.

MIND AND MATTER

When treating his patients, Hippocrates found that a healing energy radiated from his hands:

> It hath oft appeared, while I have been soothing a patient, as if there were some strange property in my hands to pull and draw away from the afflicted parts, aches and diverse impurities, by laying my hands upon the place and be extending my fingers towards it.

Magnetic Healing

Healing by magnetism was practised by the priesthood of the ancient Greeks and in Egyptian temples, where the halls of the sick were famous for their curative powers, which were kept as strictly esoteric knowledge. The oracles in Greece were the revelations of magnetized clairvoyants. Because of the secretiveness of the powers of magnetic healing, its knowledge and methods were lost to humankind for thousands of years. In the 1800s, Mesmer and Helmont developed 'mesmerism', which later became known as hypnotism. Their research concluded that animate and inanimate objects could be charged with a 'fluid', and that material bodies could exert influence over each other at a distance. This electromagnetic field, as we have seen, was further understood scientifically by James Clerk Maxwell and which, with the etheric body, can be influenced by other fields of energy.

The Etheric Body

The etheric body was discovered by Dr Kilner, who was in charge of electrotherapeutic development at St Thomas's Hospital, London. Although Dr Kilner was not interested in the curative powers of electromagnetic healing, he was interested in diagnoses by the examination of the etheric body. He discovered that a dead body did not have an aura and, further, that changes could be brought about in the aura by the concentrated attention of the person.

The etheric body is the counterpart of the physical body and resembles a matrix into which the physical cells fit. This web, or matrix, permeates the entire body, reaching a little away from the body with the edge seen as extending for about half-an-inch in width around the body. This edge is known as the 'inner etheric aura'. The etheric body should not be confused with the aura, which extends from the body as a halo of different colours that represents the emotional, mental and spiritual parts of the self. The 'aura' of Dr Kilner is a physical manifestation and is visible to almost anyone with normal eyesight, under certain conditions.

The Subtle Bodies

The subtle body is the non-physical life force that animates the physical being. In holistic health-care, we refer to the electromagnetic field and the etheric body as 'subtle bodies'. Every living thing has an electromagnetic power that attracts and repels whatever we come into contact with. This concept may answer why we like some people and not others. We take in universal energy, or life-force, in several ways: through fresh, unrefined food; by exercise, when breathing increases the intake of oxygen and which in turn stimulates the chakras by channelling the life-force through them. It is through the chakras interrelating with the auric field and subtle bodies that creates the colours in the aura and which some people can use to 'diagnose' health imbalances. The natural flow of these energies may be 'blocked' by a number of factors, such as emotional and mental and possibly spiritual stress, illness, trauma (including physical injury), pollution and tension. The most obvious existence of the subtle body is phantom limb pain. Following an amputation, the subtle body could be involved in phantom limb pain because the subtle body remains and retains the memory of the physical limb. Alternatively, this may be expressed as amputation causing a disturbance to the body's electromagnetic field.

The Aura

The research of Dr Kilner into the diagnoses of illnesses with a precise method showed that the changes in the etheric body could be brought about in the aura by the thoughts of the person. His observations further suggest that the human aura is comprised of energy waves, or fields of force. Thus, every thought consists of energy that travels across time and space.

The auric field and subtle bodies extend at a distance away from the body. With special equipment, the luminous limits of the auric field can be viewed with the colours emanating from it as an ecliptic shape. As we have seen, when there is an imbalance in a person's being, this can be detected by someone attuned to the study of the colours in the auric field and their representative meanings. Some people become 'unwell' in the auric field before the physical body without being able to pinpoint why they feel 'out of balance' and others become physically unwell, with the imbalance penetrating into the auric field over time. Whichever way we function, eventually all of the counterparts of the auric field will be affected and a general feeling of being 'under the weather', 'spaced out', 'no ground under my feet' and so on, will describe the way we feel.

Reflexology can restore the auric imbalances back to harmony, giving a feeling of calmness and of being healed with an inner security of feeling that our inner knowledge (intuition) will give us control in our lives. The word 'intuition' means in-tuition or 'inner training', where to listen with our inner voice increases our sensitivity to what presents a positive direction in a given situation. So often, we listen to our minds and cognitive thoughts; letting go of the mind and listening to our 'gut feeling' can guide us to the right solution within a situation.

SPIRIT AND MATTER

The soul can, therefore, be considered as an interaction between spirit and matter, which represents the manifestation of a prime, or divine, energy source. A picture emerges that shows that if the physical level is excluded, the 'subtle body' remains, with ill health expressing something being fundamentally wrong with the person's life. The task of a reflexologist, or any holistic practitioner, is to assist the patient in finding out what that 'something' is, so that they can take appropriate action.

The healing relationship between therapist and patient is an energetic interaction where both may experience effects that could be due to an exchange of subtle energy during a treatment. These effects can include a tingling sensation in the hands, feet and body; heat, which is channelled through the therapist's hands and which the patient may reflect back; pulsing sensations throughout the body; an increased awareness of energy flow; a 'trickling' sensation of energy throughout the body; feelings of coldness or chilliness; when stroking the electromagnetic field at the end of the treatment, the sensation of a cool breeze off the feet may be experienced; momentary discomfort or pain; somatic experience by the therapist of the client's symptoms; intuitive insight on the part of the practitioner, or 'knowing' something about the patient.

HEALTH AND WHOLENESS

The word '*holos*' is from the Greek, meaning 'whole', with the concept that the universe is greater than and different from the sum of its parts. We have seen that over the last four-hundred years, scientific validation, which has operated within strict parameters, is losing its boundaries as the advent of new physics merges the separated into the whole.

So, why is it that if a baby is healthy at birth, it develops a particular disease and health disorders? Why is it that one healthy child will develop one particular problem and another child a different problem? We know that genetic influences play a part in the overall health of the individual, but if a baby is born healthy, regardless of genetic influences, is it necessary to repeat a familial pattern of ill health? From the holistic viewpoint, we can consider genetic influences as possible weak points in the individual's make-up that predispose development of historical health conditions, if the person is unaware of what may predispose the development of a condition. Diet, exercise and attitudes to life all play a part in whether a person stays healthy or develops ill health. Reflexology is a wonderful scanning device to see where trouble spots may develop in the future, as well as those that may be present already; this is preventative therapy, which allows the body to rebalance itself before disease has a chance to get a grip.

DEFINING GOOD HEALTH

If we consider the variety of approaches to medicine and health concepts practised in Western cultures, both from holistic and orthodox philosophies, defining what constitutes good health can only be described as a subjective experience, where one patient may respond to a particular intervention and another may not. The related concepts of disease and of health cannot be viewed as separate entities but as a cohesive whole that mirrors relationships, personal perceptions and an ever-changing fluid web of life.

The mechanistic definition of disease from a clinical perspective can be described as any abnormality of bodily structure or function, other than those arising directly from physical injury, with the holistic framework defining disease as, 'looking at the patient who has the disease, rather than what sort of dis-ease the patient has' as stated by Dr William Osler over one-hundred-and-fifty years ago. The body, from this concept, is seen as being in a state of unease with rebalancing of the emotional, mental and spiritual aspects of the person taking place before the physical body can rebalance itself.

PERSONALITY, PERCEPTION AND DISEASE

Research into what constitutes 'personality', self-perception and disease is becoming increasingly enlightened. There is a growing awareness that self-help and understanding encourages the individual to take more responsibility for their life, resulting in increased control of life events. Preventatively, a self-responsible attitude to life events appears to reduce somatic symptoms that precede disease.

The human body is a self-regulating mechanism that desires to work for us as an integrated whole, and is broken down into parts with only the part that is physically damaged or broken being dealt with. For example, knee problems reflect spinal problems and to treat the knee successfully, spinal misalignment must be investigated.

Once we can relate to our perceptions and our place in the world as subjective (beneath consciousness) and individual, we can perceive the experience of health and well-being as part of the culture in which we live. The way we behave when we are ill can be viewed in the context of cultural 'norms'; for example, what do we mean by feeling healthy or sick, sane or insane, normal or abnormal? Holistic methods of treating the patient can be drawn from other cultures and do not need to be invented from scratch, where knowledge of the human mind and body and healing practices are viewed as integral parts of human philosophy and spiritual disciplines. This fundamental concept towards health and healing lends itself to be consistent with modern medical science and in harmony with traditional philosophy, where past cultural oscillations between Cartesian reductionism and holism combine to form an integrated whole.

Our perception of health, how we communicate our symptoms and who we choose to go to for care are largely dictated by our social and cultural expectations. The aim of all health-care practitioners, whether holistic or allopathic, should be to work for the patient's benefit, as a cohesive whole and not maintain two separate ideologies, where the patient is left to decide for themselves the best route to take with a particular health problem. Inadequate information concerning the disorder, and vague and sometimes misleading prognosis, leave the patient in a confused and fearful position when making a decision concerning treatment; this can leave the patient in a desperate frame of mind. With conventional medicine, rather than meeting and feeling involved in a supportive regime where all possibilities may be investigated in the production of a restorative programme, the patient often experiences dismissal when trying to discuss alternative methods of treatment.

The concept of amalgamating holistic concepts and methods of practice with allopathic medical practice creates for the patient a secure and caring environment, where there exists the best possibility that the outcome of multi-factorial treatment interventions will accelerate the healing process. Within the cultural 'split' of allopathic and holistic health-care, where the gulf between philosophies can leave the patient in a no-man's land, it becomes evident that we need a clear conceptual basis where all techniques and methods of healing are communicated and co-ordinated between health-care professionals for the benefit of the patient.

CHAPTER 4
Stress

STRESS AND THE EFFECT ON HEALTH

We need stress in our lives to function. But what do we mean by 'stress'? Most of us use the phrase, 'I feel stressed-out' at some time and usually attribute the reason for its existence to some external force for making us feel tense, anxious and exhausted physically, mentally and emotionally. Stress, it has been proved, can be a killer – coronary heart disease, high blood pressure (hypertension) and cancer providing the highest mortality rates in Western culture. Getting in touch with our stress and what it means to each one of us is very important if we are to learn how to regulate it internally and not rely on external relaxants, such as alcohol, smoking, drugs and food. Learning how to pace ourselves in the daily round and not try to cram in too much in to a day is one method of monitoring stress levels.

The medical model of 'stress' marks a major turning point in the diagnosis and understanding of disease because it introduces the factor that emotional tension is disruptive to the physical body, with, therefore, the majority of physical illnesses resulting from an overload of emotional, psychological and spiritual crises.

Within our society today, we require a constant need for a tangible proven and validated reality with which to compartmentalize health and well-being from the mind, emotions, personality and spirit. The work of Louis Pasteur, where 'one germ, one disease, one treatment' became the hypothesis for the treatment of disease. By the middle of the nineteenth century, herbs in their pure state, which had been the mainstay of curative remedies for centuries, were developed into medication – which, it could be argued, has diluted their efficacy. Pasteur's work, along with many others, has done much good in eradicating life-threatening diseases to the present day, but we are now in a position where new medication needs to be developed that will strengthen our bodies to work for themselves as we become immune to the artificial intake of substances that only debilitate the immune system further. One way of achieving this is to turn, once again, to nature in an undiluted form, to find restorative power and a deeper understanding of the psychological underlay of all health problems, with the reasons for a particular problem manifesting at a particular time in a particular person. This in-depth subject will be discussed in a second volume.

Following the work of Louis Pasteur, we now recognize that the beginning of ill health is multi-factorial, with overall lifestyle seen as important to the well-being of the individual. Our personal 'world-view' of, for example, seeing the world as being friendly and maintaining an optimistic outlook, or seeing it as a threatening, insecure place to be can create harmful stress levels.

The origination of this concept formed the foundation for the measurement of the human stress response in which 'stress' arousal can become a positive or negative influence in our life. In 1926 Hans Selye used the term 'stress' to denote 'the sum of all non-specific changes [within an organism] caused by function or damage' and in 1974 a more recent definition is 'the non-specific response of the body to any demand'. Selye chose the term 'stressor' to denote any stimulus that gives rise to the stress response. The extension of the Selyean concept of stress as a physiological response links any given stressor to a target organ with the stress response shown to inhibit or completely stop target organ systems. The depressive effects of stress arousal are sometimes the result of activation of inhibitory nerves and hormones, or acute hyperstimulation, resulting in non-function of target organs, including the mind. From this we can see that psychologically stress-related disorders can be seen as having potential target organ effects.

In earlier periods of our evolution, stress was necessary to the challenge of survival, and considerable research has been conducted into the nature of the psychophysiological response of arousal in preparation for physical activity. However, in our current time, psychosocial stimulation might be viewed as an inappropriate use of survival mechanisms by preparing the body with, for example, the 'flight or fight' response without physical activity following. Selye argued that stress can be a positive, motivating force that improves the quality of life. He called this 'eustress' (prefix *eu* from the Greek, meaning 'good') and debilitating, excessive stress 'distress'. As stress increases, health and performance and well-being have been shown to rise. As a maximum level of stress is reached, however, it becomes damaging to the body. The optimal level of stress appears to be governed by physiological, behavioural, genetic and anxiety related origins, which vary from

person to person. Treating pathological symptoms of disease falls to the physician with the traditional counsellor, psychologist, physical therapist or social worker intervening in the stress arousal process itself; for example, when treating a person suffering from excessive stress/anxiety accompanying and often exacerbating chronic infectious and degenerative diseases. The mind/body concept of stress, therefore, becomes a treatable condition with stress arousal taking the form of three interventions:

1. Helping the patient develop methods by which he or she can avoid, minimize or modify exposure to stressors, thereby reducing the patient's tendency to experience the stress response.
2. Helping the patient develop skills that reduce excessive nervous activity, mentally and physically, thereby balancing functioning and response to external stimulus.
3. Helping the patient develop methods that enable healthful expression, or utilization, of the stress response; for example, in physical activity.

These three concepts are based on self-help, awareness and understanding of how we create imbalances within the psyche and, eventually, the physical body, and methods by which we can change and grow positively through the stress response.

Because Selye used the term 'stress' to refer to a 'response' to any given situation, the term 'stressor' distinguished the stimulus or reason for the stress response. Two categories of stressor are psychosocial and biogenic: psychosocial stressors are those that are either real or imagined environmental events that 'set the stage' for the stress response but which do not directly cause the stress response; and biogenic stressors, which actually 'cause' a stress response. The nature of biochemical properties begin the stress response as, for example, intake of nicotine, caffeine, and pain-provoking stimuli. Most stressors are psychosocial, and patients are pressured by environmental events, real, imagined, anticipated or recalled, causing perception of events which lead to activation of a stress response.

PSYCHOLOGICAL CHARACTERISTICS AND DISEASE

Physiologically, it is known that the nervous, hormonal and immune systems of the body demonstrate response to stress, and individuals develop *coping mechanisms* so as to reduce or negate the stress, by acting environmentally, emotionally or cognitively. In this way, the level of arousal or activation on target organs is reduced.

Psychological characteristics that describe those who have either 'given up', or who feel like giving-up on life's problems and challenges have been shown to be significant factors in developing physical illness:

- a feeling of 'giving up', experienced as helplessness/hopelessness;
- a poor self-image, low self-esteem and self-worth;
- a sense of loss of gratification and self-fulfilment from relationships or roles in life;
- a feeling of disruption from the sense of continuity between past, present and future;
- remembering earlier periods of 'giving up'.

Through these speculations, the individual's perception of the inability to control or to cope stimulates the hypothalamus's chemical activity of the body's emergency systems, which eventually leads to illness.

CREATING OUR OWN REALITIES

The holistic concept of health and disease, or 'dis-ease', discriminates beyond the chemical, psychological and physiological study of disease with the recognition of *the human spirit as being ultimately connected with inner stresses present in a person's life*. A belief system based on the assumption that certain sensory perceptions of life events expressed in inappropriate ways, creates 'blockages' within the energy field, which create somatic symptoms, physiological illness and anxiety. Loss of meaning in one's life, grief, guilt, an unforgiving heart, hatred, loss of self-esteem and personal dignity forms fear at emotional and psychological crises, which eventually manifests as physical illness. The principle of healing, which creates and maintains health and life, is *spirituality in action*, where we create our own realities by activity, imagination and desire. The metaphor that traditional medicine represents the mind of health-care and the holistic approach the heart of health-care is concerned with systematic reasoning and logic, with the heart viewed as the energy centre for awareness of emotions, feelings and intuition. This dualistic approach results in fragmentation of the human spiritual condition.

The holistic paradigm is almost the exact opposite of the traditional medicinal model, with traditional medicine working from the *outside in* and holistic medicine working from the *inside out*. However, as we have already seen, holistic health-care should (in some cases) include traditional care in order to be considered truly holistic.

Self-Empowerment

The theory is that by expanding *an appreciation of the power of the inner self*, two things can happen:

- the person becomes receptive to learning, with attitudes and belief patterns contributing to the creation of health or a disease; and
- the individual develops a capacity of keeping healthy through being aware that negative attitudes create negative responses within the physical body.

To the extent that an individual becomes unable to process emotional, psychological and spiritual stresses, the individual becomes receptive or susceptible to the viruses that bacteria or germs present. What the holistic paradigm suggests (and this the central difference between the two models), is that the *energy* level of the human being, meaning the inner emotional and spiritual world, *precedes* and *determines* all that is experienced at the physical level of life with the success of any of the available holistic tools resting on two critical points:

- the patient's courage to evaluate *honestly* his or her life; and
- the patient's ability to *make choices* that authentically empower the inner self.

Love and Laughter

It has been shown that individuals who have strong support systems have a decreased risk of illness, regardless of dietary and other unhealthy habits. There is considerable evidence that *love* is more important than healthy living, and a sense of *humour* has been shown to enhance health – individuals who laugh regularly, show an increase in IgA antibodies. Freud is reputed to have had a better view of humour than he did of sex: 'Humour could take the sting out of bad situations'. The interrelationship of what individuals believe creates changes in the body.

Psychoneuroimmunology

Research into how the mind affects the body has produced psychoneuroimmunology (PNI), which includes the study of attitudes and social stress upon the immune, endocrine and neurological systems, and which provides the bridge between behaviour and mental processes. In addition to the effects of attitude upon the immune system, the discovery that neurochemicals correlate to anger, hostility, guilt and depression has shown the connection between biological responses and sensory stimulation. From this research, it becomes clear that the mind, brain and nervous system can be directly influenced, positively and negatively, by sensual elements in the environment. Sensorially, five major environmental factors are thought to influence physical and emotional health: colour, sound, aroma, light and touch.

Psychoneuroimmunology can be viewed as the 'bridge' between the medical and holistic models of stress and somatic symptoms, where pain and discomfort are felt without pathological disease being present.

THE PERCEPTION OF STRESS

Stress can, therefore, be seen as a *perception* of life events which promotes either an emotional reaction in positive action or thought or which leaves the individual with feelings of helplessness and hopelessness.

Use the following as a check list to see how much stress is present in your life:

- My pace of life is such that I feel unable to keep pace and feel pressured.
- My attention is directed outwards and my own feelings and emotions are ignored.
- I experience over-exertion, when my energy is over-focused either physically, emotionally or mentally or spiritually.

41

- I am unable to relax and be calm.
- I set myself, or others, unrealistic goals or expectations.
- I am always trying to conform to the demands of society.
- I have unresolved early life traumas, which have created patterns of behaviour that are harmful to me.
- I feel in pain, emotional and/or physical.
- My eating patterns fluctuate: the times I eat; eating refined foods; I don't eat and have/have had disorders such as Bulimia and Anorexia Nervosa.
- I experience feelings such as fear, guilt, unhappiness, anger and resentment a lot of the time.
- I feel a lack of control in my life, which leads to feelings of helplessness and hopelessness.
- I do not get enough exercise or physical activity.
- I feel depressed and sluggish – mentally, physically and emotionally.
- I have recently experienced dramatic personal events or changes, such as death, birth, moving house, marriage and divorce.

Ticking any one of these stress factors could indicate that your life is out of balance and action is needed to redress the balance.

Reactions, Disorders and Coping Strategies

Below are some *reactions* to stress, disease and ways of coping with stress:

- *Somatic symptoms:* headaches and migraine, tiredness, chest pains, erratic bowel movements, palpitations, insomnia, disturbed sleep patterns, indigestion, fatigue and constipation.
- *Stress-related disorders* include: asthma, skin diseases, ulcers, anxiety, allergies, heart attacks, high blood pressure, depression, migraine, irritable bowel syndrome, thyroid dysfunction.
- *Ways of coping with stress* can include: relaxation techniques, meditation, visualization, affirmations, counselling, physical exercise, a regular sex life, yoga and related martial arts, improved diet, hobbies, listening to music, a regular bedtime routine with a bath in essential oils, setting goals and working towards them, the use of Dr Bach (or other) Flower Remedies, light reading and a warm drink, pets for company and most importantly, *laughter* as the best medicine to lighten the pressure of day to day living!

Why Exercise Is Good For You

A special word about the importance of exercise and the mental, emotional and physical benefits:

- exercise maintains efficient circulation and prevents deterioration of blood vessels;
- it exercises and strengthens the heart;
- it exercises and strengthens the muscles;
- it maintains joint flexibility, reducing potential for arthritis;
- it stimulates the elimination of waste products;
- it improves the efficiency of the respiratory system;
- it promotes mental and emotional relaxation;
- it reduces stress;
- it prevents fluid build-up in the tissues;
- it uses up calories, so helping to prevent obesity;
- it reduces high blood pressure;
- it helps relieve depression.

Gentle exercise, such as walking, swimming or yoga are good for massaging internal organs to stimulate function, lighten the mood and give slight traction to the spine.

CHAPTER 5
Study Methods for the Beginner

For the student returning to study, perhaps for the first time since schooldays, learning can be a terrifying thought! There are a number of methods that aid the memory and give speedy recall. Here are a few simple methods that can help the student retain information.

With anatomy and physiology, list the *structures* of the system on one half of a page and the *functions* on the other as on the example shown below.

Mnemonics are another way of learning.

The Circulatory System

Structures	*Functions*
Heart	Provides a constant circulation.
Four heart chambers:	
right atrium	Receives blood from the inferior and superior vena cava.
right ventricle	Pumps blood to the pulmonary artery.
left atrium	Pumps blood into the left ventricle.
left ventricle	Takes blood to the aorta.
Four valves:	Stop back-flow of blood.
tricuspid valve (right side)	Pumps blood from the right atrium to the ventricle.
bicuspid valve (left side)	Pumps blood from the left atrium to the ventricle.
pulmonic valve (right side to the lungs)	Pumps blood to the lungs.
aortic valve (left side)	Pumps blood from the ventricle to the aortic artery.
Septum	Divides the right and left sides of the heart.
Apex	The lower point of the heart, on the right side of the thorax.
OTHER THAN BLOOD FLOW AROUND THE HEART	
Arteries	Carry oxygenated blood.
Veins	Carry deoxygenated blood.
Arterioles	Smaller than arteries.
Venules	Smaller than veins.
Capillaries	Exchange oxygen for carbon dioxide.

Making up a sentence from the first character of a list of words – no matter how crazy! For example, make up a sentence that is humorous or relative to you. This way, you will remember, with one word, a list of information.

Writing is the best way of learning. By repeatedly re-writing or typing information you will absorb more than just reading a book or text.

Note-taking and refining notes down to the basics will make things clearer and give you a mental process of listing important ideas and items.

Reading and highlighting text is a good way of note-taking.

Course requirements being clear about the requirements of learning at the beginning of your course will help you to plan ahead. For example, are there short essays (1,500–2,000 words), long essays (2,500–4,000 words) or projects (4,000 words plus)? Make sure you know what assignments count towards your final results.

Research material you will be expected to find out for yourself information for essays and projects. Depending on hand-outs from the tutor is unlikely to be sufficient learning material for the finished work.

Be critical about your subject. Every chosen subject has its limitations. Argue against its attributes, if appropriate in written work.

Be selective so that the content is appropriate to the subject written about. Beware of digressing from the chosen topic! Don't waffle – you will not be marked if you are not clear in your answers, which should be concise and to the point.

Essay plan write an outline before writing and submitting the finished article.

Tutor feedback is meant to be a learning curve, not a criticism. Listen to helpful insights and how you might improve your learning.

EXAMINATIONS CAUSE ANXIETY!

Preparing for your examinations is a good step in aiding confidence. Most people begin learning a professional accredited course in reflexology because they want to learn the therapy. There are always strong feelings surrounding exams but as they are a necessity, dealing with the fears beforehand will leave you feeling more in control on the day.

Take flower remedies at least two weeks before the exam date. Rescue Remedy for crisis and panic, Larch for confidence building and Mimulus for known fears (your exams!).

The imagination runs riot with, 'If I fail, will I have to do it all over again?' The answer is 'No', if you fail one part of the exam, you will only have to re-do that part. You can take examinations in a particular area of the subject as often as you wish, although it would be hoped that you pass all parts the first time.

Don't swop notes with fellow students after the exam. You may be right and they wrong in their answers. This causes unnecessary anxiety and is not helpful in maintaining confidence and motivation. If you have completed home study and completed your set course work, it is unlikely that you will fail on the day!

Unfortunately, those students who have suffered failure in school days find the ghosts of that time rearing their ugly heads! Remember that you are an adult student and in control of your future, far more than when a child, and that you have successfully completed the course work before reaching examination standard.

FURTHER ADVICE

For more in-depth help and guidance, I recommend *Learn How To Study* by Derek Rowntree for a good and comprehensive work on taking exams and study methods.

Section 2

Theory, Practice and Professional Presentation

In treating a patient, let your first thought be
to strengthen his natural vitality.

Rhazes (Ar-Razi; *c.* 865–928) Persian Physician and Philosopher
History of Medicine (Max Neuburger)

This section of the book is concerned with the theory, practice and professional presentation of reflexology. It outlines the requirements and expectations of professional practice and answers commonly asked questions by those thinking of having reflexology treatments.

CHAPTER 6
The Theory and Practice of Reflexology

INTRODUCTION

Sole Route

It is no mischance that the Chinese describe the feet as the route to the 'soul'. The word 'sole', which we use to describe the plantar area of the foot, can be viewed as a derivative of the original meaning. As we have seen in the history of reflexology, the word 'plantar' means that which is in touch with the ground. Therefore, we can use the metaphor that 'sole', or 'soul' manifests in the physical world by expressing itself as a 'personality'. The feet can, therefore, tell a story of how the soul is attempting to manifest itself, along with all its difficulties and 'blockages'.

The Three Rs

Reflexology is a powerful aid in helping the body to regain and maintain homeostasis (internal environmental balance), physically, emotionally, mentally and spiritually. The aim of any student training in the therapy will be to work with *respect* and with *responsibility* towards those who come to you for help with their health problems. By implementing respect and responsibility, *recognition* as a competent practitioner will assist you in developing a successful practice.

The Plea of Pain

The human body is the most complex, miraculous and divine creation. In fact, it is unlikely that a computer or robot will ever be able to replace it. What our bodies can and do every second of our lives is awe-inspiring – and very humbling. Most of us abuse our bodies in some shape or form and yet it goes on day after day, year after year, looking after us and serving our physical needs. Then, when we have abused it sufficiently it begins to hurt and we wonder why!

As we have seen in a previous chapter, feelings and emotions do not just go away if we ignore them – they become locked into the musculature and viscera, and can create physical problems years after an event. Pain is the last symptom in the body – a problem has existed for a long time before pain begins. Is it any wonder, then, that it takes a while for the somatic symptoms of health disorders and the physiological disorders themselves to go away?

Pain can be seen as a direct result of locked-in emotions, which can be seen in psychosomatic symptoms as well as a warning that a particular part of the body is undergoing stress. When disease appears, the blood supply to nerve endings is drying up and the life-force with it.

HOLISTIC GUIDELINES

There are four guidelines which provide cornerstones for professional practice.

1. A person exists on many levels, each of which is of equal importance in the healing process.

This refers to the subtle bodies and auric field, as well as the physical body. All parts of the self must be in balance for healing to take place.

2. The patient has systems of self-repair, which are crucial to the prevention and treatment of that particular person's illness.

This refers to the fact that the body will, most of the time and given the opportunity, heal itself. Becoming aware of the personal way in which we can aid recovery enables the person to work with their healing process. In this way, the patient prevents a somatic symptom from becoming a physiological disorder, which also includes involvement in treatment.

3. Individuals must be actively and knowledgeably involved in their own treatment.

By coming for treatment the patient is actively taking responsibility for their health disorders. With the practitioner's input in maybe suggesting supplemental therapies, at the same time as having reflexology, or adjusting their diet, exercise, and so on, the patient is involved in their own treatment. It is also the practitioner's role to explain any questions about reflexology that provide knowledge and understanding to the patient.

4. Each person is unique and must be treated as such.

We are each of us unique in our make-up, on all levels, operating as an energy field that affects and is affected by others and the external environment. Respect for individuality and methods that are appropriate for a particular person at a particular point in time must always be present in the practitioner's mind. Thus, each person needs a personal programme to aid in their recovery.

METHODS AND BENEFITS

Human beings are complex in make-up and may need help on more than one level, as we have already seen. In assessing the patient's needs at a point in time, it may be beneficial to consider parallel therapies that may be suitable for the patient to work with, which may hasten the healing process.

Reflexology is a powerful tool in helping physical, emotional and mental imbalances held within the psyche. The Ingham method

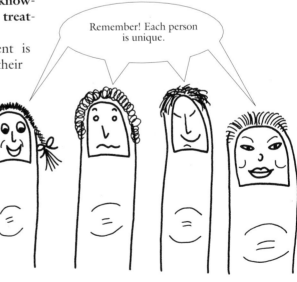

47

of working the feet has profound effects on relief from physical health problems because of its detail to specific locations. It is a system that works firstly on the physical body and, as a secondary benefit, on the subtle bodies, which comprise the auric field.

The *metamorphic technique* and *intuitive reflexology* are examples of alternative methods of working the feet that have an effect on the subtle bodies in the first instance and have secondary benefits on the physical body. Therefore, all methods are relevant and the individual must decide for themselves which type of practitioner will be of help, given the presenting problem and the psychological reason why they have developed the problem at this particular time and in a particular way. Sometimes the psychological reasons are conscious in the person and can be understood as having instigated a physiological problem with, for example, simple indigestion being symptomatic of eating too fast, or emotional stress. Sometimes the psychological reasons are largely unconscious and individuals need help in investigating what may be the cause, with, maybe, counselling and psychotherapy.

The benefits of reflexology can be described as:

- balancing and stimulating the circulatory and lymphatic (cardio-vascular) system;
- improving nerve tone by improved circulation to nerve endings;
- relaxation from tension and stress;
- healing within the subtle bodies, promoting a calmer outlook on life;
- balancing the endocrine (hormonal) system, which assists in a sense of well-being and positivity about life;
- improved energy levels, as a result of the above benefits.

LIMITATIONS

Reflexology is a wonderful therapy – but it is not the panacea for the world's ills! No matter how beneficial any holistic therapy may be at a point in time for the individual, it does not guarantee that it will work in the same way for that person at another point in time. As with any therapy, reflexology has its limitations. Knowing when you, as a practitioner, may not be able to help is as important as giving helpful treatments.

BEING IN HARMONY

All disease is caused by stress but not all stress causes disease. This statement describes stress as being an attitude and emotional response to life. The perception of life events can alter the energetic field making up the individual, which is inharmonious with the true self and 'real' life. This inharmonious way of being with the world eventually creates imbalances within the physiological functioning of the structures of the physical body.

When stress is dealt with in the right way, with a harmonious adjustment and awareness from the self of internal and external pressures, ill health is unlikely to occur.

We have seen how the emotions are the root cause of health problems, through their impact on parts of the brain involved in emotional response, known as the limbic system and the hypothalamus (refer to the Nervous System, page 251). It is by no mischance that we have developed sayings that mirror not only how we feel but reflect imbalances in our energetic system of the chakras (energy centres situated along the spine and over the body) and physiological structures of the body.

Stress can be beneficial or detrimental, depending on how a person perceives their life problems, and assisting the patient to become responsible is part of the therapist's task in assisting the route back to wholeness.

Touch and Communication

The need for human contact is through touch and communication. Sadly, in society today many people have little or no contact with their families, neighbours or the community. A sense of loneliness and isolation from the world results in debilitating the vitality of the person, with, for example, depression, somatic symptoms and insomnia.

With any one-to-one therapy that involves touch, such as reflexology, people can be helped to get back in 'touch' with themselves and the world through stimulating conversation and interest with the therapist.

For the elderly, or those living alone, this contact on a regular basis provides a therapy in its own right! If possible, encourage them to keep a pet for company so that they can give affection and feel needed by providing care and attention – and receive in return unconditional appreciation and love! Stroking a pet releases chemicals in the brain that can boost the immune system, lifts depression and relieves stress.

REFLEXOLOGY THE RELAXANT

The role of reflexology is to relax the patient, so that tension and the resultant toxicity held in muscle and internal organs and glands is released, thereby promoting healing and rebalancing of the subtle bodies and the physical body. Reflexology rebalances the person's energy field so that the wholeness of the human being can function at an optimum level. With the pressure of life in the twentieth century, who doesn't need help some of the time in coping with the stresses and strains of life!

As we have seen, there are theories explaining how reflexology works and although the physiological explanations are logical concepts, the idea of 'blocked' energy channels remain unclear in its meaning. We can consider how these energy channels are inhibited.

A Philosophy for Living

Holistic practice and living can, therefore, be described as a philosophy, as a way of life. By putting into practice, as practitioners, values, ethics and a way of being in the world we can serve as a strength and example to those who come to us in their personal aim to help themselves. From the holistic perspective, we can see how the effects of stress in the body can be released through the understanding of how our personal perception of life events have helped in creating the symptoms and illness.

Laughter – The Best Therapy!

Sometimes, with laughter, a problem can be re-evaluated in a different light. Whenever possible and appropriate, inject humour into the hour you spend with your patient. It may be the only light moment in the whole of their week! Laughter is a therapy in its own right and is severely underestimated as a part of healing for the individual. By reducing stress and tension in the body with humour we go a long way in aiding the patient back to health.

'INSTANT' HEALING

Unfortunately, we live in an instant world where the 'instant coffee ethos' provides the 'quick fix' solution. Explaining that medication suppresses symptoms and is not necessarily an ongoing solution to health problems is helpful in explaining that the body has taken a long time to become imbalanced and its cry for help is through pain and *that it will take some time for it to rebalance*, as far as it is able.

Will Reflexology Hurt?

Sensitive Reflex Points

At the beginning of treatment reflex points can be sensitive and worked with according to the patient's pain threshold. The intensity of pain can reflect the length of time the condition has existed, as in the case of 'chronic' conditions or where a condition has begun to develop. Reflexes that are sensitive can be explained by:

- a lack of energy balance in the reflex point;
- reflecting a 'blockage' or congestion of energy in one or more zonal pathways;
- uric acid crystal deposits settling on nerve endings;

- a particular area needs further attention before tension and energy blocks can be freed in out-of-balance areas in the body.

Chronic and Acute Presenting Conditions

Usually, people who come for reflexology suffer from *chronic* conditions; that is, conditions of long standing where medication does little to relieve the symptoms. Although it is highly unlikely that a patient will come for reflexology who is suffering *acutely* from a condition, if they do, ask them if they have seen their GP or hospital before commencing any consultation, as it may be in the patient's best interest for medical assistance to be a source of treatment at that point in time. An example of this may be acute lower abdominal pains, which may be symptomatic of appendicitis.

CHAPTER 7
Professional Practice and Presentation

PERSONAL APPEARANCE

The way in which you present yourself as a professional practitioner is fundamental to the success of your practice. Personal appearance with tidy hair, dress and general demeanour instils confidence, for both therapist and patient.

One of the vital requirements for a professional reflexologist is to ensure that your hands and nails are kept scrupulously clean. Nothing looks worse than dirty hands and nails, the latter, especially, when disguised with nail polish! Preferably, no nail polish should be worn as it is out of place and unnecessary for the work to be undertaken. Because of the angle and movement of the thumb technique when working the feet, caring for your nails on a regular basis will ensure that the nails are not stabbed into the foot, when reflex pain can get confused with nail pain. Sometimes the patient cannot differentiate between the two!

Remember that your hands are permanently on show and so nails should be kept clean and short with the corners filed into the shape of the thumbs and fingers. Nails should reach the tips of finger pads only, so that they cannot be seen over the tips.

Some reflex points require the use of three or four fingers and so it is essential that the nails are kept the same length. Nothing looks more untidy than nails of varying lengths – in well-groomed hands the nail length is always

the same, so apply the same principles in your professional practice!

Jewellery

Jewellery is also unnecessary on the hands and wrists; watches interfere with the electromagnetic field and gem-stone rings become instruments of torture when pressed into the feet! Bracelets are irritating to listen to and can become caught on the patient's toes – they will not be impressed! Encourage your patient in the removal of their watch, if they wear one, so that the interactive energy flow between you is unimpeded.

APPOINTMENTS

Making Appointments

It is important to give your patient an appointment card so that:

- they do not forget the next appointment date;
- they feel secure about the next appointment;
- there can be no confusion over treatment dates and times;
- they have a written record in case they need to cancel, giving at least twenty-four hours' notice.

Early Arrival

Those who arrive early for an appointment can either wait in a waiting area or wait outside your premises. For those with a waiting area, the presence of relaxing music, magazines, plenty of pot plants and a pleasing decor will begin to soothe the patient before treatment.

For those without a waiting area, interrupting a treatment to answer the door because someone has arrived early is bad practice; and for the patient receiving treatment, it can make them feel unimportant and secondary to the new arrival! Persistent early arrival can reflect control or anxiety issues in relationships and by gently exploring this possibility can save your nerves a great deal of stress!

Late Arrival

It is advisable to give patients who arrive late for appointments the same end time for their treatment as they would have expected if they had arrived on time. Giving a full treatment when the patient is late, even if it is only a few minutes, means that by the end of the day you could keep your patients waiting half an hour or more!

Non-Appearance

To charge or not to charge if a patient fails to arrive for an appointment, presents a burning question. Whether you decide to charge a fee or not can depend on the nature of the relationship that exists between you; if it's a habit to 'forget', or a genuine slip of the memory. Sometimes, people encounter delay on their way to you so that there is no time for the treatment. It is important to consider each situation, when to charge a full fee, reduced fee or none at all for the person who fails to attend their appointment time. Remember, your time and expertise are valuable and respect for you and the therapy can reflect in the patient's timekeeping!

THE PRACTICE SETTING

Decor

Providing the right 'setting' for professional practice is essential for creating a feeling of peace and calmness. The following guidelines will help you to prepare for receiving patients and for them to feel relaxed and special.

- The waiting area should be comfortable with suitable seating for those with hip, knee and spinal problems.
- The area or room where you intend to receive your patients should be aesthetically pleasing to the eye, warm, welcoming and comfortable.
- Decor should be subtle with plants and flowers giving a gentle energy.
- Plants and flowers love crystals and will grow strong and healthy with a few scattered around the room and in plant pots. Crystals grow in the earth and so planting one in a flowerpot is its natural habitation.
- Have drinking water available – lots of it!
- Angle lighting so that it is soft – not glaring or in a direct line of vision.
- Have a mirror and tissues available so that patients can rearrange their clothes, adjust make-up if they have felt upset during the treatment, or begin to discharge mucus from the respiratory passages, or even look at the soles of their feet if they ask questions about them.
- Ensure that there are bathroom facilities available for those who may need to wash their feet before treatment, feel nauseous either during or after treatment, or who wish to spend a penny! A small bowl

hidden away is useful for those who feel nauseous or who cough-up mucus from the bronchial passages.

- Ensure that the environment is hazard free, especially stairwells in your home or work place, which ideally should be covered with carpet to stop feet slipping, and have a handrail to one side.
- Have a waste bin available for tissues and soiled paper.
- A hook or hangers to hang coats should be available.
- During the consultation, it is useful to have suitable sitting accommodation so that details can be discussed in an informal way.
- A cashbox, receipt book and lockable filing cabinet in which patient records are kept, should be as unobtrusive as possible in providing an organized administration.
- Children can be induced to sit still with the temptation of a sweet at the end of the treatment! Having the availability of sweets and/or sugar lumps has the dual benefit of providing a rapid glucose intake for those who suffer from low blood sugar (hypoglycaemia) or who may be diabetic.

Equipment

Ideally, a couch or relaxation chair where the back reclines and lifts the feet and legs should be used. If using a couch, have a footstool to assist your patient onto the couch.

The subject of whether to invest in a couch or relaxation chair depends on your pocket and available space. A couch should have adjustable legs, a backrest and be wide enough for a 130kg (20-stone) person to sit on! I suggest a 65 or 75cm (26 or 30in) width couch, with aluminium legs and frame so that the person's body size can be safely supported and with adjustable legs so that the height of the couch is set for your body height in a sitting position.

The health of the practitioner is equally as important as that of the patient! Necks, backs and shoulders suffer if you are seated at an angle that puts strain on to the shoulder girdle and spine. Ideally, a gas chair with a good, high back support should be used when working. An office chair is good for adapting to knee height, so that the shoulders and trunk are relaxed. If you have a busy schedule, the correct sitting and working position is essential in maintaining your own health. Never sit in a slumped or crouched position as this will cause skeletal misalignments and muscle tension – and take a great deal of money to be corrected!

Ensure that couch covers are clean and that you have sufficient towels and pillows to hand. The room should be a comfortable temperature with adequate ventilation, with a blanket available to cover those who feel vulnerable, unwell or who are chilled. The foot not being worked on should be 'parcelled' at all times to keep it warm. Covering the body with a blanket and parcelling the feet can give a feeling of safety for the patient.

Musical Harmony or Disharmony?

The availability of music can be relaxing for the patient – providing they enjoy what they are hearing! Always check with your patient whether or not they want music played and if so what type of music. There is nothing more irritating than being enforced to listen to music that we do not enjoy – especially since the patient is paying to be relaxed! Sometimes people need to talk about their problems, and fighting with music, no matter how soft and gentle, can stop this necessary process.

Health and Hygiene

Hygiene standards are equally important as the general decor and ambience of the therapy room. The risk of cross-infection, either to the reflexologist or patient, is likely to occur unless equipment and surroundings are scrupulously clean. The following guidelines will help you to get into good habits from day one of working with the public.

- Personal hygiene is essential – especially hands and nails! Grimy nails and hands are not professional and do not look appealing from the other end of the feet. Have hand and foot cream available for massaging the patient's feet at the end of the treatment and for the reflexologist's hands. Constant washing of the hands dries the skin, leaving skin rough and uncomfortable.
- Hair should be kept away from the face as far as possible – hair that is unkempt can impede clear vision and looks untidy.
- Ensure that any abrasions on the hands are covered with a plaster and that hands are washed after each treatment with an antibacterial liquid soap. If the patient has infectious complaints, appointments should be postponed until recovery.
- Working clothes should be suitable for the place of work. For example, if working in a clinical environment a less intimidating 'white coat syndrome' would be more appropriate. Clinical environments go hand-in-hand with white coats of health care professionals and have a reputation for raising blood pressure! On the other hand, if working from home or a less clinical environment, wearing 'whites' may be more appropriate in creating a professional image. Make sure that your clothes are clean, fresh and appropriate!
- Have a well-stocked availability of clean towels and covers to protect the therapist, to wrap the foot not been worked and to cover the pillow under the feet. Towels should be replaced after each treatment.
- Paper towelling should also be replaced after the completion of each treatment.

- Hygiene standards for equipment are essential and storage should be clean, dry and regularly disinfected.
- Use sterile wipes or surgical spirit as a disinfectant on the patient's feet before beginning treatment and on the practitioner's hands after finishing treatment.

Clock Watching

It is a good idea to have a small clock within your vision so that you can check the time as you work. Treatments should take one hour from start to finish, with an additional half-an-hour for the initial consultation. If you have a number of patients booked you will not be able to afford to run over the allotted time. Removing clothing and then dressing again after the treatment takes time as does paying your fee and making a further appointment.

THE THERAPIST–PATIENT RELATIONSHIP

Building the Relationship

An essential part of treatment is to encourage the patient to feel safe with you. With professional practice, good listening skills and accurate assessment of treatment, the patient will be more receptive to treatment. Building a good relationship with your patient is the foundation of good practice.

It makes no difference whether your patient believes in the therapy or not; reflexology will work whether they do or whether they don't. To illustrate the point, I remember a male patient who had been coming for some time to help his regular bout of hay fever in the spring. One night, he got onto the couch, folded his arms and said, 'Of course, I don't believe in this [reflexology]'. I said, 'Are you better?' He said, 'Oh, yes!' That's male logic for you!

Focusing on the patient's predominating state of well-being in the initial consultation is essential for the assessment of how to commence a treatment plan and encourage the patient in communicating their feelings. An example of a client who may have emotional problems predominating physical disorders may present symptoms such as obesity, excessive alcohol and caffeine intake, smoking, has eating disorder patterns and who has hard, impacted skin on the balls of the feet (where the heart and respiratory system reflexes are found), with hard skin over the chakra reflexes on the spinal pathways. These presenting symptoms may indicate high stress and/or anxiety levels, which are not communicated. An initial treatment plan in this situation would involve encouraging the client to talk about their feelings as a route to improved self-esteem, self-image and self-worth so that their harmful and addictive habits would lessen or cease altogether. Eventually, as the client begins to release held-in feelings and emotions, the subtle bodies have a chance to rebalance and the physical and psychological problems may take on a different perspective, leading to positive action in dealing with addictive behaviour patterns.

Clients who present physical imbalances as a predominating factor require concentration on rebalancing the physical being, in the first place. As their awareness of physical well-being increases over a period of treatment sessions, the Subtle Bodies are re-balanced as a secondary benefit, leaving the client feeling calm and generating a sense of integration on all levels of their being.

Being a Good Listener

Being a good listener is one of the major skills of any complementary therapist. Working in a one-to-one relationship with your patient develops trust, communication, empathy and a genuine caring for the person coming to you for help.

Unless qualified as a counsellor, never assume the role of a would-be counsellor. What is more important in your role as a reflexologist is that you have true *empathy* and can *listen* without giving advice, making judgements or imparting your worldly advice!

Sympathy is different from *empathy*, in the former you engage in the feelings and emotions of the individual concerned, which may serve a purpose for the patient but leave you feeling tired and drained over a situation about which you can do nothing. Empathy is the skill of listening and reflecting back to the patient their concerns, without becoming emotionally involved.

As a therapist it is easy to get hooked-in to a sense of power and authority, as your patient may expect you to be the local oracle for all their problems. All this will do, however, is to confuse you as their therapist and if 'advice' you have given doesn't work out, you will be the one to receive the blame!

The components on the medical form will give you an idea of the client's awareness of any imbalances in their life-style and provide you with questions about them. You will also find out if they have made efforts to seek help from any other source, with any possible outcomes.

In the confidential setting of patient and therapist, relief from talking about a problem

---

Emotional Balance and Physical Well-Being

Focus On	*Focus On*
The Subtle Bodies	Physical well-being
Emotional well-being	

with an opportunity to air fears, grievances and life events in a non-judgmental atmosphere helps the patient to feel valued. To those who live alone and who may not have any or little social contact, their hourly session of reflexology may be the highlight of their week. Make it a pleasurable experience as a therapy in its own right. Talking may also help the patient to become aware of unrecognized or unacknowledged feelings by bringing them into focus.

Unique Response

It is important to explain to your patients that if somatic symptoms have been present for some time, then it will take a while for them to improve. Never state a number of treatments – you don't know how many your unique patient will need! It may be three or it may be twenty-three. Remember, *each person is unique and needs to be treated as such*!

Recommend that a course of six treatments is likely to see some improvement with a view to extending it to twelve. Within that time, improvement should be experienced and, if not, then a review of whether reflexology is the right treatment for that particular person at that particular point in time should be considered, with recommendation of other therapies, if possible and appropriate, within the complementary therapy spectrum that may be suited to their problem.

Over the years, with this method of working, people's problems can improve dramatically, and even though they may only be receiving reflexology for a relatively short space of time, they always come back in the future! Genuineness and goodwill go a long way to reassure the patient that you have their welfare at heart and that you are trying your best to aid their recovery.

CONSULTATION RECORDS AND CONTRAINDICATIONS

To assist the reflexology practitioner in providing safe, confident and reassuring treatments, keeping records ensures that the reflexologist has a memory aid to refer to later in the course of treatment. It can also act as a reference point for patients who present with similar conditions, and as a means for collecting data for research. In the case of any dispute arising between the patient and practitioner, the record can be used for insurance purposes.

The following guidelines will ensure that records are adequately safeguarded.

- Use a metal and lockable filing cabinet to store records.
- Ensure that no one has access to the filing cabinet but yourself.
- Confidentiality, honesty and integrity and the patient's overall relationship with their reflexologist are essential components of the therapeutic relationship and under no circumstances should discussion of the patient's personal details, reflexology treatments or any possible research be divulged to another party.
- Discussion with another health-care professional should be carried out in anonymity. Any breach of confidentiality will lose the trust of the patient and could cause undue pain and embarrassment.
- Research or completion of case studies with students in training and clinical experience should be reported as honestly as possible.
- It is easy for misunderstandings to arise during or on completion of treatments and the patient's views as to benefits received and their general progress may be at variance with the practitioner's. To ensure that there is a reduced chance of this

happening, follow the guidelines for completing medical questionnaires outlined in this chapter.

The Data Protection Act 1984

If you intend storing personal data with client records on a computer, compliance with the Data Protection Act 1984 will be required. Information on individuals stored in a computer or similar equipment operating automatically in response to instructions from the user for the purposes of recording information must be lawfully registered to meet the requirements of the Computer Protection Act.

The main provisions of the Computer Protection Act are to:

- Ensure personal data is obtained lawfully and fairly;
- Ensure data is held for one or more specified purposes;
- Ensure data is held for purposes compatible to specified purposes;
- Ensure data held should be adequate, relevant and not in excess of the purpose required;
- Ensure data should not be held for any longer than is necessary;
- Ensure individuals are entitled to enquire whether the data user holds personal data on them;
- Ensure access obtained by the data user;
- Ensure that, if appropriate, data is corrected or deleted;
- Ensure appropriate security measures to prevent unauthorized access, alteration, disclosure or destruction or accidental loss of data held on an individual.

Individuals may sue for compensation in the event of associated stress or damage suffered as a result of:

- Inaccurate data which is misleading or incorrect;
- Unauthorized disclosure;
- Loss of data;
- Unauthorized destruction of data.

For more information contact the Registrar's Office at The Office of the Data Protection Registrar, Wycliffe House, Water Lane, Wilmslow, Cheshire SK9 5AF. Tel. 01625 545700.

Completing the Consultation Record

Completing a consultation record will give an overview of the lifestyle of the patient, their stresses and environmental problems, which may have a direct bearing on the patient's health. A comprehensive record should be maintained from the initial consultation throughout the course of treatments so that you can refer to it years later, if required, when the patient returns and expects you to remember every detail of their health problems, and also to monitor the progress of treatments over a period of time. Asking relevant questions provides the patient with an opportunity to talk about their life and their perception of life events.

The following information is vitally important to include in a consultation record.

Demographic Information

This includes the patient's name, address, telephone number, date of birth, marital status, children, occupation. The GP's name and telephone number, in the event of an emergency should also be included.

Psychosociological Factors and the Consultation

Information gathered during the initial consultation will give you an overall picture of the patient's lifestyle and possible stressors. This information gives the psychosociological background of the individual. Where they live can tell you about environmental and social pressures. For example, a single parent living in a high rise block of flats who is unemployed and smokes and drinks alcohol heavily will literally have 'sky high' stress levels. The emphasis here is on the person's psyche, where the subtle and physical bodies interrelate with the environment; this can create somatic symptoms due to stress in the body.

General Health/Life Awareness/Imbalances

This includes questions concerning: blood pressure (if known); allergies; sleep patterns; alcohol/cigarette consumption; relationships; spiritual outlook/awareness; financial problems; any special diets (diabetic, vegetarian, vegan, red-meat eater, etc.); stress factors; medication; digestion; bowel movements; exercise; interests; weight and height (to ascertain if the patient is either under- or overweight for their age and height, or to allow them to talk about any eating disorders they may have); reactions to treatment and reflexes that were found to be sensitive; the emergence of new symptoms; changes in body processes after treatment; any 'homework' or aftercare given to the patient and finally, changes in the condition of the feet.

Psychological/Emotional Status

Importantly, how does the patient feel emotionally and mentally at the time of the consultation? What is happening in their life to have brought them to you? This information can include current physical health problems – remember, the emotional response to life events will also have an impact on part of the patient's overall health pattern.

Past Medical History

This may shed light on current conditions, establish a reason for treatment and can help build the jigsaw puzzle of the individual's lifestyle and stress factors and possible causes of health disorders. Its usefulness also includes establishing presenting symptoms, assisting and understanding the reflex findings and gives a foundation on which to base progress over a period of time.

Under the Medical History section of the consultation record, include:

- Details of what the client has had wrong with them in the past – going all the way back to childhood, so that you can check the relevant reflexes for any imbalances at the present time.
- It is important to leave plenty of space for taking medical details – you may have a client who has suffered from ill health for years and who has experienced a number of health problems.
- Memory can distort remembered symptoms or disorders experienced in the past, especially in the elderly; forgetting health problems completely is not uncommon. However, the precision of reflexology ensures that the forgotten problems will be found – much to the amazement of your patient!
- List all systems of the body and leave plenty of room to record disorders over the patient's lifetime.

Unidentified Disorders

There are additional circumstances where the patient may need to contact their GP or seek other medical advice when there appears unidentified and prolonged or reoccurring pain. For example:

- The appearance of growths or lumps.
- A medical condition outside of the practitioner's experience or knowledge.
- Psychological changes, either through medication or fluctuating mood changes without medication.

Genetic Influences

These can give vital clues with regard to health patterns and weaknesses in the body that tend to run in families. If a baby is born healthy there is no reason why it should develop the same health problems as the parents, siblings or relatives. Unconsciously, patterns of emotional holding are adopted by the family and, as sometimes happens, are passed on from generation to generation with the result that certain conditions tend to reoccur in the family.

Ask the patient if their parents are alive and healthy and if the answer is 'no' to one or both questions, ask them what condition(s) they have, or what they died of, which will assist in getting a 'feel' for the type of personality and attitudes. Genetic influences do not predict that your client will develop the same set of health problems. However, parental and close family health problems can indicate genetic weakness in a part of the body.

Anything Else?

Completing the consultation record is a form of preventative health-care, where the patient is helped to become aware of what may happen if they don't reapportion their life in some way, or become aware of repeating family tendencies in regard to lifestyle, emotional response to life situations and mental attitudes.

Finally, asking if there is anything else that may prove helpful in relation to the patient's health pattern that you haven't asked gives the patient the opportunity to talk about anything important which may be peripheral to their health problems.

Good Note Taking

Making good, detailed notes with sensitive reflex points will help you to place the pieces of the puzzle together until you have a good idea of where the person holds tension in the body. Reflexology is a way of scanning the whole person, on all levels, as the feet mirror how that person is thinking and feeling at a point in time as well as what disorders may be present.

Contraindications

Included in the medical history are contraindications, which are health disorders, relevant to reflexology that must either be approached with extreme caution, or not worked with at all.

Contraindications are predisposing factors that are included in an assessment of a patient and their suitability for treatment; they can also affect the length and depth of working the reflexes.

In all cases, when any doubt is present with regard to the welfare of the patient, the practitioner should contact the patient's GP.

Present or Subsequent Contraindications

Attention to the presence of contraindications, either during the consultation or which occur during a course of treatment, will alter the length and depth of the treatment. For example, a diabetic or epileptic patient who in between treatments has suffered a hypoglycaemic coma or epileptic fit will need to be reassessed with the possibility of medical or other professional advice being sought.

High levels of medication can leave the patient feeling unwell after treatment as the liver is stimulated and a detoxifying process begins. It is advisable to check the side-effects of medication in a drugs handbook. The practitioner is advised to weigh up whether the strength of medication may be contraindicative and contacting the patient's GP may be the safest way forward before planning and beginning a course of treatment. Conditions that may affect the viability of giving reflexology because of medication include: epilepsy, diabetes, heart problems, extremely high or low blood pressures, thrombosis or thrombophlebitis.

Recent surgery, especially deep tissue surgery, can promote bleeding or haemorrhage if treatments are given too soon. It is advisable to wait for four to six weeks for healing to have taken place in the case of deeper internal tissue before beginning treatment. This is because the external skin may have healed but not internal tissue. It is important to check thoroughly with the patient that they have not suffered any complications after surgery. Adhesions and infections may require referral to the patient's GP, if they have not been already consulted.

Arthritis in the elderly. Although not life-threatening, elderly patients who have suffered from arthritis for a long period of time and have received high levels of medication, will have a weakened constitution, making the detoxifying process of the build-up of medication over the years debilitating and weakening for the individual. Giving reflexology treatments on the hands is a good alternative and is soothing. Massaging the feet with essential oil-based creams, especially with lavender, will calm, soothe and relax. Sometimes, with arthritis, the joints bend so that the toes and fingers become inflexible. If this is the case, work referral areas or cross reflexes on the arms and legs.

HIV/AIDS: both conditions should be worked with care. As with any viral infection, working with a patient who is in the midst of an infection can leave them feeling worse rather than better. Allow an infection to burn itself out and then treat to help boost the immune system.

Care should also be taken for the practitioner's self-protection if a patient who has developed AIDS or is HIV-positive has any abrasion on the feet; if the practitioner also has an abrasion on the hands, the risk of cross-infection is increased. Cover any open areas on the patient's feet and the practitioner's hands with a plaster, or wait for the abrasion to heal.

Explaining to new patients the need to ask whether they are HIV-positive should be carried out sensitively. As a general rule, those patient's over the age of 60 years are unlikely to have contracted the disease as it generally affects those of younger years. Deciding whether or not to ask a patient of an older generation if they have been HIV tested should be considered carefully.

Thrombosis and thrombophlebitis are contraindicative because of the risk of blood clots lodging in or near to the heart. It is important to check that the patient has been discharged from the hospital before commencing treatment.

Fever, infectious and contagious diseases. It is advisable to wait for the condition to improve before commencing treatment. Giving treatment whilst the patient is suffering from a high fever and other symptoms can over-stimulate the already stressed systems of the body, which is trying to fight the invader in a natural way.

Pregnant patients should avoid therapy for the first trimester (first three months of pregnancy), so that the embryo has securely implanted itself in the uterine wall. Giving reflexology before this point could implicate the practitioner in the unfortunate event of a miscarriage, where blame could be attributed to the reflexology treatment. Pregnancies that are unstable should be discussed with the patient's GP before giving treatment.

When treating a full-term pregnancy, the treatment should be adapted in the following ways.

- Provide adequate support and comfort, especially with the lower back and knees.
- Take special care in helping the patient on and off equipment, supporting them from the back.
- Increase work on the urinary system, small intestine and large colon reflexes to ease elimination.
- Work reflexes that assist possible associated problems of pregnancy, such as digestive discomfort with heartburn and indigestion, backache and fluid retention, caused by inadequate emptying of the bladder.
- Avoid heavy pressure on the uterus, pituitary gland, hypothalamus and adrenal glands until the end of pregnancy, as these important glands could stimulate labour before full-term. If possible, show the mother's partner or attendant how to work the relative reflexes extensively during labour or, if permitted, treat her yourself. Reflexology is very helpful in assisting uterine contractions and in a speedy disposal of the placenta.
- Increase work on ankle-loosening to aid circulation and lymphatic drainage and increase working the pelvic reflexes and lymph drainage.
- Avoid recounting stories of pregnancy and labour that could cause anxiety, especially when it is the first experience of childbirth.

Continuing extreme negative reaction. Where the patient feels consistently worse after treatment it is advisable to reconsider the suitability of reflexology for the patient. Very often, if reflexes become progressively tender after several treatments then there is a likelihood that there is a condition which has wors-ened. Advise your patient to consult their GP as soon as possible.

Cancer is a difficult and contentious area when working with reflexology and there are various thoughts as to whether it is wise or unwise to treat the cancer patient. It is helpful to consider what happens with cancer cells and how they are spread round the body through the lymphatic system and the role that reflexology plays in stimulating the body systems.

Although there are many different forms of cancer and the practitioner can never be sure what effect the reflexology treatment may have on that particular person at that particular time, in general, a good 'rule of thumb' is to be guided by the medical prognosis.

If the prognosis is unclear, it is unwise to work with the individual as the stimulating effect of reflexology on the lymphatic system could, conceivably, make the condition worse by spreading cancer cells round the body. With self-awareness, the patient may be able to help themselves, perhaps with visualization and other methods of complementary medicine that do not have such a powerful effect on the physical body, which with medical intervention may assist the patient's recovery. It is advisable to wait for discharge of the patient from the hospital before commencing treatment.

Reflexology and the Terminally Ill

If the medical prognosis indicates that the patient has no chance of survival, receiving reflexology can be a great comfort and pain killer, and will give quality of life for the remaining time left to the individual. When treating someone with a terminal illness you should adapt your reflexology session in the following ways:

- increase time on pain relief;
- increase frequency of treatments;

- increase working eliminatory systems;
- give special attention to comfort;
- give shorter treatments;
- spend more time on relaxation and reassurance;
- adjust the treatment to work on subtle energy levels so that the vital, etheric, mental, emotional and spiritual counterparts of the person are balanced – by working the reflexes lightly and 'holding' them with the thumb, using a light pressure, visualize the *whole* person being healed;
- give healing at the end of the treatment and allow time for the client to express their feelings or spiritual needs.

Continuing with Medication

If your patients are on medication, *never tell them to stop taking it or to cut it down* unless either the patient or yourself has spoken to the GP; doing so may be harmful and even life threatening.

Never claim to be able to help a condition that is beyond your scope, knowledge or ability – this leads, inevitably, to disastrous consequences and is unprofessional for you and devaluing for reflexology as a therapy.

When to Complete a Disclaimer

As with any condition when working with reflexology, the responsibility of the practitioner ensures the safety and welfare of the patient. As a professional practitioner you will have considerable trust and confidence placed in your ability to help the patient. Make it a habit of being conscious of this at all times!

In the event of a patient either being unable to complete the consultation record or when, despite your reluctance to treat them because of contraindications, the person insists that they want you, and no one else, to give them treatment, then ask them to complete a dis-

claimer and sign and date it so that they take full responsibility for the results of any treatments given. It may also be advisable to have a relative present if the information given by the patient cannot be guaranteed to be correct; in this way, they are a witness to information given and recorded.

A disclaimer also provides the practitioner with protection in the event of any dispute concerning the effects of treatments given. The reflexologist has the right to refuse to give treatment if they feel that the patient's health condition, mental stability, commitment or other pertinent reason could have adverse reactions for the patient, or which may become apparent in disruptive or threatening behaviour towards the practitioner.

A disclaimer should be provided at the end of the treatment record and worded to include the following:

Disclaimer

I agree that the above information is correct and I give my permission for treatment. I take full responsibility for the results of any treatments of reflexology given by Ima Nicesole.

Signed . . . .

Dated . . . .

PROFESSIONAL NEGLIGENCE

As a professional reflexologist you will wish to safeguard your reputation as a skilled and accomplished practitioner. By taking out adequate professional indemnity/malpractice insurance, staying within the limits of your training and competence and telling your patients in the initial consultation that you are not medically trained and are not qualified to give a medical diagnosis, will ensure that the interests of both patient and practitioner are safeguarded.

Never practise a therapy unless you are qualified to do so. You may not have insurance and legal proceedings could destroy your confidence and reputation. Adequate public indemnity/malpractice insurance cover for one million pounds is an essential item for the professionally trained reflexologist and students in training should consider taking out insurance cover immediately training commences, so that should any problems occur in the early days of training, confidence and motivation are maintained.

CHECKING CREDENTIALS

If we experience unsatisfactory treatment with a health-care professional we seek a second opinion from another source. Generally, when a person receives an unsatisfactory treatment with reflexology they tend to dismiss the therapy completely and do not consider changing to another therapist. Checking training credentials before risking your feet to the 'home-taught' practitioner without any formal qualification is a wise precaution. If you are not happy with the results of treatment or the professionalism of the practitioner, change to another – today! *See* Organizations for a list of reputable accrediting bodies for a variety of complementary therapies who will be able to refer you to a professionally trained therapist in your area.

The following questions will help you to ascertain whether your chosen reflexologist is suitably qualified to help with your problems:

- Where did they train – was it an accredited course?
- How long was the training course (it should be a minimum of one year)?

- What are their qualifications?
- How long have they been practising?

TAKING A BREAK BETWEEN PATIENTS

It is advisable to allow at least 15–20min between patients, in order to:

- wash your hands and prepare the room before their arrival;
- collect the patient's records, paper towels, tissues, talcum powder or cornflour, foot cream and clean towels;
- complete the patient's treatment notes;
- allow time for patients to prepare for treatment and dress at the end;
- make the next appointment and possibly wait for the patient to write a cheque for your fee;
- allow for overlap if the next patient is a few minutes late;
- have some recuperation time, with a drink, meditation or taking some fresh air.

FIRST AID

The aims of administering first aid are to:

- promote recovery from the presenting condition;
- limit the effects of the condition and to preserve life.

As a reflexologist practitioner it is advisable that a first-aid certificate should be obtained, so that adequate insurance cover is available if operating a clinic from your home. If you wish to practise from a complementary medicine clinic or GP practice, check that insurance for the administration of first aid is in place. Failure of insurance cover carries risk of legal

63

action if the patient is harmed through first-aid interventions whilst on your premises.

When practising first aid, follow these guidelines:

- assess the situation;
- ensure the area is safe;
- assess the condition of the patient;
- give emergency aid;
- get help.

Items that should be available in a first-aid kit, kept in the treatment room in case of medical emergencies, are as follows:

- scissors for cutting dressings to size;
- sugary drinks, glucose tablets or sugar lumps in case of diabetic/hypoglycaemic attack;
- plasters and dressings to cover abrasions;
- triangular bandages for use as slings;
- roller bandages to secure dressings;
- tubular support bandages to support limbs and hold any dressings in place;
- an eyebath to wash irritants out of the eye and to secure contact lenses;
- disposable gloves for use when dressing abrasions or disposing of waste;
- safety pins to secure dressings and bandages;
- antiseptic for cleansing abrasions;
- sterile gauze dressings to cover existing wounds;
- a paper bag to aid hyperventilation.

The A, B, C of Resuscitation

- **A** is for Airway – tilt the client's head back and lift the chin to open the airway.
- **B** is for Breathing – restore breathing with mouth-to-mouth resuscitation by blowing your own expelled air into the casualty's lungs.
- **C** is for Circulation – apply compression to the chest to restore circulation to the heart and body.

The Recovery Position

This is used when the client is breathing but unconscious and the heart is beating. This ensures that the airways remain open with the head, neck and spine aligned. The tongue cannot fall back and block the throat and the body is supported in a stabilized position. This position also allows vomit or other substances to drain from the mouth.

Fainting

In the case of a patient fainting whilst in your place of work:

- lay them down on the floor;
- loosen tight clothing;
- reassure as they recover;
- offer water to drink;
- if in doubt, seek medical aid;
- raise and support legs, if possible, or put the head between the knees and suggest that the patient grips the knees to stop from falling sideways;
- increase ventilation;
- look for and treat, if possible, any injury sustained from the fall.

Nosebleeds

Those suffering from nosebleeds should have the soft part of the nostrils pinched together, with the head forward. Encourage the patient to breathe through the mouth, and release pressure after ten minutes, reapplying if it reoccurs. Advise them not to blow their nose for as long as possible to allow for the blood to clot. Nosebleeds can be symptoms of other conditions in the body and the patient should seek medical advice if they are frequent.

Epilepsy

Experiencing or being present when someone has an epileptic attack can be frightening. The following actions should be taken when a patient suffers a *'grand mal'* fit:

- if possible, support the patient to ease the fall;
- ensure privacy and space for the patient;
- ensure that the patient cannot damage themselves, others or objects whilst suffering the attack;
- loosen clothing round the neck;
- if possible and appropriate, remove false-teeth but *do not to prise the mouth open*;
- protect the patient's head;
- once the convulsions have ceased, place the patient in the recovery position;
- stay with the patient to reassure and monitor recovery until fully recovered.

Diabetic Attack

In the case of a diabetic attack the following procedures should be taken:

- help the patient to sit or lie down;
- give sweet food or drink;
- on improvement, give more sweet food or drink;
- allow to rest until recovered;
- contact their GP.

Loss of Consciousness

In the case of finding your patient unconscious and lying on the floor, the following actions should be taken:

- check patient response to calling their name;
- check for danger and provide safety precautions if necessary;
- check that their airway is free;
- check the pulse at the carotid artery, next to the 'Adam's Apple'.

No Heartbeat or Breathing

If the patient has stopped breathing and there is no pulse, the following action should be taken:

- dial 999 for an ambulance;
- clear the airway;
- perform mouth-to-mouth resuscitation with two breaths, then 15 chest compressions;
- alternate between mouth-to-mouth resuscitation and chest compressions until arrival of the ambulance or the patient recovers consciousness.

See Bibliography for a recommended first aid book.

Treating a Nervous Client

When giving treatment to a very nervous client, a reassuring atmosphere and practitioner are essential in the relaxation process. The following allows time for the patient to become acclimatized to you, the environment and in learning what you will do to them during the treatment session:

- ensure that the atmosphere is non-intimidating and quiet;
- allow more time and make extra effort to establish a rapport with the patient;
- take time to answer questions and give reassurance;
- give a clear explanation of what to expect during treatment;
- demonstrate the working technique on the patient's hand;
- work more often throughout the treatment on areas for tension-release and calming,

for example, the solar plexus, diaphragm, brain and toes;

- give reassuring information about possible after-effects;
- suggest to the patient that they phone you if they are feeling anxious between treatments.

Hyperventilation

People who are very stressed can suffer from hyperventilation, which is an abnormally fast rate of breathing, gasping or deep breathing. Symptoms include:

- tingling hands;
- trembling;
- dizziness and faintness;
- cramps in the hands and feet;
- acute anxiety, terror and fear, causing hysteria, panic attacks or shock;
- a precursor of asthmatic or other bronchial dilatation disorders;
- acute cases can lead to tetany (*see* Systemic Disorders: Muscular System).

It is vital that the client is aided in calming their anxious and fearful state by:

- speaking gently but firmly to them in a reassuring way;
- removing them from the cause of distress, if possible;
- asking them to do something to take their mind off the cause of the anxiety;
- if symptoms persist, ask them to breathe their own expired air out of a paper bag so that more CO_2 enters the brain;
- encourage the client to do a *grounding exercise* by placing their feet firmly on the ground, the reflexologist holding the client's hands, whilst the client breathes slowly;
- if symptoms persist, call the client's GP.

Nausea

A patient who begins to feel nauseous or faint should also be attended with emergency first-aid procedures and the treatment curtailed with a gentle massage. If necessary, call for help to take the patient home or call their GP if in doubt about the reason for their adverse reaction to treatment.

BECOMING AN EXPERT

Take time to develop your expertise in reflexology before deciding on further training. Rushing from training in reflexology to training in another therapy will not give you time to assimilate knowledge gained and to become a well-rounded practitioner. Once experience has been gained, ongoing personal and professional development are the hallmarks of a dedicated and genuine therapist. Patience is a virtue – it is best to wait for any additional therapies, which you feel may be suitable for you to train in, to appear naturally, in their own time! Experiment by receiving therapies to see what feels natural to you before committing your time and financial outlay with training. Training in more than two therapies can mean a loss of impact with building a reputation as a good reflexologist as the energy field will become too scattered, and develops a therapist who is a 'Jack of all trades and master of none'!

ADVERTISING YOUR SERVICES

In any advertising material, ensure that the nature of your services as a reflexologist are described *appropriately and accurately*. Claiming to cure, diagnose or guarantee the effectiveness of treatment is misleading and is illegal under the Trade Descriptions Act 1968.

CHAPTER 8

Caring for the Practitioner and Patient

GREETING THE PATIENT

The way in which you greet the patient can have long-term effects on the relationship. Be friendly and polite and try to establish a rapport with them when introducing yourself, without gushing! You will be building an intimate relationship with this person over a period of time and the way the foundations are laid for this will become part of the therapy for the patient.

To assist in the building of the relationship, projecting a sensitive manner when taking personal details for a confidential medical questionnaire will instil confidence in your ability.

- Assist the patient onto the couch and adjust the pillows for them so that their head is well supported and offer the cover of a blanket, if appropriate.
- Ensure that their knees and back are supported adequately and, in normal circumstances, that you can maintain eye contact with them. This is important in allowing the patient to talk if they need to.
- Laying flat is not helpful in holding a conversation and so a back support is essential in angling the body so that the patient is comfortable and relaxed but can see and speak to you at the same time.

I have had two patients who suffered from severe migraine, with one even attending the treatment sessions wearing sunglasses. Neither of these ladies could bear any light and sitting aggravated the condition; they wished to lie flat for the treatment, with the curtains closed and any lighting in the room as low as possible. Feeling as unwell as they did at the beginning of the treatments, they had no desire to talk. This is a good example of when lying down is preferable to the half-sitting position.

Giving Support

It is important to assist, or offer to help, your patient on and off the treatment chair or couch for the following reasons:

- to avoid any accidents;
- in case they feel disorientated;
- for insurance purposes;
- in case they are unable to do it for themselves.

Financial and Personal Circumstances

Those who are genuinely in financial hardship very often forego the benefits of reflexology because they cannot afford the treatments. Offering payment of a fee that is within their scope will allow them to feel valued and offer a chance for them to improve their health. It is important to state or negotiate your fee before treatments begin so that there can be no confusion about fee paying.

TREATMENT SCHEDULE

A question commonly asked is: 'How many treatments will I need?'

Very often the patient needs to have an idea of how many reflexology treatment sessions will be required. This information is important to them, maybe because of holiday plans or other commitments and any financial constraints.

It is important to discuss with the patient during the first consultation your fee structure and any concessions that you may be able to offer, and the importance of regular weekly or more frequent treatments, if they have a presenting health condition.

Frequency of Treatments

The frequency of treatments will vary from person to person and unless the patient wishes to have reflexology for relaxation purposes, weekly treatments provide good support and gradual improvement. It is important to explain to chronic sufferers with conditions such as asthma, sinusitis and back and bowel problems, that twice weekly treatments will impact all levels of the person with conditions that are long established. Working in this way for approximately one month, then reducing to weekly treatments once the condition begins to improve, will speed the body's healing process.

Generally, the following check-points can answer the patient's question of how many treatments they will need.

- It depends on the client and their individual needs.
- Each person is unique and responds differently to treatment.
- A treatment plan will be discussed after the first treatment.

- A review, after a number of treatments, will give the patient and therapist an opportunity to express their views on progress made.
- It may depend on the seriousness of the condition and how long the patient has had the condition.
- It depends on individual commitments and financial circumstances.

The Length of Treatments

The length of the treatment session may be influenced by the presenting condition, if there is any.

- What is the presenting condition?
- The age of the client (children and the elderly need special attention, *see* later in this chapter).
- What is the client's overall condition and state of health from your observation of them?

Commitment to Treatment

Encouraging the patient to commit themselves to treatment over a period of time develops the idea of taking more care of the self and taking responsibility for their health.

Reducing Treatments and Maintenance

Those patients who reach their optimum level of improvement can reduce treatments slowly over a period of time until, maybe, monthly treatments provide a top-up to keep energy levels and a sense of well-being at their optimum.

Remember that your intuition will give you vital information about the patient's needs, which may not be obvious to the patient.

PATIENT PARTICIPATION

Discuss the treatment with your patient either during or at the end of a session – the patient will feel empowered if given knowledgeable advice and information of what you have found from the feet and how they may be able to adopt simple restorative measures in their own time. If appropriate, teaching some hand-reflexology or, where they can, foot reflexes also helps them to feel involved in their treatment and boosts the effectiveness of self-healing during treatments with you.

Feet Belong to a Body!

Reflexology is a very physical and energetic way of working with people and may look easy to the patient sitting at the other end of the pair of feet! Remember to constantly check your patient's facial expressions – those who feel that showing pain is a sign of weakness will tense their facial muscles unconsciously and those who are more obviously gripping the side of the chair or couch and clenching their teeth need to be monitored constantly for their personal pain threshold.

I often ask people to 'scream quietly', or 'just bite onto a piece of leather' to inject some humour into the treatment! When it is the first treatment, nerves, anxiety and 'What is he or she going to do to me?' are the primary concerns of the patient.

In the first treatment, ascertaining the level of sensitivity of reflexes is vitally important in finding a patient's pain threshold, and makes future treatment a pleasant and a relaxing experience.

ASSESSING SENSITIVITY OF REFLEXES

Assessing the sensitivity of reflex points may require the method of working the feet to be adapted to the needs of the patient. Remember to listen to your intuition constantly when working with your clients and let your thumbs go where they want to go on the feet and hands – they have an intelligence and knowledge that the logical brain interferes with!

There are various reasons why reflexes may be sensitive.

- The emotional or mental state of the patient.
- The presence of medication in the body.
- Weakness or somatic symptoms, which may develop into pathological problems in the future.
- Temporary tension or stress in an area.
- A memory held in a particular area that relates to a past condition but is no longer present.
- Ongoing chronic problems that may have their origins in previous acute conditions or which have been newly diagnosed.

The Pain Threshold

The pain threshold is very important to judge when working with someone who has a low pain threshold or a chronic problem. In the first treatment, the pain threshold is ascertained by *gently* exerting pressure with the thumb or index finger until pain is felt. At this point, lessen the pressure until it is comfortable. In this way, you will build an accurate picture of where energy imbalances are in the body and which in future treatments you will be able to monitor by applying appropriate pressure for the patient's comfort.

Remember, *it is not good practice to use a hard pressure on painful feet.* Finding your patient stuck to the ceiling means that they won't return and your reputation as being a good practitioner will suffer! Eventually, the feet will feel no pain at all and, by this happy time, you know that the patient's whole being has rebalanced itself to an optimum level and can, in future, enjoy the pure relaxation of treatment without sensitivity.

Sometimes, people come solely for relaxation without health-related disorders and quite naturally they do not have any sensitivity on the feet at all. Although this may not be helpful whilst you are training, when sensitive feet are more interesting and a better learning aid, you will still learn a lot about the person from, for example, where they store tension in the body; how toxic they are or maybe how emotionally 'up-tight' they are.

The *amount of pressure* applied when working the reflexes can vary from person to person and from one treatment to the next.

Sensitive reflexes benefit from the following methods which can be incorporated into the full treatment.

- Work the reflexes in several directions (*see* Section 3).
- Change the angle of working with the thumb.
- Work over the area several times, being careful not to overwork reflexes, which can cause adverse reactions.
- 'Hold' reflexes under the thumb, remembering to monitor the patient's pain threshold.
- Work the reflexes for a longer time and return to them throughout the treatment.
- Show your patient how to work the sensitive reflex points on the hands and, where possible, on the feet.
- Work complete systems of the body as represented on both feet.
- Provide pain relief with areas giving distress.
- Supporting and strengthening surrounding areas before working the main area of energy imbalance.
- Increase time given to relaxation techniques.

- Adjust pressure as first aid. For example, in the case of the client fainting where a lighter pressure 'holding' the reflex will assist recovery.
- Work cross-reflexes, especially in cases where it may be unsuitable to work the feet.

Below are some guidelines where pressure applied should be lighter than normal.

- During the first treatment, so that any adverse reactions and overload to the body are minimized.
- When accessing the subtle bodies.
- For the terminally ill, the elderly, young children, recent surgery and general debilitation.

TREATING SPECIAL PEOPLE

When treating the very young, the elderly, those who have recently had surgery, patients who are nervous or who have psychological problems, extra care should be given. Remember to work lightly and gently in all cases.

Treating a Young Child or Baby

When treating a young child or baby you will find that they are either expert wrigglers or will appear so mystified by what you are doing that they sit quite still! In either event, adapting the session assists giving treatment. Many years ago, a little four-year-old girl who came for treatment because of mucous congestion used to call me 'the tickling lady'! Children are a constant source of amusement and, on the whole, I have found that they thoroughly enjoy treatment. Generally, the following methods of working with them will be helpful.

- Use lighter pressure and give a shorter treatment.

- Have mother present for reassurance and comfort.
- Have toys or books available.
- Modify equipment to child's size or allow the child to sit on mother's lap.
- Work briefly to give light stimulation of reflex points.
- Build a relationship to help the child get used to treatment.
- Provide a relaxed, informal atmosphere.

It is an offence in law not to seek adequate medical aid for a child under the age of sixteen and the professional reflexologist should ensure that the following information is given to the carer before embarking on treatment with the child. A failure to do so could result in aiding and abetting the parent or guardian by not advising them of the need to seek medical advice

The parent or guardian should sign a statement to the effect that they have been advised to contact their GP concerning the health of their child, which should also be witnessed before treatment commences.

A statement can be added with a disclaimer at the end of the confidential medical form and can be phrased as shown below.

Disclaimer for Use when Treating Patients under Sixteen Years Old

I have been informed by . . . . that in accordance with the law I should consult a doctor concerning the health of

. . . .

who is my . . . .

Signed: . . . .

Dated: . . . .

Witnessed by: . . . .

Sometimes it is advisable to give the mother treatment before the child, when the mother may be stressed or anxious about her child. Children are emotional sponges and will soak up subconsciously the mother's feelings and so by helping the mother to be more relaxed, her child will be more relaxed. Some childhood illnesses can be caused by family tensions and if this is the case, telling the parent to contact their GP about the Family Guidance Clinic, where the whole family can find support and understanding, may mean that the family's health improves as a whole.

Treating the Frail or Elderly Person

When treating the frail or elderly person, adapting the treatment session builds confidence, possibly with someone who has never heard of reflexology and who may be anxious as to what the treatment involves. It has been my experience that the elderly sometimes have difficulty in understanding how the feet can affect the body, or that it is a medical method of 'treatment'. It is a good idea to explain a little of the history of reflexology without going into too much detail, which can confuse the patient and is not helpful in letting them know of the likely benefits of receiving treatment. The following guidelines serve to gently reassure and leave the patient feeling that they have a role to play in their treatment.

Remember! Work lightly and gently with young, elderly or nervous clients.

- Gentle, light treatments take into account thinning skin and osteoporosis.
- Using a slow, gentle rhythm is relaxing and comforting.
- Allow time to talk – remember, it may be their only contact with anyone during the week.
- Have available additional padding for comfort, for example, with the elbows, neck, knees and ankles.
- Give more time for relaxation techniques.
- Give shorter treatments as over-stimulation can easily occur.
- Work with the natural shape of the toes and do not attempt to straighten curled toes. Hand reflexology may be preferable if the toes are painful or inaccessible.
- Take special care when helping the client on and off equipment. Support them from behind with one arm and use the other hand to support the arm nearest to you.
- Work lightly over broken capillaries as thin skin means that bruising can occur more easily.
- Keep massage light and massage the hands as an extra relaxant.
- Do not work reflexes for too long or too often during the treatment.

The Mental State of the Patient

If the patient has psychological problems and is on medication, treatments should be arranged with a view to relaxing them and gently working the reflexes, especially the endocrine glands, which play a key role in personality and mood changes.

Very often, patients cathart (a release of emotional tension through crying, screaming and sobbing), which for the newly qualified reflexologist can be a frightening and perhaps unexpected experience. The following guidelines will be helpful in situations of this kind.

- Don't try to make it 'better' by comments such as 'It will be all right' – it may *not* be all right in the case of bereavement, relationship problems, terminal illness and financial stress.
- Allow the patient to release their feelings and ask permission to touch before assuming that they want to be comforted. Remember their personal space and intimate zones when touching any part of the body from the knee upwards.
- Explain to them that they are experiencing a healthy release of tension, which has been held in the body and would eventually lead to somatic symptoms and possible pathological disorders.
- Encourage them to go into psychotherapy and counselling to help them explore their feelings and to receive healing from someone who is professionally trained in other methods of healing, such as crystal healing, biodynamic massage, rolfing and bio-energetics, all of which work on releasing feelings stored in the body and on healing the 'sick' spirit.

Surgery, Scars and Adhesions

For those who have recently undergone extensive surgery, encourage them to rest properly – there is nothing clever about going back to work too soon, doing the domestic chores or digging the garden because guilt sets in about 'doing nothing'. In fact, we can never 'do nothing' as while we exist in a physical body we are moving and changing, whether consciously or not! Proper rest will prevent adhesions forming and possible complications arising after surgery, and your doctor will not tell you to rest unless necessary – so slow down and give your hard-working body a chance to recover!

Scar tissue and possible adhesions may leave tender reflexes, so do not be surprised if the patient explains that they have had a part of their body removed or repaired. The surrounding viscera (organs and glands), muscle, tendons and tissue move around to fill the empty space – nature always adapts herself, given the chance.

After surgery or illness, the patient's vital energy may be low and the following observations will give clues if this is the case:

- a dull or no response on reflexes;
- a numbness or loss of feeling;
- coldness, possibly indicating poor circulation;
- dampness or clamminess, possibly due to medication, a hormone imbalance, anxiety;
- 'empty' or degenerated areas indicate poor blood supply or 'holding' of energy;
- slack muscle tone may be due to lack of exercise or of emotional debility;
- sponginess or puffiness can be multi-factorial and individual to the patient;
- pale colour can indicate poor circulation or energy which is 'held in';
- an intuitive awareness of low energy field can encompass all of the above, including tension in the cavities of the body.

Remember to monitor the pain threshold of the patient constantly!

ADVERSE REACTIONS TO TREATMENT

Very often, patients experience adverse reactions after the first treatment or during a course of treatment. In the first instance, advise the new patient that they may feel slightly unwell or 'off colour' or nauseous, faint or weak. (For further reactions *see* Section 3.)

Forewarning your new patient of what *may*, but not necessarily *will* happen, will allow your patient to become involved in their treatment, which encourages trust and confidence.

Encourage your patients to drink plenty of water – at least one glass whilst they are with you and to drink five pints per day at home, if they can manage it. This will help the liver and kidneys detoxify and the bowels to function more efficiently, thereby getting rid of toxic waste that would otherwise stay in the blood. It is amazing that once we take simple steps, like drinking plenty of water (filtered or bottled – never tapped, the chemicals in the water and repeated human recycling negate any benefits of drinking it!) how much better we feel. The benefits of 'Adam's Ale' have been much demeaned and derided for far too long.

As a nation, we do not drink enough pure water and it is no wonder that our kidneys and digestive system protest! Get into the healthy habit of drinking a glass of water every time you reach for the kettle to brew tea or coffee. See how much clearer your skin becomes and how much more efficiently your body rids itself of excess body fluid and aids the adrenal glands by reducing the amount of adrenaline and sympathetic nerve stimulation.

Nurses and clinical staff who have come for training always have spine and kidney sensitivity on the reflexes. The repeated reply to my questioning has been that they don't have time to drink water because they don't have time to go to the bathroom! Spinal problems with them occur because of lifting patients. The result is that the kidneys have a hard time in keeping pace with a high concentrate of toxins and the spine suffers without

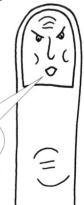

Remember! Advise your client that they might experience an adverse reaction to the treatment.

regular realignment of the skeletal frame. Adverse reactions may indicate a need for a change in the treatment plan.

Below are some positive, negative and eliminatory reactions, which patients may experience after treatment.

Positive effects can include:

- feeling very relaxed;
- increased energy;
- improved sleep pattern;
- feeling elated or 'on a high';
- feeling as though they are 'floating on air';
- feeling more in control of their lives;
- relief from pain;
- manipulation of the foot itself;
- human touch and interaction between the patient and therapist can give caring contact;
- a feeling of balance in body, mind and spirit.

Negative effects can include:

- pain from reflex points;
- temporary worsening of presenting and/or the underlying condition;
- a feeling of being generally unwell;
- headaches;
- needing to sleep a lot;
- feeling very tired and listless;
- feeling emotionally upset, irritable or restless;
- feeling depressed;
- feeling cold or hot.

Eliminatory effects can include:

- increased urination and/or defecation;
- slight constipation or diarrhoea;
- increased sweating, especially from the hands and feet;
- nausea or dizziness;
- a skin reaction;
- a runny nose.

The following are possible reasons for a reaction to treatment.

- As part of the *healing crisis*, where the condition may appear to worsen for a short time, with either new or worsening of existing symptoms before a positive response to treatment.
- As an elimination and release of toxins and waste products.
- A chronic condition moving into an acute phase, when the patient's GP should be consulted.
- The body replays a memory of past conditions or symptoms not yet resolved, which are of an emotional origin.
- A rebalancing of energy pathways, which leaves the patient feeling 'off balance'.

Newly Occurring Conditions

Sometimes, new conditions occur whilst the patient is receiving treatment, which can change the course of treatment. How treatment is affected will depend on what the new condition is and whether it is contraindicative or the patient is receiving newly prescribed medication, which reflexology may interfere with by detoxifying the body so that it doesn't have time to take effect. Treatment may need to be rearranged to fit the new circumstances.

No Presenting Conditions

Regular treatments can act as a prevention to disorders developing and periodic treatments, for example, on a monthly basis, can help maintain relaxation well-being on all levels of the psyche. Patients attend treatments as desired and it is a good exercise in self-nurturance, where time spent on the self is a healthy way of loving the body. Very often, people feel it is 'selfish' to spend time on themselves.

They couldn't be more wrong! We cannot love and respect others if we cannot love and respect ourselves!

PROTECTING THE ENERGY FIELD

One of the wonderful benefits for the working reflexologist is that the energy interaction between the patient and practitioner gives healing to *both parties*! I have found, when feeling under the weather, that if I give a treatment, I feel much better. So we can view giving treatment as a two-way benefit, most of the time. Sometimes, however, individuals can drain your energy field and can leave you feeling like a limp rag!

Most of us at some time or the other have the experience in day-to-day life of people who we try to avoid because we know how depleted of energy we feel when we leave them. Protection of the solar plexus chakra is essential when working with individuals who may do this. Visualization is a very powerful method of keeping your energy for yourself and will help you to monitor energy levels throughout the day. There are many methods of visualization that can be used to protect the energy field against 'invaders'.

The first is to imagine entering a metal egg, which is comfortable and warm, lock the door once inside and settle down to enjoy the feeling of being surrounded by warmth and comfort. Another method is to imagine a band of gold encircling your body, which is flexible but impenetrable. Imagine keeping *love* in the heart centre so that you can give out to others, but they cannot penetrate your gold band of protection. Alternatively, imagine a mirror placed over the solar plexus, so that whatever someone gives out towards you, will reflect back through the mirror to themselves. It is best to visualize for yourself a method that feels natural for you – and remember to do it whenever you are with anyone who you feel is draining your energy field! It is easy to forget to practise protection when someone may be talking at you nineteen-to-the-dozen!

THE DISADVANTAGES AND ADVANTAGES OF SELF-TREATMENT

Advantages of Self-Treatment

There are advantages to self-treatment between attendance at professional treatments. The additional stimulation to the reflex points provides extra support in the healing process, as symptoms can be eased immediately in stimulating sensitive reflexes. However, it is wise to check with your reflexologist before any additional working of reflexes, as over-stimulation could create adverse reactions. One of the major benefits of self-treatment is that your feet are instantly available – and without cost to yourself!

Disadvantages of Self-Treatment

Working on your own feet is difficult and uncomfortable to perform with only a limited number of reflexes able to be worked. It is always best to receive a full treatment, so that the whole body receives balanced stimulation. The inadequacy of self-treatment means that vital reflexes will not be worked. Underlying health problems may not respond to self-treatment unless the whole foot is worked, due to an absence of the interactive energy field of the practitioner, who has knowledge of your condition and understanding as to how the reflexes should be worked.

Reflexology is meant to aid relaxation – having your foot and leg twisted at an unnatural angle is not conducive to feeling relaxed!

CHAPTER 9
Making Connections

THE HUMAN JIGSAW PUZZLE

We can relate, metaphorically, to reflexology resembling a jigsaw puzzle. Imagine that you have a jigsaw puzzle with which to make a beautiful picture. Some parts of the puzzle are easier to find than others, some need considerable time to find where they fit, some pieces begin to give you a good idea of the overall picture and some pieces are obscure and blend into the background. All pieces are necessary for the completion of the picture, and even with one piece missing the picture feels incomplete. So it is with the art and science of reflexology. Try to imagine the reflexes on the feet as pieces of a jigsaw puzzle which, when integrated with anatomy and physiology, and the theory and practice of reflexology, will give you a picture of the person's overall health and well-being.

This chapter is designed to enable the reader to check reflex point areas, and to give information on areas of special interest, such as where to find the reflexes. The directions of how to work the reflexes will be found in Section 3.

3-D HUMANS AND THE LAYER EFFECT OF REFLEXES

Our bodies are arranged in three layers and the human body can therefore be described as being three-dimensional. If our bodies were arranged in one layer, we would be three

times as wide or high! So we need to bear this in mind when working the feet. Correspondingly, the reflexes in the feet are found in layers and the direction in which we work means that we are contacting different reflexes. It is therefore important to follow the angles and directions of thumb and index finger movements to ensure that you gain an accurate picture in your mind of where about you are in relation to the body.

With some reflexes, *altering the angle of the thumb changes the intensity of sensitivity* (if any) and so do not be afraid to try for yourself different angles of working. Remember to work in the immediate area surrounding the text book reflex point – no one person's body is identical to another and, therefore, reflexes can be found in an approximate area.

ZONES AND BLOCKS

We can imagine zonal energy and energy blockages in the body like a road system – where there may be roadworks that block the road off completely, or which has limited access, or is a 'stop' and 'go' system. Where the road is blocked completely, there is no movement and can be likened to the body becoming completely blocked in one area, where disease has developed. Where there is limited access, there is still some movement and this can describe restricted energy movement in the body caused by stress and tension.

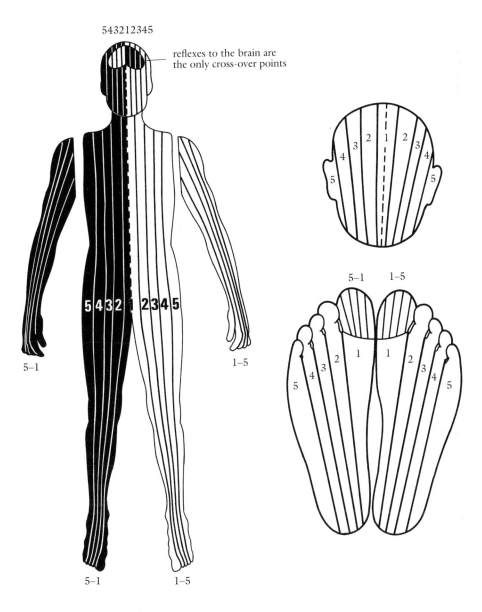

543212345

reflexes to the brain are
the only cross-over points

5-1

1-5

5-1   1-5

Fig 1. The ten zones of the body.

This is the kind of situation where psycho-somatic disorders can develop. Finally, 'stop/go' means that sometimes there is movement in the right direction and sometimes it becomes contraflow! In the body, this means that there are energy imbalances with corresponding see-sawing somatic symptoms.

If we imagine the five zones of energy either side of the spine, as described in Chapters 1 and 2, the word 'blockage' can be interpreted as feelings. When we fail to express our feelings and 'swallow' them down into the body, they become locked into the viscera and musculature, thereby constricting blood supply to nerve endings. Thus, the pain of disease or somatic symptoms can be interpreted as the body crying out for help to be stimulated back to health.

The subject of emotional anatomy and how we create our body shape through our perceptions and responses to life situations has great relevance in the philosophy of holism. Emotional holding in the body of unexpressed feelings and emotions ('*e-motion*' means energy in motion), which eventually disturbs physiological functioning and homeostasis, is a most important concept to understand in holistic practice as all disease and physiological disorders almost always have a psycho-emotional reason for developing.

Energy Movement

A little should be said about the flow of energy, which moves from left to right around the body. I have found over the years that patient's who block out external thoughts, feelings and emotions from others completely, with expressions such as 'I don't want to know', 'turn the other cheek', or who simply put their head in the sand, tend to develop imbalances on the *left side* of the body, which are reflected in the *left foot*. Based on Yin/Yang principles, the left side of the body is the Yin, the feminine, passive, receptive side. By blocking these out when we feel we have had enough input, we can create a 'blockage' that can reveal itself through skeletal misalignments, physiological dysfunction and somatic symptoms.

Conversely, when the right foot is more tender than the left, the Yang side of the body, which relates to the masculine, outgoing, expressive element, is blocked and is caused by the person taking on board the thoughts, feelings and emotions of others but then doing nothing with them! In other words, these thoughts, feelings and emotions are not communicated and stay 'stuck' in the middle of the energetic field of the individual.

By working the left foot first of all, the patient's resistance and defence mechanisms to outside stimulus are dissolved and, with a course of weekly treatments, leaves them feeling energized to cope with life's problems, which gives a feeling of being in control in their lives.

Dense Energy

The 'density' of working blocked energy zones can be described as trying to swim against the tide. If you have ever tried to swim against a strong current, you will know how hard it is to move forward. The same principle can apply to working the feet. Chronically held energy resulting from deeply held emotional tension results in the physical holding, reflected in the feet. After a few treatments, this deeply held tension will begin to break down and the feet will become easier to work. Energy that is moving freely will give the reverse feeling – you swim easily with the tide!

The feet are a mirror of the whole individual, on all layers of being, and so never dismiss your intuitive feelings about them or how it feels to work on the feet.

DEVELOPING THE INTUITION

Imagine that your fingers and thumbs are antennas, which are highly sensitive and attuned to the person you are working with. With practice and by allowing your thumbs and fingers to go to reflexes without using your mind to interfere with the process, you will find that your hands know more about the patient's needs than your head!

Eventually, you will 'see' and 'feel' the reflexes on the feet without putting your hands on them. When I teach students this amazing therapy, I 'see' if they are on the centre of the reflex point, on the edge of it or nowhere near it. My palms and head tingle, telling me that the student needs to reposition their hands. The sensation can be described as a laser beam coming from the centre of the palms of the hands.

When giving healing at the end of the treatment, 'seeing' with the third eye, the person's energy field and where they are holding imbalances in the body can aid in recognizing the extent of the imbalance reflected in the physical body. These imbalances have been shown to be grey, heavy or symbolized in such a way as to be intimately connected with that person.

For example, a patient had a 'wondering' mind! This was accurately confirmed by her as she had been 'wondering' about her career change – I picked up the words, 'I wonder…'! The interaction between the patient and reflexologist appears to work in a different dimension to the physical and, by opening the third eye to 'see' unspoken areas of the patient's psyche, can help them to focus on mental thoughts.

The experience of 'seeing' into a student's body, to the muscle and bone, when a student complained of bad shoulder problems has also occurred. After examination at the hospital, she confirmed that the area 'seen' was clinically defined and connected to a spinal problem in the upper thoracic area.

These experiences have led me to the conclusion that we *look* with our *eyes* and interpret with the brain various stimuli, and that we *see* with the *third eye*, where we can interpret, physically, unseen dimensions of the human being. Equally, we *hear* with our *ears* but we *listen*, selectively, to those things which have import for us personally.

Continual working with the therapy heightens sensitivity to patients and all relationships! This sensitivity to the energy field of the human being also enhances counselling skills when 'feeling' the patient's somatic tensions and emotions occurs simultaneously with my own.

Everyone has the ability to develop this kind of sensitivity – there is nothing spooky or special about doing it! Do not be disheartened if you cannot achieve energy sensitivity immediately – it takes a time to develop but, like swimming or riding a bicycle, once developed it never leaves you. With confidence, perseverance and experience of working with those who come to reflexologists for help, you will achieve heightened perception.

The First Treatment

One of the main functions of reflexology is to relax and reduce anxiety and stress levels and to respect the individual's emotional, mental, spiritual and physical symptoms. Usually, with the first treatment the patient is somewhat nervous and tense as they have no idea what you are going to do to them. By giving a brief explanation of reflexology, its history, benefits and how we believe it works, the patient can begin to form a picture in their mind and to feel that you know that you are professional in your approach.

SUPPORTIVE REFLEXES

Supportive reflexes are additional reflex points to be worked in conjunction with the main reflex(es). As well as supportive reflexes, a cross reflex or referral area refers to the principal of zone therapy, where the upper limbs directly reflect the lower limbs. There are six cross reflexes or referral areas:

- hand to foot;
- hip to shoulder;
- fingers to toes;
- knee to elbow;
- ankle to wrist;
- arm to leg.

In the case of injury or trauma, one part of the body can be helped by working the cross reflex, with the ripple movement of the thumb over the alternative part of the body. This is useful where, for various reasons, direct treatment cannot be applied, such as amputation of a limb, congenital abnormalities, or break, sprain or fracture of the foot or hand. For example, if the left foot cannot be worked, work the left and the right hand (remember that nerves cross over as they enter the base of the brain). If the hands and feet cannot be worked, work an appropriate area of the body as detailed above.

MUSIC AND MOVEMENT

I liken learning the skill of reflexology to that of learning a musical instrument – precision, sensitivity and constant practice are prerequisites to good practice and should consistently be attended to, no matter how experienced or knowledgeable the practitioner. Like music, reflexology is an art form as well as an accurate science and so smoothness of movement, dexterity when working the reflexes and imagining that you are 'hugging' the feet in a caring way, helps the patient feel nurtured and cared for. It is, therefore, essential for novice students to practise every day on a pair of feet or, failing this, on their own hands. Without constant practice, the hands cannot gain the strength required to work a pair of feet. Many students feel like putting their thumbs in splints to support them after their first lesson! The more you practise, the more

perfect your practice will be and the stronger your thumbs.

Thorough Practice

Thorough practice is the keystone of good reflexology. Working every centimetre of the feet and ankles ensures good benefits for the patient, good practice and a good professional reputation. Skimping the reflexes with finger movements that are wide apart or 'skimming' across the foot reflects a sloppy attitude, as does rushing the treatment; the latter is stress-inducing for the patient and actually more tiring for the practitioner. A good, steady forward movement of thumb and finger pressure takes less energy and gives what the patient has come for treatment for – relaxation!

Walking or Working the Feet?

Never push implements into the feet to stimulate reflex points. Pure reflexology uses only the hands of the practitioner and the patient's feet! I am often asked if reflexology sandals are as beneficial as reflexology treatments – the answer is 'No'! Although this kind of footwear may stimulate the circulation to some extent and may, in some cases, reach the reflexes, becoming a professional reflexologist includes the emphasis on human interaction on all levels between practitioner and patient as a primary concern, and the stimulation with pressure applied precisely to the reflexes provides relaxation and a sense of calm, which is impossible to experience when walking! Adverse effects of over-stimulation of sensitive reflex points can also occur if footwear presses constantly on the reflexes.

Observations and Clues

Observation of the feet before beginning treatment is essential in 'reading' the patient's overall stress levels and possible energy imbalances within the anatomical and physiological systems of the body. By holding the foot between the thumb and fingers, and flexing each anatomical cavity (the cranial, thoracic, abdominal and pelvic), the presence of tension indicates where the patient is holding tension in the body. A common area for finding tension in the feet is the diaphragm line, which indicates breathing that is too shallow. This can coincide with sensitivity with the solar plexus, where emotional tension may be present. Practise this method and check with your patient if they are aware of holding tension in the relevant area of the body.

The patient's well-being is important to assess before commencing reflexology treatments, as well as the condition of the feet. Body language and any physical disabilities give vital clues as to how to work with the patient. The following guidelines will allow you to process information rapidly, so that you do not stare at the patient for an undue amount of time, or look as though you are interrogating their every move!

Does the patient have:

- a physical disability;
- ease of movement;
- good/poor posture?

Are they:

- under- or over-weight for their age and height;
- breathing correctly or hyperventilating?

What is:

- the condition of their skin, hair and eyes;
- their skin colour and texture;

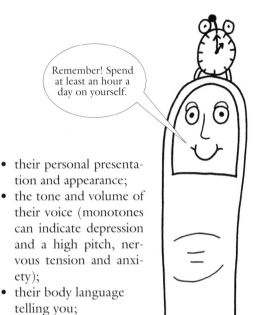

- their personal presentation and appearance;
- the tone and volume of their voice (monotones can indicate depression and a high pitch, nervous tension and anxiety);
- their body language telling you;
- their manner and attitude telling you about how they feel about themselves, others they may be discussing or you as a reflexologist?

Thumb Power

A little should be said about the reasons why we sometimes work with the thumbs and sometimes with the index fingers. The thumbs are power tools – the 'Black and Deckers' of your hands; the index fingers are for sensitivity when reflexes and corresponding parts of the body are relatively small and need tiny

Regular thumb press-ups strengthen the thumbs.

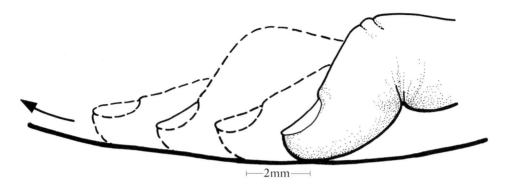

├──2mm──┤

Fig 2. 'Ripple walk': bend and straighten the first joint of the thumb, gradually creeping forward. Always use a forward movement and ensure that the thumb/finger joint remains flexed as above when massaging or hooking reflexes.

movements to find the reflexes. Throughout treatments on both feet, you will find you need to swap from the thumb to the index finger for certain reflexes.

To work the reflexes, use the medial edge of the pad of the thumb and the full pad of the thumb and index fingers.

The thumb and index finger movements are very important for two reasons.

1. The angle of the thumb has great bearing on the smoothness, accuracy of finding the reflexes and relaxation. Additionally, if the angle of the thumb is too steep then the thumb joint will receive considerable strain over time with the possibility of developing arthritis, carpal tunnel syndrome or repetitive strain injury (RSI), or other problems. Fig. 2 shows the correct angle of the thumb, which can be practised on your own hands as well as on feet.
2. The index finger joint may need to become more flexible, which it will with time and practice.

Consistent Pressure

The pressure worked with on the reflexes should be *consistent at all times.* A regular and constant pressure is a keynote of successful practice. It is tempting to continue working across the width of the foot, even though the hand span is not broad enough to reach; for example, when working from the medial edge of the foot to the lateral edge the thumb can become strained and ineffective. By swapping the working hand so that the lateral edge can be worked with the correct pressure and working back into the middle of the foot or where the hands were changed, the reflexes are worked with constant pressure.

Messages the Feet Can Give

The soles and tops of the feet can vary in colour and skin texture. How we project ourselves into the world may sometimes

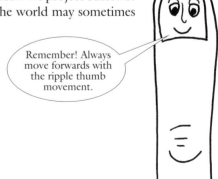

Remember! Always move forwards with the ripple thumb movement.

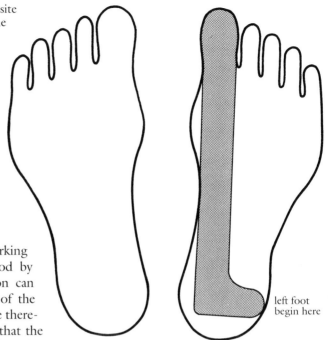

Fig 3. Because you are sitting opposite the patient, remember to reverse the right and left sides. This hint might help you to remember.

left foot
begin here

be at variance with how we are really feeling and so the tops of the feet can indicate how we project ourselves into the world and the soles, how we are really feeling!

Foot Friction

Because of the method of working the feet with the ripple method by moving across the foot, friction can occur between the fleshy pad of the thumb and flesh on the foot. We therefore need to soften contact so that the thumb and fingers can move easily without sliding across the foot. Talcum powder, if used, should be done so sparingly as it has been found to be a carcinogen (cancer forming), and when the dust is inhaled regularly it can put the practitioner at risk. Cornflour is an ideal substance as it doesn't dust. To apply, dip the fingers into a dish filled with cornflour so that a little adheres to spread on the soles, tops, and sides of the feet. Equally, oils used on the feet mean that the ripple technique of moving across the foot becomes a sliding action, resembling massage. Although this can feel very relaxing, some reflexes are deeply imbedded in the feet and sliding across them means that some vital reflexes will be missed

The Importance of Hand Positions

One of the most important aspects of professional practice in reflexology are good, caring hand positions. The patient's comfort is of paramount importance and with gently 'hug-

ging' the feet they will feel truly cared for. To demonstrate this, ask a friend or reflexologist to hold your feet casually, tightly or roughly and see for yourself how uncomfortable this is – and uncaring!

We begin the treatment on the left foot. This is partly because of the energy flow around the body, which moves from left to right, and the physical reason that the heart is on the left side of the body. As we aim to improve nerve response and stimulate the circulatory system, the heart reflex is the most important reflex to be worked, physically, and maybe emotionally. The heart chakra is the feeling centre of our being and, as we have seen, our emotional response to life events has a profound effect on our health.

Wherever possible, *the working hand should be placed over the supporting hand*, and the fingers, when not in use, either held together or tucked underneath the palm. When working the areas of the thoracic, cranial, abdominal

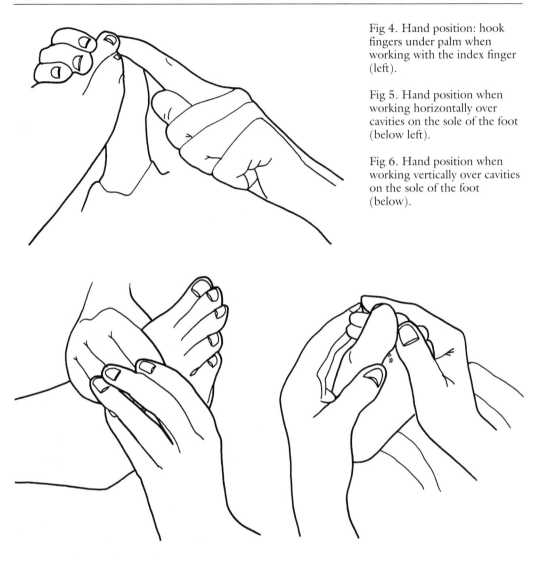

Fig 4. Hand position: hook fingers under palm when working with the index finger (left).

Fig 5. Hand position when working horizontally over cavities on the sole of the foot (below left).

Fig 6. Hand position when working vertically over cavities on the sole of the foot (below).

and pelvic cavities (not the pelvic extension), always have the working hand over the supporting hand. As an experiment, try reversing this on your patient and ask them to tell you how differently it feels. If the working hand is on the foot with the supporting hand pressed on the top, not only will the working hand fingers be squeezing the foot but the additional pressure of the supporting hand may give added discomfort, thereby distorting the information gained from the feet. Study Figs 4–6 as you work the reflexes.

Never grip the toes from above, or squeeze them together – a patient with arthritis in the feet will suffer agonies and will not thank you for causing them unnecessary additional pain! The following points should be integrated into your practice from the first day of training to ensure that bad habits don't have a chance to creep in!

- *Always* support the foot from the base of the toes to ensure that the toes are not squashed together.
- *Always* place the supporting hand on the foot and place the fingers of the working hand over them whenever possible.
- *Always* place the working hand *under* the supporting hand when working around the heel area of the foot.
- *Always* place the working fingers on the top of the foot. Never curl them under the palm of the hand. Curling fingers lessens pressure and control of movement.
- *Always* work thoroughly from edge to edge of cavity boundaries and the medial/lateral edges of the feet. This ensures that every possible reflex has been worked and a good, thorough treatment received by the patient.
- *Always* work slowly and methodically. Working slowly is relaxing for yourself and the patient – *never* rush a treatment, or your patient will leave in a more tense state than when they came in!
- *Always* ensure that your fingernails are not only short but that the corners are filed into the shape of the finger. The corners of nails impaled in the flesh is bad practice and painful for the patient.
- *Always* be polite and courteous to your patient – even if you find them hard to relate to or be at ease with. They are paying you for a service and therefore deserve to be treated politely. From my experience, those who I have found difficulty in relating to tend to drift away.

Working the Cavities in Sequence

A common question asked by students is, 'Why do we begin working the thoracic cavity in an upwards movement and not the cranial cavity, so that we work down the foot and therefore the body?' The answer is that the diaphragm, lungs and heart are intimately connected. The diaphragm muscle aids blood and lymph fluid movement back to the heart and increases the blood supply round the heart and to the lungs, where fresh oxygen is taken in and carbon dioxide given off. The diaphragm muscle is the key reflex for relaxing the breathing and allowing the lungs to expand so that more vitalizing oxygen is taken in, which in turn aids the efficiency of the heart. As one of the main functions of reflexology is to stimulate the blood supply around the body, it becomes clear that working the lungs and heart are vital in the overall treatment.

Finding the Cavity Boundaries

It may be helpful to draw the anatomical cavity boundaries on a pair of feet so that you can visualize parts of the body contained in them when working the feet. The cavity boundaries are found as follows.

The cranial cavity boundary is found at the root of the toes, across the width of the foot. Draw a line across the foot as shown in Fig. 7, point 1.

The thoracic cavity boundary is found at the base of the ball of the foot and extends across the width of the foot. It extends upwards to meet the cranial cavity boundary. Draw a line across the foot as shown in Fig. 7, point 2.

The abdominal cavity boundary is found from the top of the cuboid notch (or 5th metatarsal notch) and across the width of the foot. It extends upwards to meet the thoracic cavity boundary. This boundary line is of the utmost importance in constantly checking where you are working. For example, the transverse colon reflex point is on the waistline. Above it, in the abdominal cavity are the digestive organs and beneath it lie the reflexes of the pelvic cavity. Constantly check the waistline when in the area so that you can monitor which cavity may be related to sensitivity. Draw a line across the foot as shown in Fig. 7, point 3.

The pelvic cavity boundary is found across the width of the top of the heel line, where the flesh of foot dips into the instep. It extends

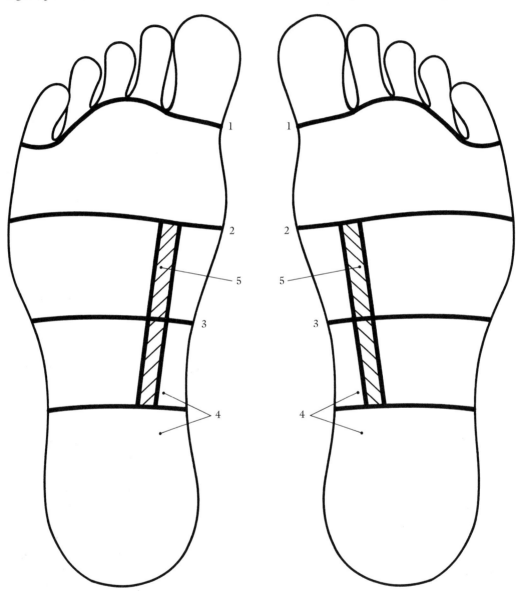

Fig 7. Anatomical boundaries: finding the cavity boundaries on the right foot (left) and left foot (right). 1. cranial/thoracic cavity boundary; 2. thoracic/abdominal cavity boundary; 3. waistline: abdominal/pelvic cavity boundary; 4. pelvic cavity and pelvic cavity extension; 5. plantar tendon (or longitudinal ligament).

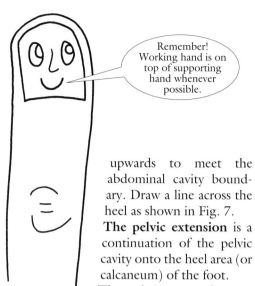

Remember! Working hand is on top of supporting hand whenever possible.

upwards to meet the abdominal cavity boundary. Draw a line across the heel as shown in Fig. 7.

The pelvic extension is a continuation of the pelvic cavity onto the heel area (or calcaneum) of the foot.

The plantar tendon or main ligament on the sole of the foot descends from the base of the ball of the foot down to the heel line. Draw a line on the lateral edge of the ligament as shown in Fig. 7, point 5.

In order to work the five energy zones from the base of the big toe to the tip, with the thumb pointing in an upward direction, work with the ripple movement from the base of the great toe to the tip. Repeat this movement across the width of the toe.

Working Laterally to Medially Across the Width of the Foot

The *lateral edge* of the foot is the outside edge, where the shoulder and hip are found in the body. The *medial edge* of the foot is the inside edge, where the spine is found in the body.

When working the cranial, thoracic, abdominal and pelvic cavity, left foot on the medial edge, the right hand should be the supporting hand and when working the medial edge on the right foot the left hand should be the supporting hand.

When working the left foot on the lateral edge, the left hand should be the supporting hand and on the right foot, the right hand should be the supporting hand.

Relaxation Techniques

To aid in the patient's 'letting go' and relaxation, we begin treatment with five relaxation techniques: ankle agitation, metatarsal massage, phalange rotation, spinal spiral, working the diaphragm and massaging the solar plexus. Although the diaphragm line is worked to aid relaxation, it has been included in Section 3 as a main reflex point.

The purpose of each relaxation technique is given below.

- **Ankle agitation:** this stimulates the blood supply to feet, thus warming them up – and the practitioner's hands!
- **Metatarsal massage:** this loosens the metatarsal joints, thereby assisting in finding the reflexes.
- **Phalange rotation:** this loosens the base of the phalange (toe) joints and massages the metatarsal joints.
- **Spinal spiral:** this gentle twisting movement loosens the medial (middle) side of the foot where the main arch of the instep takes the pressure from body weight.
- **Working the diaphragm:** this reveals tension held in the diaphragm muscle and is a key movement for assisting relaxation and improved breathing. This reflex is the first to be worked with the ripple thumb movement.
- **Solar plexus:** this reflex is found in the centre of the diaphragm line, usually where an inverted 'v' can be seen. It is a guide for the practitioner in assessing how much emotional tension is being held, which needs to be released in communication, either with the practitioner or in someone the patient can trust.

These relaxation techniques should be worked for three to four minutes at the beginning of treatment when working both feet and brought into treatment if the reflexes are very painful. Remember, pain tenses muscle and so these techniques can counteract tension and keep the patient in a relaxed state. Working with these relaxation techniques will loosen the hands and, for the novice student, be a good starting point for strengthening the hands, especially when working the diaphragm line. Work them frequently throughout the treatment if your patient finds the reflexes painful.

Spinal Innervations

The spine and brain are vital for the functioning of organs and glands and movement in the world. Special consideration should therefore be given to the spinal innervations that extend from the spinal cord to the viscera and the periphery of the body. The spine affects every part of the body through the three functions of each part and so we work the spine and brain automatically with each specific health problem, as well as the overall treatment.

To aid the student in visualizing where the innervations would be on the spinal pathways on the foot, individual innervations are given with each reflex point. Refer to the nervous system in Section 3 to find out more about the functions of nerves.

By studying the foot charts in the colour section, the sequential order of working the reflexes is shown with a numbering system for easy reference.

The Cardio-Vascular, Nervous and Muscular Systems

Blood vessels, nerves and muscles are everywhere in the body and so by giving a complete treatment, all the muscles, nerves and blood vessels are automatically worked. There are, however, specific reflex points for the cardio-vascular system, which include the heart and lymph nodes and lymph ducts, the brain and spinal cord for the nervous system and the diaphragm muscle for the muscular system. A complete treatment on both feet should always be given to ensure that these vital systems have had a chance to help the body to rebalance.

Reworking the Reflexes

Once both feet have been worked, it is good reinforcement to go back to systems affected by a disorder(s). For example, if there are digestive problems, work all of the reflexes on the left and right foot related to the digestive organs and glands. If someone has a problem with the large colon, then begin working the ileo-caecal valve, then the ascending colon, transverse, descending colon (on the left foot), sigmoid flexure, pelvic extension and rectal area. If the skeletal system requires reinforcement, work all of the reflexes on both feet related to the skeletal frame and joints. In this way, problem areas gain more support *but this method of working is not meant as a substitute for working both feet individually first of all*. Remember the reasons for beginning to work on the left foot:

- Energy flow moves from left to right around the body and the heart is situated mainly on the left side of the thorax. Blood is life-giving and energizing as it carries vital nutrients to all cells in the body and so the heart is the muscular organ we need to assist in improving the circulation.

Once your hands are on the foot, they should not be removed unless in an emergency situation. Moving across from foot to foot is disjointed and unsettling for the patient. Patient comfort, relaxation and a soothing calmness received from the treatment will not be obtained if your hands are jumping around like a grasshoppers!

Care should be taken when practising in this way to provide additional time to carry out reinforcing systems, as your next patient may be kept waiting for some time unless additional time is allowed. It is therefore a good idea to arrange for the extra time during the next treatment session with your patient.

Overworking the Reflexes

Following on from reinforcing reflex points by working individual systems of the body, we should consider the possibility of overworking the reflexes. When reflexes are found to be sensitive during a treatment, do not be over zealous and think that by working with deep pressure you will be helping the body – quite the reverse, in fact! Over-stimulation of the reflexes can have adverse effects with the particular reflex being worked and can lead to the patient maybe not continuing treatment with you, or worse, requiring medical attention. Working the reflexes as outlined in this book requires good training and expertise – reflexology is a powerful tool and misuse can devalue the therapy by inappropriate treatments and thus turn away those who may benefit from a series of good professional treatments.

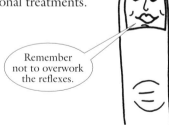

Remember not to overwork the reflexes.

Keeping Contact with the Feet

One of the most important factors of good practice is to never take your hands away from the feet once treatment has begun, unless in an emergency. The interactive energy flow between the client and yourself is vital as part of the self-healing process and interrupting this flow means that you may lose concentration with where you were working on the feet or hands and the energy link will have to be re-established in the remaining time available.

Leaving the patient's feet while you answer the telephone or taking your hands away if the patient has drifted off to sleep, may leave the patient feeling insecure and may break the healing atmosphere. Leaving the client so you can deal with interruptions can also leave the client feeling less important than the distraction!

FINISHING THE TREATMENT

Once all reflexes have been worked on both feet and any sensitive reflexes reworked, your patient should be relaxed and possibly sleepy. Spending a few minutes to finish the treatment will leave your patient floating on air, calm, relaxed and feeling that they have received an enjoyable treatment – even if some of the reflexes initially felt tender.

Rounding off the treatment with a foot massage is the next step towards completing the treatment and by soothingly applying foot cream preparations, preferably with essential oils such as lavender and tea-tree if there are fungal infections or abrasions on the feet, gently massage from the back of the ankle from the top of the Achilles tendon, downwards towards the base of the calcaneum. This movement has the double benefit of stimulating the related large colon reflexes. Then massage the whole foot, massaging around the ankle joints slowly and caressing the whole foot.

To 'cleanse' the auric field round the feet, with the tips of the fingers placed at the ankles, stroke in light movements up the foot towards the toes and shake your hands once at the toes to shake off auric debris which may have accumulated round the feet. Repeat this movement on both feet several times.

Stroking the electromagnetic field towards the therapist takes away negativity from the lower limbs by stroking downwards from the knee to the tips of the toes. Then sweep up from the toes to the knees to re-energize the EMF. This important field encompasses the whole body but as you will not have time to re-energize it all, working from the knee down will leave the legs and feet feeling lighter and the person 'floating on air' as they leave you.

Deep breathing is an important education at the end of the treatment in bringing into focus how badly we normally breathe! By breathing in deeply through the nose and pushing out the stomach as far as possible, the rib cage and lower lobes of the lungs have a chance to expand as the diaphragm muscle is stretched and tension released. Hold the breath for two to three seconds, then release slowly through the mouth until the chin drops onto the chest and the rib cage collapses. At the same time suggest to your patient that they visualize tension leaving the body as they expire air. Repeat the in and out breath several times, depending on the amount of tension present and how comfortable it feels for the patient to practice.

Finally, giving healing with the palms of the hands placed on the soles of the feet can generate calm and tranquillity before the person leaves you. Methods of visualization can open the practitioner as a channeller for universal, or divine energy, to channel through their hands and into the patient. This will help to rebalance the therapist as well as the patient and leave you ready for the next patient.

The average time for giving a treatment should be one hour from beginning to end, unless additional time has been allowed to give a deeper and/or more extensive treatment.

It is important to give your patient a glass of water before they leave and encourage them to drink plenty more once they are at home and, ideally, to put their feet up for an hour to allow the body to detoxify. Remember that the liver, kidneys, bowel, skin and lungs are the organs of elimination and by drinking plenty of water after a stimulating reflexology treatment, the body will have a chance to expel harmful substances through these organs.

After making a further appointment, which should be written down to save any confusion, assist your patient off the chair or couch, escort them to the door and see them safely off the premises.

It is important to wash your hands with an antibacterial soap before completing the treatment record and beginning the next treatment.

Once they have left, write up your notes and give yourself a break to disengage from them, leaving you fresh for the next patient's arrival.

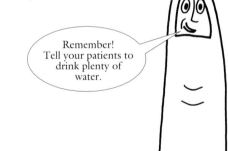

Remember! Tell your patients to drink plenty of water.

Section 3

Directions for Working
the Reflexes

*We ourselves are our own bodies, and those must be made happy on earth.
It is our bodies that should be in glory …*

The Upanishads, Chandogya Upanishad

This section of the book is concerned with the structures (anatomy, meaning 'I cut up') and functioning (physiology, 'phys' meaning 'nature cure') of the human body, systems, reflex points, common disorders and a special-interest section related to each system of the body, hand positions, how to work the reflexes, and hand reflexology. Refer to Chapter 26, Systemic Disorders, for a comprehensive guide to disorders related to each system.

> Remember to begin working on the left foot, then work the right foot; finally re-work sensitive reflexes as complete systems of the body, for example, all digestive organs and glands in the case of gastric problems.

CHAPTER 10
Adverse Conditions and Anatomy of the Feet and Hands

More often than not, patients apologize for their feet – stating that they are ugly, they can't 'stand' them (an interesting word to use!) and how ashamed they are of them! Our poor feet suffer more abuse and neglect than any other part of our bodies and yet when they hurt and we find it difficult to walk, how important they suddenly become!

Make it a habit to cream them regularly and treat yourself to a pedicure every once in a while for the sheer pleasure and pampering they deserve!

Common conditions that the elderly develop, who may not have worn well-fitting shoes as children, or those who have worn high-heels and 'winkle pickers' in the 1960s are: bunions, calluses, deformity of the feet, dropped arches and hammer toes. Friction caused by footwear that is too loose and 'slops' up and down, or which is too tight, where the feet are crammed into the shoe, play a part in structural foot deformities in later life.

Immobility and poor circulation will create foot-related problems because blood in the veins has to fight against gravity on its way back to the heart. Those who are infirm or bed-ridden and therefore immobile will need to be worked on very gently and regularly to aid their general blood circulation. Make a check with those who are ill that they are eating a well-balanced diet, as poor nutrition will cause skin and muscle tone to deteriorate and bones to become more brittle, making walking or standing painful. Working the reflexes on the hands as well as the feet is a good support or alternative with those who find the feet too painful to be handled.

Hormonal imbalance and exposure to the elements can affect skin texture, soften the nails or cause conditions which with awareness and care may be avoided.

Skeletal problems with the pelvic bones or spinal vertebrae can create callouses on the lateral or medial edges of the feet. If these are in evidence, recommend to the patient that they receive gentle manipulation to realign the spine and innominate bones (the pelvic bones). *See* Chapter 23 The Skeletal System for more information on skeletal misalignments.

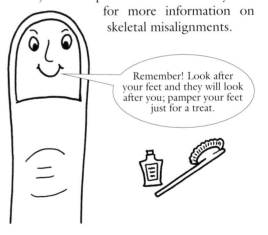

Remember! Look after your feet and they will look after you; pamper your feet just for a treat.

VISUAL EXAMINATION OF THE CLIENT'S FEET

The following conditions may be present on a visual examination of a client's feet (*see* Chapter 26, Systemic Disorders, for causes and information on specific conditions):

- **Inversion/eversion:** when the feet are either inverted or everted, psychological holding of tension in the pelvic cavity is expressed as anal retention or anal expulsion. In the former, anal retention, eversion grips the buttocks in tightly together and this represents a fear of letting go. When the feet are inverted and the buttocks relaxed outwards, anal expulsion represents an inability to hold on emotionally to inner feelings of security. Thus, both inversion and eversion can be seen as deep-rooted insecurity.
- **Dry, rough or cracked skin round the heel** can indicate bowel disorders and problems in the pelvic cavity generally, deeply held emotional problems, exposure to the elements, such as walking barefoot, or hormonal imbalance, especially an underactive thyroid gland. With this condition, the shins of the legs and ankles can also appear dry and flaky. *See* Chapter 18, The Endocrine System for symptoms of an underactive thyroid. Sigmund Freud's psychological theory of anal expulsion and anal retention can also be related to dry, cracked skin round the heels. When found on the medial edge of the foot, the foot is inverted, giving the appearance of 'knock-knees', which is symbolic of anal expulsion. When found on the lateral edge of the feet, this is symbolic of anal retentiveness.
- **Peeling skin** can be caused by the elements, as well as medication, hormone imbalance and systemic disease.

- **Warts** can appear without obvious cause, as they can anywhere on the body, and can disappear overnight. Recommend medical intervention, which may reduce or cure the problem.
- **Unusual hair growth** can be treated by a practitioner qualified in body-hair removal.
- **Protruding veins** can be associated with various disorders connected with the circulatory, digestive, reproductive, lymphatic and urinary systems of the body.
- **Texture of skin** can indicate medication and use of narcotic drugs – especially 'pot' (marijuana). *See* Chapter 20, The Urinary System.
- **Swollen areas and puffiness** can indicate medication, chronic conditions, fluid retention, the presence of diabetes mellitus and other systemic disease.
- **Bone growths** can include spurs, which are mineral deposits, and are extremely painful as they tend to form around the weight-bearing bone of the calcaneum (heel bone).
- **Ulcers and sores** can be caused by systemic disease, poor circulation and sitting or standing for too long a period of time. Where possible, encourage your patient to move about to keep their circulation moving.
- **Scar tissue** found on the feet may result in desensitization of nerve endings, if the nerves have been severed through injury or surgery. Sensitive reflex points may or may not be found round such an area. Adhesions that form in the body as a result of injury or surgery can leave very sensitive reflex areas, even when a part of the body has been removed.
- **Wrinkles, folds and hard patches of skin** can indicate emotional and psychological trauma. Dependent on where the hard skin is found, for example, over the heart, which represents the feeling centre of the human being, is where emotional defences are

developed. As a general rule, if hard skin is removed regularly and regrows within a couple of weeks, then the root cause has a psychological origin.

- **Sweating or 'wet' feet** can indicate the presence of toxins, caused by obesity, digestive disorders, fear, hormonal and fluid imbalance, such as hyperthyroidism, stress, fever, bacterial infection, fluid imbalance, hypothalamus dysfunction, stress, dietary deficiency, energy release during treatment (especially with shock or fainting), footwear or medication, hypersensitivity to treatment, footwear, energy release during treatment.
- **The colour of feet** can tell a story about stress levels, presenting health conditions, medication and the health history, going back to childhood.
  - **Red:** areas of the feet which are varying shades of red, tell of stress levels including rushing to keep the reflexology appointment! Many people explain away redness for this reason, until they reflect on the fact that there may be other reasons, which may have created the redness.
  - **Yellow:** a yellowish colour can represent past or present liver conditions, the presence of medication, or simply hard skin.
  - **Blue** feet tend to indicate bad blood circulation and the possibility of heart problems and the experience of a stroke –

Remember! Begin a treatment by carefully observing the feet. Note the colour, texture and temperature, and look for any puffy areas.

the latter showing round the head and especially the brain area of the big toe. In this case, study both big toes and see which one appears to be affected, remembering that the *left side* of the brain affects the *right side* of the body and vice versa.

- **Purple:** a purple colour can indicate poor circulation, drug abuse and medication levels.
- **Green:** a greenish hue can indicate the presence of poisonous or toxic substances, chronic or acute digestive problems or travel sickness.
- **Pale skin** can indicate a lack of blood flow to capillary endings in the feet and certain medical conditions, emotional trauma, fainting and drop in body temperature.

CONDITIONS OF THE FEET

We balance on the feet and it therefore becomes perfectly clear how we can rebalance the body through reflexology. If our feet are 'out of balance', through disease or structural problems, then so too probably will be our body. As part of the observation of the patient, foot disorders can give an important clue to the overall health of the individual. Badly fitting shoes, injury, emotional blockages, systemic disease, structural problems and infections will be reflected in the feet and can aid the practitioner in the initial consultation to assess how to work the feet.

The use of drugs, such as steroids and anticoagulants, can lead to problems with the skin because of complications with the circulatory system, and requires various methods of working the feet. Skin diseases may mean that the hands or cross-reflexes will need to be worked if the skin of the feet is contagious or impossible to work because of conditions such as ulcers which restrict working the reflexes.

Some conditions may mean that the method of working the feet may need to be adjusted, or that the hands or cross-reflexes will need to be worked instead. For example, with diabetes mellitus, where degeneration of the peripheral nerves results in a wasting of the skin due to loss of nerve reaction and nourishment, flaky and peeling skin, spongy, odorous and perspiring feet, and eventually gangrene can mean that an alternative approach must be found, such as working the reflexes of the hand.

Ageing can lead to rheumatism, osteoarthritis, skin atrophy (deadness), melanoma (cancer of the skin), osteomalacia (painful softening of the bones caused through lack of vitamin D) and general lack of mobility.

Other common groups of infections and conditions of the feet are given below. It is important that the feet are thoroughly checked before beginning treatment. If the feet are badly affected, they should not be worked, as infection could spread to the next patient, or to yourself!

If, however, the condition can be worked round, or covered, then avoid working over the area and give light, short treatments over the rest of the foot until the condition has healed when normal pressure and length of treatment time can be given. There are three main causes of infection in the feet:

- **bacteria** can cause inflammation and sepsis (pus-forming bacteria);
- **viral** infections can cause verrucae;
- **mycotic** infections are those such as athlete's foot and fungal infections of the nail-bed.

Specific conditions are detailed below:

- **Athlete's foot** is a fungal skin eruption, which gives the following symptoms:

- white, wet, flaking areas between the fourth and fifth toes;
- skin at the base or between the toes is itchy and sore;
- in severe cases, cracking, peeling and blisters may be present;
- an unpleasant odour may accompany the condition.

Infection is usually found between the toes and is caused by ring-worm, excessive sweating of the feet caused by inadequate ventilation in footwear, and allergic reaction to drugs, sweat, dyes and leather; inadequate drying between the toes and/or using infected towels or bath mats. Recommended allopathic treatment is the use of antifungal powder, ointment or gel on the affected area. The essential oils of tea-tree and lavender have powerful antiseptic and wound-healing properties and are suitable for general external application of skin disorders.

Advise your client to dry between the toes carefully, wear open, well-ventilated shoes or sandals, avoid sharing towels, flannels and bath mats, walk barefoot whenever possible, disinfect floor space frequently and change socks, tights and stockings frequently. Refer to tinea pedis as an associated condition of the feet.

- **Tinea pedis** is an infection that involves principally the toe webs or soles of the feet. Rubber-soled shoes and shoes that inhibit circulation of air encourage infection. Swimming and athletics venues, where the feet become damp or tread in infected water, can also spread the condition.
- **Tinea unguim** affects the big toes but may include several nails. It causes discoloration and chalky deposits. Unusual trauma, occupations or hobbies, congenital changes or misalignment may also produce misshapen

95

toenails. When several toenails are affected, psoriasis will be present.

- **Hyperkeratosis** is a form of psoriasis, where there are no other symptoms of the disease and the nail-bed, affecting the toenails. It can be difficult to distinguish from fungal infection.
- **Hyperidrosis** is caused by excessive sweating of the feet.
- **Bromohidrosis** is the odorous excretion of perspiration, which may be caused by long-term medication.
- **Erythema pernio, or chilblains,** is an inflammation of the skin on the hands and feet, caused by poor circulation and health disorders.
- **Plantar warts** have a flat top and are found on the plantar area of the feet.
- **Onychauxis** is caused by thickened nails.
- **Onycholysis** is a separation of the nail from the nail-bed.
- **Onychia** is an inflammation affecting the nails.
- **Onchogryphosis** is a distortion of the nail in which thickening, overgrowing and the nail twisting back on itself is caused by inflammation and chronic irritation. More commonly known as ram's horn or Ostler's toe.
- **Onychomycosis** is due to a fungal infection of the nail plate.
- **Verrucae** are a form of wart and consist of small, solid growths on the surface of the skin. They belong to a group of viruses that are highly infectious and are spread by walking barefoot and where damp and wet conditions exist, such as swimming baths.

STRUCTURAL FOOT DEFORMITIES

Structural deformities can be caused by mechanical and congenital reasons. Specific disorders are given below:

- **Bunions** are common conditions, caused by badly fitting footwear; they are found over the joint at the base of the big toe due to thickening of the skin and the metatarsal bone becoming pressured to bend outwards. The cause is short-fitting or pointed toe footwear. Bunions can also indicate neck, thyroid or shoulder problems and when surgically removed, can lead to depression as the position of bunions is placed on the spinal reflexes, where the seventh cervical vertebrae leads into the medulla oblongata (brain-stem).
- **Callosities** on the tops of the toes can represent chronic sinus problems and catarrh.
- **Corns** are caused by a thickening of the epidermis, which develops as an inward-growing conical shape, known as the 'eye' of a corn. When thickening of the skin occurs over a wider area it is called a callosity.
- **Fallen arches** can indicate spinal problems, especially the longitudinal arch on the medial edge of the foot.
- **Ingrowing** toenails can indicate headaches as the placement of the nail is close to the brain reflex point.
- **Spurs** are due to a mineral build-up at the edges of bone, commonly found at the back of the calcaneum (heel bone). By gently massaging around the affected area every day, the deposits will break down and be swept away in the blood circulation. As the spur becomes less painful, increase pressure until the spur itself can be worked over.
- **Hammer toe** affects the second toe, and is caused by wearing too short shoes.
- **Metatarsalgia** – pain affects the metatarsal area of the foot and is often associated with adolescents and flat feet. In adults it is a manifestation of rheumatoid arthritis.
- **Pes planovalgus** is the medical term for flat feet and can be caused by a deformity of the feet in which the arch on the inside of the foot sinks until it rests on the

ground. Mostly occurs in young people where the ligaments remain soft but can also occur in the middle-aged, who have to stand a great deal without moving the muscles of the feet.

- **Pes cavus** is the medical term for claw-foot, which forms an abnormally high arch that causes shortening of the foot, leading to inversion of the foot and heel. This can result in a stiff gait and aching pain.
- **Hallux valgus** is an outward displacement of the big toe and is associated with bunions. The cause is the pressure of footwear on broad feet and loss of muscle tone. Bunions are formed by the pressure of footwear on the protruding base of the toe.
- **Calcaneal bursitis** is a pain in the heel and can be associated with the formation of spurs.
- **Dropfoot** is caused by an inability to flex the foot at the ankle, causing the foot to hang down and to be swung when walking. Its cause can be damage to the popliteal nerve or the peroneal muscles.

ANATOMY OF THE FEET

Bones of the Feet

Each foot consists of twenty-six bones. All the bones of the feet are movable and have strong muscles and ligaments, which are necessary in maintaining the strength, resilience and stability of the feet. The tarsal bones develop from the sixth month of foetal life until after puberty. The metatarsal bones develop from about the ninth week of foetal life and are fully formed by 18–20 years of age. The phalanges begin development in the tenth week of foetal life, and are fully formed by 18 years.

The tarsal, or ankle bones, form the back part of the foot. These bones are: one talus,

one calcaneus, one navicular, three cuneiform and one cuboid.

The furthest extremity of the tibia forms the ankle joint with the talus and the fibula. The medial malleolus (bony prominence) lies to the middle of the ankle joint. The talus articulates with the tibia and fibula at the ankle joint. The other bones articulate with each other and with the metatarsal bones.

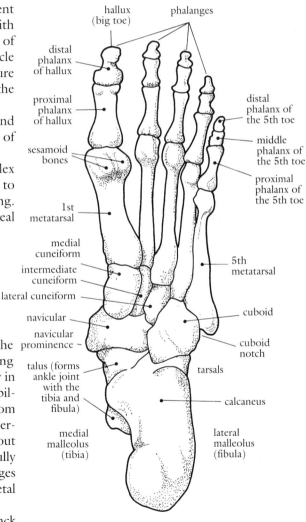

Fig 8. The bones of the left foot, plantar aspect.

There are four important ligaments strengthening the ankle joint: the anterior, posterior and lateral ligaments and the deltoid, a very strong medial ligament. Muscle movements of the ankle joint include flexion (dorsiflexion) and extension (plantarflexion). The gastrocnemius and soleus muscles in the calf are assisted by the muscles that flex the toes.

There are five metatarsal bones on each foot, which form the greater part of the dorsum (top) of the foot. At the upper end, they articulate with the tarsal bones and at the furthest point with the phalanges (the toe bones). There are fourteen phalanges on each foot, arranged in a similar manner to those in the fingers, for example, two in the great toe and three in each of the other toes. The arrangement of the bones of the feet facilitate movement and support; this can be illustrated by comparing a normal foot with a flat foot, which has no arches. The main weight bearing bones in the feet are the calcaneus, talus and the first metatarsal head.

The two main functions of the feet are to support the weight of the body in an upright position and to propel the body forwards. The ligaments found supporting the feet are called the plantar (spring), short and long. The plantar ligament or spring ligament is very strong and thick, and stretches from the calcaneus to the navicular. It plays an important part in supporting the medial longitudinal arch and structures that support the lateral and transverse arches of the feet.

Tendons

Movements are produced by muscles in the leg, with long tendons that cross the ankle joint and by the muscles of the foot. The tendons crossing the ankle joint are held close to the bones by strong, transverse ligaments; they move smoothly within their sheaths as the joints move. In addition to moving the joints of the foot, leg muscles support the arches of the foot and help to maintain body balance. The Achilles tendon is attached to the calcaneus and calf muscles called the gastrocnemius and the soleus.

Four Arches of the Feet

There are four arches on the medial edge of the foot, which reflect the four arches in the spine. The bones have a bridge-like arrangement and are supported by muscles and ligaments, so that four arches are formed: a medial and lateral longitudinal arch, and two transverse arches.

The medial longitudinal arch is the highest of the arches and is formed by the calcaneus, navicular, three cuneiform and the first three metatarsal bones. Only the calcaneus and the furthest point towards the toes of the metatarsal bones should touch the ground.

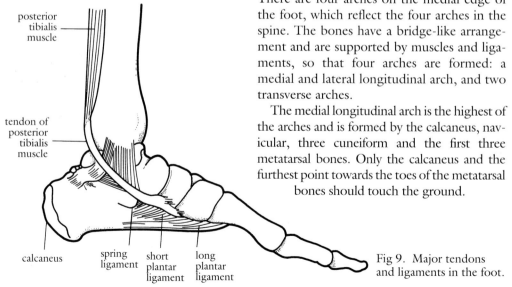

posterior tibialis muscle

tendon of posterior tibialis muscle

calcaneus   spring ligament   short plantar ligament   long plantar ligament

Fig 9. Major tendons and ligaments in the foot.

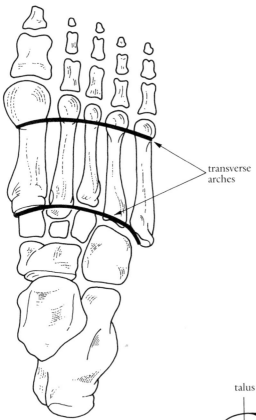

The lateral longitudinal arch is less marked than its medial counterparts. The bony components are the calcaneus, cuboid and two lateral metatarsal bones. Only the calcaneus and metatarsal bones should touch the ground.

The transverse arches run across the foot and can be easily seen by examining the skeleton. They are marked at the base of the phalanges and at the level of the three cuneiform and cuboid bones.

The posterior tibialis muscle acts as a sling for the arch and is the most important muscular support for the medial longitudinal arch. It lies to the back aspect of the tibia and fibula with its tendon passing behind the medial malleolus where it is inserted into the navicular, cuneiform, cuboid and metatarsal bones.

The short muscles of the feet are a group of muscles mainly concerned with the maintenance of the lateral longitudinal and transverse arches. They make up the fleshy part of the sole of the foot.

transverse arches

Fig 10. Upper surface of the right foot (above).

Fig 11. Bones and medial longitudinal arch of the right foot (right).

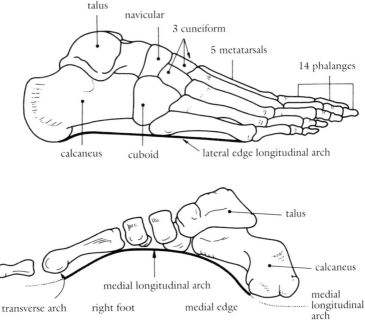

talus

navicular

3 cuneiform

5 metatarsals

14 phalanges

calcaneus   cuboid   lateral edge longitudinal arch

talus

calcaneus

medial longitudinal arch

medial longitudinal arch

Fig 12. Medial longitudinal arch of the right foot.

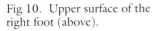

transverse arch   right foot   medial edge

medial
longitudinal
arch

Joints of the Feet

The joints of the feet and toes are synovial joints and are, therefore, moveable. They are found between the tarsal bones and metatarsal bones, and between the metatarsals and phalanges. The movements of inversion (turning the feet into the middle of the body) and eversion (turning the feet to the lateral edge of the body) occur between the tarsal bones and not at the ankle joint. There are two types of joint: hinge joints, which are found in the ankle and toes, and gliding joints, found between the tarsal and metatarsal bones.

The movements of the foot consist of dorsiflexion, plantarflexion, inversion, flexion, extension, eversion and circumduction.

Muscles of the Feet

All of the muscles of the foot act upon the toes. They are described as abductors, adductors, flexors and extensors. The muscles in the plantar region of the foot may be divided into three groups, similarly to those in the hands.

- Those of the internal plantar region are connected with the great toe, and correspond with those of the thumbs.
- Those of the external plantar region are connected with the little toe and correspond with those of the little finger.
- Those of the middle plantar region are connected with the tendons intervening between the two former groups.

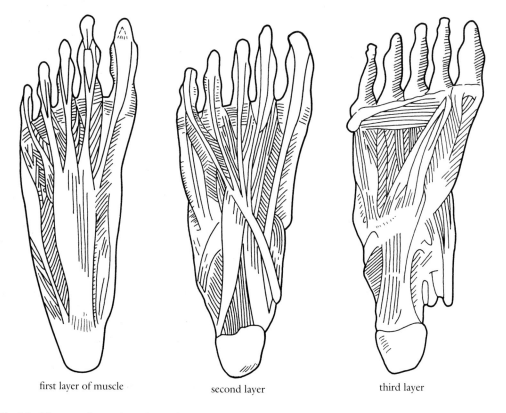

first layer of muscle   second layer   third layer

Fig 13. The muscles and tendons of the feet.

The extensor brevis digitorum is a broad thin muscle, which begins at the upper and outer surfaces of the calcaneum and then passes obliquely across the top of the foot and terminates in four tendons. The action of the extensor brevis digitorum is accessory to the long extensor, allowing extension of the phalanges of the fourth toes but acting only on the first phalanx of the great toes.

The second layer are called the flexor muscles and are separated from each other by the long plantar ligaments. The innermost, which is the largest, is inserted into the dorsal surface of the base of the first phalanx of the great toe, crossing the dorsal artery.

Four muscles comprise the third layer. The first muscle, called the flexor brevis hallucis, begins from the inner part of the under surface of the cuboid bone, the cuneiform bones and the tibialis tendon. The muscle divides and inserts into the inner and outer sides of the phalanx (small bones) at the base of the big toe, where a sesamoid bone develops in each tendon.

A large, thick muscle called the adductor obliquus hallucis, passes obliquely across the foot and occupies the hollow space between the four inner metatarsal bones. It begins at the second, third and fourth metatarsal bones and the peroneus longus (a muscle on the outside of the leg). The adductor obliquus hallucis is inserted, like the flexor brevis hallucis into the base of the first phalanx of the big toe. The flexor brevis minimi digiti begins at the base of the metatarsal bones of the little toe and the sheath of the peroneus longus and inserts into the base of the first phalanx of the little toe.

The fourth muscle called the adductor transversus hallucis is narrow and flat and stretches transversely across the heads of the metatarsal bones and between the flexor tendons. It begins at the metatarso-phalangeal ligaments of the three outer toes and inserts into the first phalanx of the big toe

There is a fourth layer of muscles called the interossei muscles, which are similar to those in the hand with the exception that they are grouped around the middle line of the second toe, instead of the middle of the third finger in the hand. There are seven in number, which consist of two groups: the dorsal and plantar.

The anterior tibialis muscle originates from the tibia bone and is inserted into the middle cuneiform bone of the foot by a long tendon. It provides dorsiflexion of the foot.

The soleus muscle is the main muscle of the calf of the leg, lying beneath the gastrocnemius. It originates from the heads and upper parts of the fibula and the tibia. Its tendon joins that of the gastrocnemius, so that they have an insertion into the calcaneus by the calcanean tendon. It causes plantarflexion at the ankle, and helps to stabilise the joint when the individual is standing up.

The gastrocnemius, as described above, is a powerful plantarflexor.

Blood Supply of the Feet

The dorsal pedis artery passes over the dorsum (top) of the foot, supplying arterial blood to structures in this area. It finishes by passing between the first and second metatarsal bones into the sole of the foot where it forms part of the plantar arch. The peroneal artery supplies the leg, passing into the ankle joint, then into the sole of the foot where it continues as the plantar artery. The plantar artery supplies the structures of the sole of the foot. As it branches, it forms an arch from which it branches and supplies the toes. Veins of the foot accompany the arteries.

Nerves of the Feet

The sciatic nerve descends from the buttock and back of the thigh and divides at about the middle of the femur where it forms the tibial and common peroneal nerves. The tibial nerve supplies muscles and skin of the sole of the foot and the toes. A branch of the tibial nerve supplies the heel, the lateral side of the ankle and a part of the top of the foot. The common peroneal nerves divide and become the superficial and deep peroneal nerves that supply the dorsum (top) of the foot and the toes.

ANATOMY OF THE HAND

Bones of the Hand

Each hand consists of twenty-seven bones. There are eight carpal bones or wrist bones arranged in two rows of four. These bones are closely fitted together and held in position by ligaments that allow a certain amount of movement between them. Some bones are associated with the wrist joint; others form joints with the metacarpal bones of the hand. Strong fibrous bands hold tendons of muscles lying in the forearm that cross the wrist firmly in place.

The metacarpal bones, or bones of the hand, are five in number and form the palm of the hand. They articulate with the carpal bones and at the furthest ends with the phalanges (fingers).

There are fourteen phalanges: three in each finger, and two in the thumb. They articulate with the metacarpal bones and with each other.

Joints of the Hand

The joints of the hand comprise gliding, hinge, condyloid and saddle joints, all of which are grouped as synovial or freely moveable joints.

Muscles of the Hand

The muscles of the hand mostly originate from the radius and ulna bones of the forearm. Some insert on the carpal bones of the wrist and others, which have long tendons that cross the wrist, insert on the bones of the hands and fingers. The muscles responsible for movements of the hands are the flexor carpi and the extensor carpi muscles. Finger movements are produced by several flexor digitorum and extensor digitorum muscles. There are special groups of muscles in the fleshy part of the hand which allow intricate movements to be performed by the thumb and fingers. In humans, the thumb has evolved considerable freedom of movement and allows the movements of gripping and holding.

There are many ligaments and tendons in the hand which together provide the movements of gripping, pinching, squeezing and wringing. The hands are more versatile in their range of movements compared with the feet. Joint movements consist of extension, flexion, circumduction, abduction, and adduction.

Drop wrist is an inability to extend the hand at the wrist, which is caused by damage to the radial nerve. This nerve serves the extensor muscles.

Blood Supply of the Hand

The radial artery passes down the forearm into the wrist. The pulse in the wrist is felt at the radial artery. It continues between the first and second metacarpal bones and enters the palm of the hand. The ulnar artery also passes into the hand. Deep and superficial arches form the palmar metacarpal and palmar digital arteries that supply the hand and fingers. Veins follow the same route as the arteries.

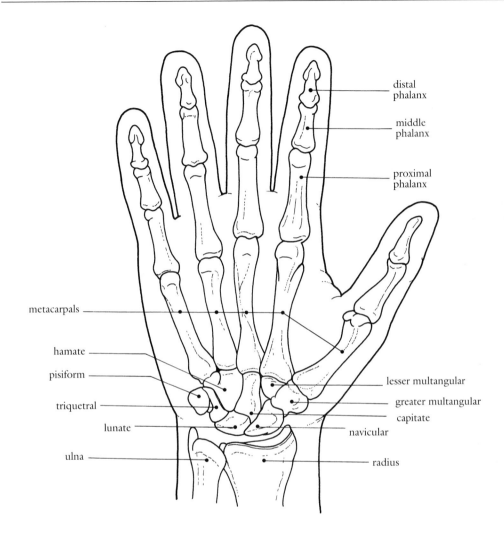

Fig 14. The bones of the right hand (palm up).

Nerves of the Hand

The radial nerve branches from the brachial nerve and supplies the wrist and finger joints. It continues into the back of the hand to supply the skin of the thumb, the first two fingers and the lateral side of the third finger. The median nerve supplies small muscles and the skin of the front of the thumb, the first two fingers and the lateral side of the third finger. The ulnar nerve supplies the palm of the hand and the skin of the little finger and the medial side of the third finger.

103

CHAPTER 11

Directions for Working Relaxation Techniques

Finding Tension in the Cranial, Thoracic, Abdominal and Pelvic Cavities

Supporting the foot from under the heel and holding each cavity between the thumb and fingers, flex the foot towards the patient (dorsiflexion) and towards yourself (plantarflexion) and sense the tension held in each cavity.

Wrapping the Foot not Being Worked

To keep the foot not being worked on warm and comfortable, wrap it securely in a towel as follows:

- Lay a good-size hand-towel on the supporting pillow under the foot and ankle not

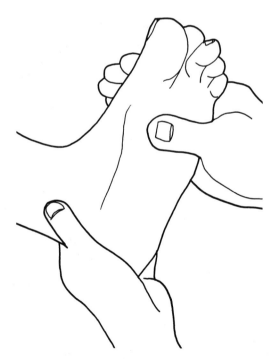

Fig 15. Finding tension in the cavities (1).

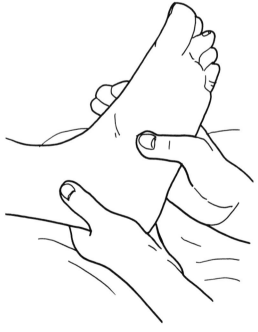

Fig 16. Finding tension in the cavities (2).

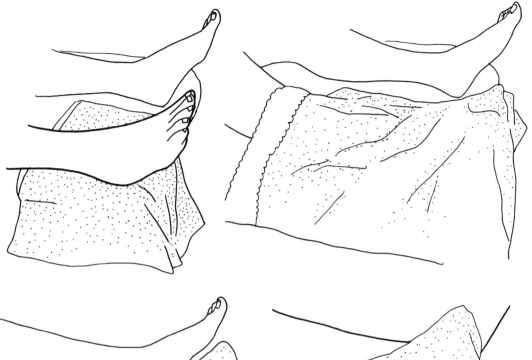

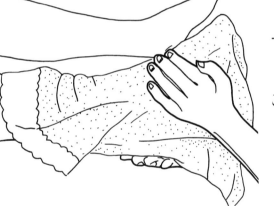

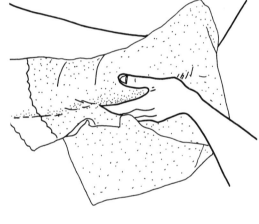

Fig 17. (top left) Place towel under the foot to the base of the calf muscle.

Fig 18. (top right) Fold towel over the top of the foot/ankle.

Figs 19 & 20. (middle left and right) Fold towel either side of the leg/foot in both directions.

Fig 21. (right) Tuck the remaining towel under the ankle.

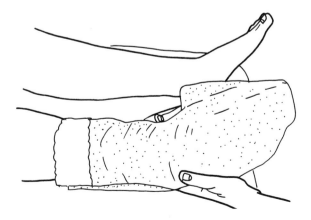

being worked on, just a little way up behind the ankle to the base of the calf muscle.

- Fold the towel either side of the leg and foot in both directions over the foot and leg, making sure that the top fold is securely tucked underneath the leg and ankle.
- Tidy the remaining towel by tucking under the ankle.

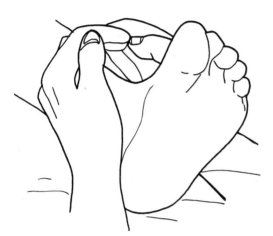

Fig 22. Ankle agitator (first movement).

Ankle Agitator Relaxation Technique

Grip the ankle joints with the base of the palms and shake the foot with fingers moving towards the body, so that the foot wobbles from side to side. Move the middle of the palms to the middle of the foot and shake from side to side. With both techniques, keep the fingers relaxed and loose so that the muscles of the upper arm are worked. If the fingers are stiff, muscles in the forearm are used which limit the benefits of this movement.

Phalange Rotation Relaxation Technique

Grip the lateral edge of the foot with the base of both palms and imagine that you are rolling across the foot in circular movements on the ball of the foot. You should see the toes move from side to side. It is important to keep your hands at the base of the toes, as squeezing toes can be very painful with joint-related problems.

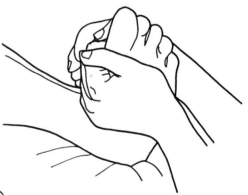

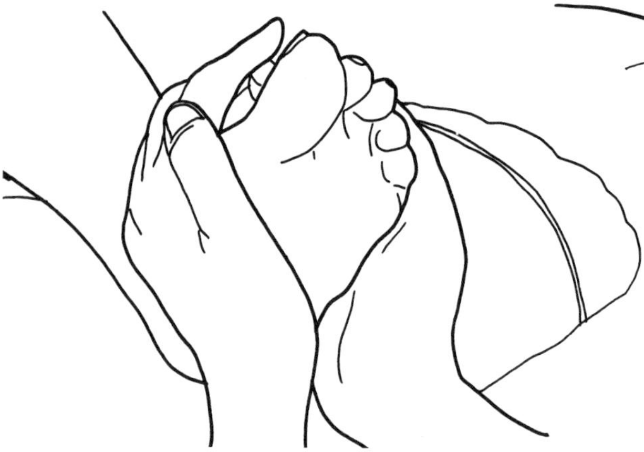

Fig 23. (above) Phalange rotation.

Fig 24. (left) Ankle agitator (second movement).

106

Metatarsal Massage Relaxation Technique

Make a fist with the supporting hand and place over the ball of the foot. Grip with the base of the palm over the edge of the foot, keeping the fingers together. Make sure the fingers are at the base of the toes so they are not squashed together. Push in and down-

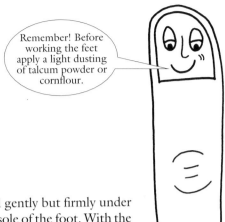

Remember! Before working the feet apply a light dusting of talcum powder or cornflour.

held gently but firmly under the sole of the foot. With the top hand only doing the work, twist the foot keeping the index fingers of both hands in contact on the sole of the foot. Use the supporting hand to follow the working hand up to the top of the toes keeping the index fingers in contact. Once at the top of the toes, the top hand then works down towards the ankle, gently pushing the bottom hand from above. This reverses the upward movement. Twisting with both hands results in a Chinese burn!

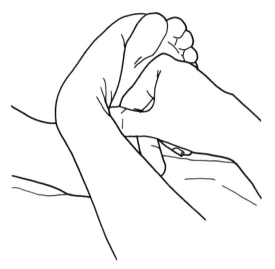

Fig 25. Metatarsal massage.

wards with the fist exerting pressure on the ball of the foot so that the metatarsal joints open on the dorsal part of the foot. Then, keeping your hand in contact with the ball of the foot release the pressure. As you release the pressure, with the hand on top of the foot, squeeze the metatarsal joints in together. The combination of these movements creates a pushing and squeezing massage.

Spinal Spiral Relaxation Technique

Grip the medial side of the foot with both hands over the ankle. Grip firmly with thumbs

Fig 26. Spinal spiral.

CHAPTER 12
The Human Body

The body comprises ten major systems, which are interdependent, one with the other. The circulatory and lymphatic systems are jointly called the cardio-vascular system.

- **The nervous system** is the electrical wiring system, as in a house, which sends electrical impulses to and from the brain.
- **The digestive system** processes food to provide energy for cells to keep them healthy and strong.
- **The lymphatic system** prevents infection and cleanses the blood.
- **The circulatory system** is the major transport system and communicator between all systems and is life-sustaining.
- **The endocrine system** sends hormones around the body as chemical 'messengers', which are sent to target organs.
- **The excretory system** cleanses the blood by elimination of toxins and includes the respiratory, urinary, integumentary and digestive system.
- **The respiratory system** feeds cells with oxygen (O_2) and eliminates carbon dioxide (CO_2).
- **The reproductive system** is concerned with propagation of an individual's genes into the next generation.
- **The skeletal system** provides support and enables movement and leverage of the human frame.
- **The muscular system** gives leverage and enables movement of the human frame.

In addition, five special senses give us information about our external surroundings through sight, hearing, taste, smell and touch.

Homoeostasis is the internal environmental balance of the body. An example of this process is sweating, when the body overheats and returns to normal temperature with a reduction in water levels in the body, which in turn stimulates thirst.

CAVITIES OF THE BODY

There are four main cavities of the body.

- The **cranial** cavity consists of the brain, the surrounding skull bone and associated structures.
- The **thoracic** cavity is the upper part of the trunk of the body and lies between the root of the neck and the diaphragm muscle. The thoracic cavity contains the organs of the heart, lungs and associated structures.
- The oval-shaped **abdominal** cavity is the largest cavity in the body. It is situated in the main part of the trunk and its boundaries are the diaphragm, which separates it from the thoracic cavity, and the pelvic cavity. The abdominal cavity contains organs and glands involved in the absorption and digestion of food.
- The **pelvic** cavity is triangular and narrows towards the lower end. The boundaries

extend downwards from the abdominal cavity to the pubic bones, sacrum, coccyx, innominate bones, and ends at the muscles of the pelvic floor. It contains the pelvic colon, the rectum and anus, some loops of the small intestine, the urinary bladder with the lower parts of the ureter, the urethra and the reproductive organs and glands.

HEAT COMBUSTION

Human beings are warm-blooded and in health the body temperature is maintained at an average of 36.8°C (98.4°F). If the temperature exceeds the average, the metabolic rate rises, and if it is lowered the metabolic rate is reduced. The body is able to generate heat internally or lose heat to the environment in order to maintain a constant level. The most active organs chemically and physically that produce the most heat are:

- The **muscles** – muscle movement generates heat, the more strenuous the exercise, the more heat is produced. The body's reaction to extreme cold is to produce involuntary muscular movements, that is shivering.
- The **liver** produces large amounts of heat as a by-product of chemical action.
- The **digestive** organs involved in digestion produce heat by the contraction of the muscles of the alimentary tract.
- The **respiratory organs**, by chemical action.

Most heat loss occurs through the skin, with small amounts lost in urine, expired air and faeces. Skin is the only organ which can regulate and maintain a constant body temperature.

CELLS OF THE BODY

The most amazing thing about human cells is that every cell has a 'memory' and knows exactly what it has to do within the body. All cells ingest nutrients, digest them to provide energy and the needs of the body, and excrete waste products from cellular activity.

A cell needs oxygen and nutrients to survive, and 99 per cent of cells are composed of hydrogen, oxygen, carbon and nitrogen, with minerals and salts of calcium, sodium, potassium, chlorine, magnesium, phosphorus and sulphur making up the remaining 1 per cent.

Human Cell

Every new human being develops from a single cell called a *zygote*, which develops from the fusion of the ovum from the female and the spermatozoa from the male.

Cell Structure

Human cells have a cell surface membrane, which is semi-permeable. This means that some molecules, like nutrients, can pass through the membrane whilst others can not.

Living cells are made up of protoplasm, which is a jelly-like substance composed of water and organic and non-organic substances. These substances can either be dissolved or held in suspension (meaning molecules in a solid state or those which have been diffused). The materials from which these compounds develop are carbohydrates, fats (lipids), amino-acids and minerals. Substances pass into and out of the cell across the membrane in a variety of ways.

The inside of the cell contains cytoplasm, which has very small structures called organelles present. Certain chemical reactions occur only in or on these organelles. Inside the cell, the central area shown in Fig 27 is the nucleus. It

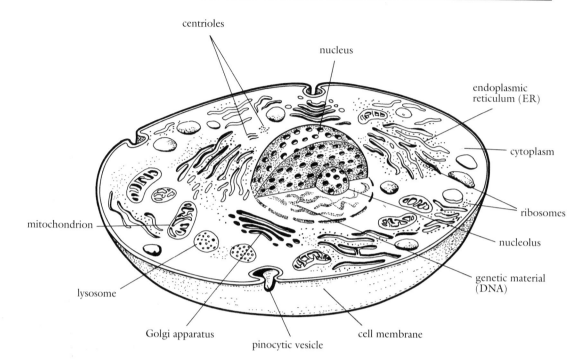

centrioles

nucleus

endoplasmic
reticulum (ER)

cytoplasm

ribosomes

nucleolus

mitochondrion

genetic material
(DNA)

lysosome

Golgi apparatus

pinocytic vesicle

cell membrane

Fig 27. Diagram of a typical cell showing the main organelles.

controls the chemical reactions occurring in the cell and is therefore a store of information.

Our bodies are made up of millions of cells that work together as a cohesive whole.

Some proteins on the surface of cell membranes are associated with the individual's immune response. These antigens are responsible for individual factors, such as the compatibility of transplanted organs, or blood groups.

Cell Function

The functions of the cell are to:

- protect the contents of the cell;
- allow porous substances in and out of the cell;
- convert oxygen and nutrients into energy in the metabolic process.

The breakdown of nutrients inside the cell membrane and subsequent release of energy requires organelles called mitochondria.

With the exception of erythrocytes (red cells), all cells contain a dark staining mass of deoxyribonucleic acid (DNA) in the nucleus, enclosed in the nuclear membrane. DNA acts in the manufacture of proteins within the cells and carries genetic information. The actual formation of proteins occurs on small bodies called ribosomes, which may be loose in the cytoplasm or attached to a network of membranes throughout the cell. Also contained in the nucleus are molecules of ribonucleic acid (RNA), which are responsible for the synthesis of proteins.

Within the cytoplasm are small spherical bodies called centrosomes, which are involved in cell division. Vacuoles are the clear, circular spaces inside the cells, which contain waste materials formed by cells.

Cell Regeneration

Cell regeneration occurs when the original cells are replicated by cell division. The extent to which regeneration is possible depends on the normal rate of physiological turnover of particular types of cells. The only cells in the body that do not replicate are nerve, skeletal and cardiac cells.

A cell-dividing process known as meiosis takes place in the reproductive glands, the ovaries and testes. These so-called gonads produce eggs and sperm cells, known as gametes. The process of cell division resulting in growth and repair is called mitosis.

Types of Cell

The cell must be able to pick up information like electricity and pass it on. Examples of different cells in the body are:

- erythrocytes or red cells, present in plasma;
- thrombocytes or platelets (blood clotting cells), present in plasma;
- leukocytes or white cells, present in plasma;
- sperm cells;
- nerve cells;
- osteogenic cells;
- Exocrine glands are groups of cells that release their secretions onto the surface of an organ either directly or through a duct.
- Endocrine glands are other groups of cells that have become isolated from surfaces and release their secretions into the bloodstream and lymph. These are also called ductless glands and their secretions are hormones.

- Plasma cells are derived from B-lymphocytes and secrete specific antibodies into the blood when foreign material or microbes are present.
- Mast cells are found in the liver and spleen and around the blood vessels. They produce serotonin and histamine, which are released as a response to injury or disease. They are also involved in inflammatory reactions, the development of allergies and hypersensitivity.
- Fat cells vary in size and shape and may occur singly or in groups, especially in adipose tissue under the skin. The hormone leptin, contained in fat cells, is involved in appetite control.
- Some cells have small hair-like projections from the surface called cilia, which wave to create movement around the cell. Examples are the cells that line the passages of the respiratory and reproductive tracts.

Movement of Nutrients across the Cell Membrane

There are four methods by which the cells receive nutrients: diffusion, osmosis, active transport and filtration. In these ways cells take what they need from fluids and nutrients and release waste materials from the cell into the plasma.

Diffusion

Diffusion is the movement of a *higher* molecular content into a *lower* molecular content. For example, imagine a jelly cube put in to a jug of boiling water. The jelly cube has a much higher molecular content than the water, so when boiling water is poured on to the jelly cube it melts and the molecular structure of the jelly cube becomes equal to that of the water.

Osmosis

Osmosis is only concerned with the movement of water through a cell membrane. To keep our body in a state of balance, or homeostasis, the water content inside a cell must be equal to that outside a cell membrane. Water moves from a *less* concentrated solution to a *more* concentrated solution until the concentration inside the membrane is equal to that on the outside of the membrane. For example, if cells are dehydrated, they will 'pull' water in through the cell membrane.

Active Transport

This is where a molecule is energetically *carried* across the cell membrane by a transmitter called adenosine triphosphate (ATP). This is a protein in the cell membrane that acts as a carrier of nutrient molecules.

Filtration

Filtration is a method where molecules are 'pushed' through the semi-permeable membrane of the cell. Larger solids cannot get pushed through a sieve but because of pressure behind filtration some substances get pushed through the small holes and others, which are too big, stay within the structure.

Membranes

Mucous membrane is a name given to the lining of the respiratory tract, alimentary tract and urinary tract. The latter, together with the reproductive system, is known as the genito-urinary tract. Organs lined by mucous membrane are lubricated and this protects the lining membrane from injury or friction. Foreign particles are trapped by the sticky mucus surfaces in the alveoli of the lungs.

Serous membranes consist of two layers, separated by a watery or serous fluid. It enables an organ to move without being damaged by friction between it and adjacent organs. Serous membranes are found in the thoracic cavity, the pleura surrounding the lungs and the pericardium surrounding the heart. The peritoneum surrounds the abdominal organs. **Synovial membranes** secrete clear, oily synovial fluid and are found lining the joint cavities and surrounding tendons. The fluid prevents injury to the tendons by rubbing against bones, for example, over the ankle joints.

TYPES OF TISSUES

Groups of specialized cells together form tissue. The main types of tissue are listed below:

- **Epithelial tissue** is found in the heart, blood vessels, alveoli of the lungs and the lymph vessels.
- **Connective tissue** is found in all organs supporting specialized tissue. Examples are hard connective tissue found in bone and the soft connective tissue of blood.
- **Areola tissue** is found widely throughout the body and its function is to connect and support other types of tissue.
- **Adipose tissue**, or fat, has a mesh-like structure which is either distended by several small drops or by one large drop of fat. This tissue replaces fibrous tissue when the amount of food taken in is in excess of the body's requirements.
- **Aponeurosis** is a white fibrous membrane, which forms muscle sheaths that extend beyond the muscle to become the tendons that attach the muscle to bone.
- **Lymphoid tissue** produces highly specialized cells called lymphocytes, which are found in blood and in lymphoid tissue.
- **Cartilage** is a stronger, more solid tissue than any of the other connective tissues.

There are three types:

- **Hyaline cartilage** is found on the surface of parts of the bones that form joints; forming the costal cartilages, which attach the ribs to the sternum and forming the larynx, trachea and bronchi.
- **White fibrocartilage** forms pads between the bodies of the vertebrae called the intervertebral discs, between the articulating surfaces of bones of the knee joint, and on the edge of the bony sockets of the hip and shoulder joints.
- **Yellow elastic cartilage** forms the support for the pinna, or ear lobe, the epiglottis and part of the blood vessel walls.
- **Muscle tissue** – there are three main types of muscle tissue:
  - **Cardiac muscle**, which is specialized groups of cells found only in the heart;
  - **Smooth or involuntary muscles** found in internal organs or viscera;
  - **Striated or voluntary muscles**, which give us movement and leverage.

SYSTEMS AND ORGANISMS

Groups of specialized cells become tissues. Groups of tissues formed together become an organ. Groups of organs composed of the same specialized cells become a system. The ten systems of the body which are interdependent with each other as a whole are called an organism.

THE INTEGUMENTARY SYSTEM

The word 'integument' means covering. It includes the skin and its appendages – the hair, the nails, the sweat and oil glands. The skin itself has two main layers different from each other in structure and function.

The skin is the largest organ *of* the body, whereas the liver is the largest organ *in* the body. The skin is referred to as an organ because it contains several kinds of tissue, including epithelial, connective and nerve tissue. It is known as the integumentary system because it includes glands, vessels, nerves and a subcutaneous layer that work together as a body system.

Most substances put onto the skin will be absorbed into the body over varying amounts of time. The skin completely renews itself by cells constantly dividing and pushing upwards until the top-most layer is shed. Skin has two main types of tissue: the epidermis, or surface layer; and the dermis, the underlying layer. The subcutaneous layer is the deepest and has an abundant supply of lymph and blood capillaries, and sensory nerve endings.

Skin varies in thickness, from thin over the eyelids to thick on the soles of the feet and palms of the hand. In $1cm^2$ it contains an estimated three million cells, thirteen oil glands, nine hairs, one hundred sweat glands, 1m of blood vessels and thousands of sensory cells.

Skin is a guide to the state of physical, mental and emotional health.

Functions of Skin

- Skin protects the deeper tissues against drying and against invasion of organisms or toxins through chemical means. Cells are composed of keratin and form an interlocking pattern that prevents penetration by organisms and water. They are constantly shed, causing removal of harmful substances.
- Skin regulates body temperature by evaporation of heat to the surrounding air. The epidermis acts as a water barrier and is vital in providing the wet environment required by cells in the dermis and underlying structures.
- Nerve endings in the periphery of the body

Overview of the Integumentary System

The largest organ of the body which can be described as an enveloping membrane

Structure	Function
Epidermis (outermost layer of skin)	Surface layer of cells die from lack of nourishment and develop large amounts of protein called keratin, which thickens and protects the skin.
Dermis or true skin (connective layer)	Contains blood vessels, nerves, hair follicles, sebaceous glands, collagen fibres, apocrine glands, sweat glands and elastin fibres.
Subcutaneous layer (no clear boundary between dermis and subcutaneous layer)	Consists of elastic fibres and connective tissue as well as adipose tissue which serves as an insulator and a reservoir store of energy. Continual bundles of elastic fibres connect the subcutaneous tissue with the dermis. Major blood vessels that supply the skin run through the subcutaneous layer. Also present are blood vessels concerned with temperature regulation, sweat glands and hair roots which extend into the subcutaneous layer where there is an abundance of nerves and nerve endings. Skin renews itself here and reaches the dermis layer in 3–4 weeks.
Erector pilli	Muscles attached to hair follicles that contract in response to cold and fear.
Sebaceous glands	Secrete sebum.
Sensory nerve endings	Provide sensations of pain, touch and temperature. Superficial blood vessels help regulate body temperature.
Nails	Outgrowths of the epidermis.
Adipose tissue	Fat deposits.
Sweat glands (two types): Apocrine Eccrine	Secrete water, salts, urea and other waste products. Produces sweat but decomposition by bacteria gives rise to perspiration and odour. Regulate body heat and disperse large quantities of water. Sweat consists of water, small amounts of minerals and other substances.

LINKS TO: muscular, nervous, circulatory, lymphatic, endocrine, urinary and digestive systems.

provide sensory information about the external environment.

- Sensory information has a protective function, for example, it enables withdrawal from harmful stimuli, such as a hot oven. Nerve receptors give sensations of pain, touch and temperature and are involved in immunological reactions in the body.
- Skin pigmentation prevents injury from ultraviolet light.
- Vitamin D is synthesized by sunlight in the epidermis.

Structure of Skin

Epidermis The epidermis contains nerve endings but no blood vessels. It is the outer layer of skin and is nourished by tissue fluid derived from the dermis. The epidermis is where cells are constantly lost through wear and tear. Since there are no blood vessels in the epidermis, the only living cells are found in the deeper layer of the dermis, where nourishment is provided by capillaries. The cells in the epidermis layer are constantly dividing and produce daughter cells, which are pushed upward towards the surface. As surface cells die from the gradual loss of nourishment, they undergo changes and become flat and horny forming the top layer of the epidermis. Skin may have additional layers between the stratum, corneum and stratum germinativum. Cells in the deepest layer of the epidermis produce melanin, the pigment that gives skin its colour. We call irregular patches of melanin freckles.

Dermis Sometimes called the 'true' skin, the dermis is a thick layer of connective tissue. The dermis layer of skin comprises hair follicles, sebaceous glands, blood vessels, collagen fibres, apocrine glands, sweat glands, nerves and elastin fibres. The word 'cutaneous' also refers to the skin. The integumentary system consists of skin and the subcutaneous layer, which contains structures extending from the skin.

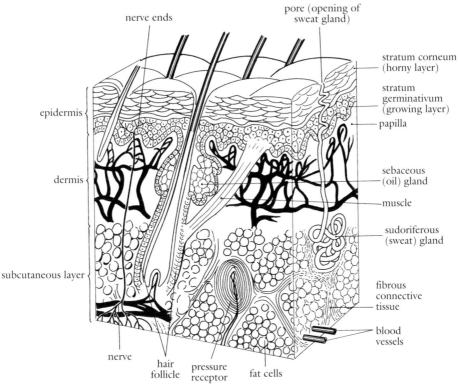

Fig 28. Cross-section of the skin.

Subcutaneous layer The dermis rests on the subcutaneous layer, which connects the skin to the surface muscles. This layer consists of elastic and fibrous connective tissue, as well as adipose (fat) tissue. The fat serves as insulation and a reserve of stored energy. Bundles of elastic fibres connect the subcutaneous tissue with the dermis, so there is no separation between the two.

The major blood vessels that supply the skin run through the subcutaneous layer, and are concerned with temperature regulation. Some of the appendages of the skin, such as sweat glands and hair roots, extend into the subcutaneous layer where tissue has a plentiful supply of nerves and nerve endings. The sweat glands are coiled and tube like structures located in the dermis and subcutaneous tissue. The erector pilli muscles are attached to hair follicles, which contract due to cold and fear. Nerves and nerve endings also supply the dermis and the varying thickness of the subcutaneous layer in different parts of the body. The thinnest layer is found on the eyelids and the thickest in the abdomen.

Sweat Glands Sweat consists of water, small amounts of mineral salts, urea and other waste products. There are two types of sweat glands.

- **Apocrine glands** are considered to be more social as they are found in the axilla (armpit) and genital area. These glands develop in puberty and enlarge premenstrually. Fresh sweat is sterile, but decomposition by bacteria gives perspiration an odour.
- **Eccrine glands** provide millions of sweat glands over the body and excrete diluted salt and water and control heat regulation of the body, providing a constant internal temperature of 36.8°C. These glands disperse large quantities of water, which can reach about 2 litres per day.

Each gland has an excretory tube that extends to the surface and opens at a pore. The point at which an excretory tube joins the skin acts as a valve and provides regulation of body temperature through the evaporation of sweat from the body surface.

The wax glands in the ear canal and the ciliary glands at the edges of the eyelid are modifications of sweat glands, as are the mammary glands.

Sebaceous Glands These secrete sebum and open into hair follicles. Sebum consists mainly of fatty acids and cholesterol and is secreted into the hair follicles. These glands lubricate the skin and hair and prevent drying. They appear over all the skin, except the palms and the soles of the feet. They are most numerous on the scalp and the face and may become blocked by dirt and sebum and cause blackheads and pimples or cysts to form.

Hair This is composed mainly of keratin and is not a living substance. Each hair develops in a sheath called a follicle, and new hair is formed from cells at the bottom of the follicle. The hair follicle is richly supplied by nerves and blood vessels and contains melanin, which gives hair its pigmentation. There are three types of hair:

- coarse hair, for example, on the scalp, moles, beard, eyebrows and pubic hair;
- vellus hair is short, fine, downy hair, for example, on the face of women and pre-pubescent boys;
- lanugo hair, which covers the foetus.

Attached to most hair follicles is a thin band of involuntary muscle. When this muscle contracts, the hair is raised forming goose-pimples on the skin, and when the muscle presses on the sebaceous gland associated with the hair follicle, it causes the release of sebum. Hair colour is determined by the amount of melanin present; white hair has no pigmentation as pigment has been replaced by tiny bubbles of air.

Nails These are an appendage of the skin and form outgrowths of the epidermis. Nails on the fingers and toes are protective structures made of hard keratin produced by cells that originate in the outer layer of the epidermis. New cells form continuously at the nail root. A fingernail takes up to six months to replace itself and its growth can be affected by disease or malnutrition. Nails on both the toes and the fingers are affected by general health. Changes in the nail structure include abnormal colour, thickness, shape or texture, grooves or splitting, and can be caused by chronic diseases, such as heart disease, malnutrition and anaemia.

Ageing and the Skin

Due to the loss of fat and collagen in the underlying tissues with increasing age, wrinkles or crow's feet develop around the eyes and mouth. The dermis layer of skin becomes thinner and may become transparent and lose its elasticity, giving the effect of 'parchment skin'. Hair does not replace itself as rapidly as before and thus becomes thinner with increasing age.

The formation of pigment produced by melanin also decreases with age, causing hair to become grey or white. However, there may be areas of extra pigmentation in the skin that form brown spots on the skin especially on areas exposed to the sun.

Sweat glands decrease in number, so there is less output of perspiration. The fingernails may flake, become brittle or develop ridges, and toenails may become discoloured or thickened.

Emotions and the Skin

Emotional trauma can sometimes upset the skin and be a reflection of inner feelings that are not being dealt with. It is important to observe the patient's skin before embarking on reflexology treatment. The first indication of serious systemic disease may be a skin disorder.

Pigmentation of the Skin

Melanin is a dark body pigment, produced by the pineal gland. It is found in the hair, the iris of the eye and the skin. The function of melanin is to protect the body from the harmful rays of the sun. The skin may change colour through sun-tanning (browning), liver disease (yellowing), emotional changes in the circulation from the skin, such as fear (blanching), anger (reddening), cold (a blue appearance) or embarrassment, for example, with blushing.

Darker people have much larger quantities of melanin in their skin. A yellowish discoloration of the skin may be due to the presence of excessive quantities of bilirubin (bile pigments) in the blood. Another cause of a yellowish discoloration can be an excessive intake of deeply coloured vegetables, for example, carrots. In many disorders, discoloration of the skin appears and the student is advised to study this further in conjunction with a particular illness.

CASE STUDIES WITH SKIN DISORDERS

Excema

Nicola is a young woman who came for reflexology treatments complaining of excema, which extended to her scalp, ears, eyes, arms and chest. She had been receiving homeo-pathic treatment for some time and, although she had received relief from the complaint, she felt that reflexology may provide the additional boost her system needed.

We discussed creams and shampoos used and decided on trying tea-tree essential oil rubbed into the affected parts, with a few drops in the bath to see if it would have any effect. It didn't make any difference to the condition, which also appeared to become aggravated with alcohol and stress generally. We then decided to try lavender essential oil and, with regular weekly treatment of reflexology, she found the condition improved dramatically.

Nicola now attends reflexology sessions on a monthly basis as she finds that she has stabilized and the excema has cleared.

Psoriasis

Some years ago, Linda came for treatment complaining of tiredness, stress, bowel prob-lems and a small patch of psoriasis on the tarsal bones of her left foot. I have often found that grape-seed oil rubbed on to skin conditions creates a healing crisis, after which the condition disappears. I advised Linda to rub the oil onto her ankle and to persevere until the condition improved. Combined with regular weekly treatments of reflexology and the grape-seed oil, she went through the healing crisis where the affected area of psoriasis looked far worse for a short time, then cleared completely. With regular weekly treatments, Linda's problems began to improve and in a relatively short time had improved to a point where she felt able to reduce treatments.

Linda had a good sense of humour and in many sessions we would both cry with laughter about a recent situation in her work. I feel that this release for her became part of the healing process – and probably helped myself, as well!

The result was that she was so impressed with her overall improvement that she decid-ed to train in reflexology.

CHAPTER 13

The Muscular System

Overview of the Muscular System

Gives movement and leverage, and aids in internal functions of viscera (organs and glands).

Structure	*Functions*
VOLUNTARY OR STRIATED MUSCLE *Isotonic* muscular movement requires a muscle to contract (prime mover) and a muscle to relax (antagonist) *Isometric* muscular movement promotes tension between muscles and no contraction	Movement, leverage and weight bearing
Controlled by the cerebrum of the brain – the central nervous system (CNS)	Functions under the conscious control of the will
INVOLUNTARY OR SMOOTH MUSCLE Controlled by the cerebellum of the brain and the medulla oblongata (brain stem) – the autonomic nervous system (ANS)	Internal visceral (organ/gland) functioning Functions beneath the level of consciousness
CARDIAC MUSCLE The heart The medulla oblongata	Provides a constant circulation Can be stimulated by hormones or sympathetic nerve action as a part of the autonomic nervous system

LINKS TO: nervous, endocrine, urinary, special senses, respiratory, cardio-vascular, skeletal/joints, digestive, reproductive and integumentary systems.

INTRODUCTION

There are 640 named muscles in the body. Muscles are a group of specialized cells bundled into fibres, which are capable of contracting and relaxing. Muscle cells can be excited by chemical, mechanical or electrical means.

Muscles are attached to bone, ligaments, tendons and skin. Muscle names are dependent on their shape, the direction of the fibres, the position of the muscle and their function.

MUSCLE FUNCTION

The major functions of the muscular system are to:

- provide movement for the skeletal structure of the body;
- give shape to the body and enable it to remain erect;
- pump blood from the heart through the arteries;
- move food through the alimentary canal of the digestive system;
- expand and contract the thoracic cavity to enable breathing;
- open and close orifices in the body;
- generate body heat;
- provide expression through facial muscles.

Substances required for muscle action are: glycogen, oxygen, calcium, sodium and potassium. By-products of muscle action are lactic acid and carbon dioxide. Waste products are removed from muscles and eliminated by the body through the veins, lymphatics, lungs, kidneys, urine, and skin.

Tendons

Tendons are an extension of muscle and are composed of strong fibrous tissue. They are flexible and only slightly elastic and form cords or sheets that enable muscles to move bones. When tendons become broader sheets of tissue attached to bone, they are called aponeurosis.

INVOLUNTARY MUSCLE

Muscles that work beneath the level of consciousness are called 'involuntary'. Involuntary or smooth muscle is found in the internal organs: stomach, intestine, uterus, bronchi, bladder and blood vessels.

Cardiac Muscle

Involuntary muscles are under the control of the autonomic nervous system. Cardiac muscle is found in the heart only and is under the control of a part of the brain stem called the medulla oblongata.

VOLUNTARY MUSCLE

Muscles that work within conscious decision-making are called 'voluntary'. Voluntary or striated muscles give leverage, movement and the ability to stretch. Voluntary muscle is comprised of specialized cells bundled into

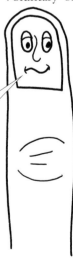

Remember! The ripple movement is always made with the medial edge of the thumb.

fibres that are capable of contracting and relaxing. It is found in the arms, legs, back, face, chest, diaphragm and abdomen. Muscle contraction is the ability of muscle to change its shape and shorten itself, when it becomes thicker. Voluntary muscles work in pairs:

- the *prime mover* contracts;
- the *antagonist* relaxes, allowing bones to move at the joints.

When muscles shorten, movement is called *isotonic contraction*. When muscles tense but do not shorten, muscle tension is called *isometric*.

Voluntary muscle is under the control of the central nervous system. A sphincter muscle is a circular muscle that surrounds an opening or passage in the body, and it contracts to close the opening or relaxes to allow passage of substances. Sphincters are found in the anus, bladder, urethra, stomach, duodenum and the common bile duct.

Abdominal Muscles

The abdominal muscles consist of four pairs of muscles attached to the front of the abdominal cavity, which form a strong muscular wall and keep the human frame in an upright position. When the muscles contract together, they:

- compress the abdominal organs;
- flex the vertebral column in the lumbar region.

Respiratory Muscles

The respiratory muscles are divided into:

- eleven pairs of external intercostal muscles, attached to and filling spaces between the ribs;
- eleven pairs of internal intercostal muscles, attached to and filling the spaces between the ribs;
- one diaphragm muscle.

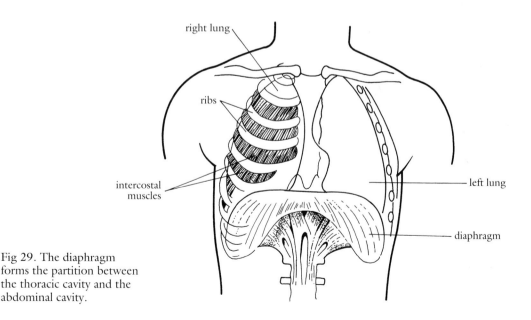

Fig 29. The diaphragm forms the partition between the thoracic cavity and the abdominal cavity.

The diaphragm is attached to the spine, ribs and breastbone and is the main muscle of respiration.

Muscle Glycogen

Muscle glycogen provides the glucose requirement for muscle activity, with adrenaline and glucagon being the main hormones associated with the conversion of glycogen to glucose. Carbohydrate in excess of that required to maintain the blood glucose level and glycogen levels in tissues is converted into fat and stored in the fat deposits.

Healing of Muscle Fibres

Damage to muscle fibres may be accidental or caused through surgery. The extent of the damage determines the way healing takes place. Damaged tissue is removed by phagocytosis and replaced by fibrous tissue, which can leave a scar or adhesions.

Lactic Acid

Muscle fatigue is caused by an accumulation of lactic acid in the muscle. Oxygen is needed to oxidize lactic acid and rebuild it into glucose.

SPECIAL INTEREST

Working the Diaphragm

This reveals tension held in the diaphragm muscle and is a key movement for assisting relaxation and improved breathing, and blood and lymph circulation. It is the first reflex to be worked with the ripple thumb movement.

Emotional tension held in the solar plexus can affect breathing and the digestive tract, plus circulatory and lymphatic efficiency will be impaired by decreased stimulation to the movement of blood upwards towards the heart from the lower limbs.

Encourage deep breathing with your patient at the end of the treatment with your thumbs placed on the solar plexus. As they inhale, press in on the reflex point and as they exhale, release the pressure. Suggest that they try and make a habit of it whenever tension is present.

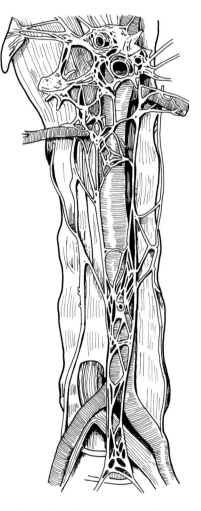

Fig 30. The solar plexus nerve ganglia.

The Muscular System

System(s)	Associated Reflexes	Disorders
REFLEX POINT 1: THE DIAPHRAGM		
Muscular	Whole foot	Diaphragmatic fatigue
Respiratory	Lungs, sinuses, nose, trachea	Respiratory disorders
Nervous	Solar plexus, brain	Emotional and physical tension
Cardio-vascular	Lymph nodes and heart	Cardio-vascular disorders
Digestive	Stomach, oesophagus	Hiatus hernia, peptic reflux, oesophagitis

Nerve Innervation: 5th Thoracic

See Chapter 26 for a description of disorders related to the Muscular System

WORKING THE REFLEXES

Diaphragm and Solar Plexus – Reflex Point 1 – Respiratory, Nervous and Muscular Systems

To work the diaphragm, keep the working hand over the supporting hand on top of the foot. Look for the base of the ball of the foot where the sole changes colour and work from the lateral edge to the medial edge across the width of the foot using the ripple movement. Swap hands and work from the medial edge to the lateral edge. Each time the centre of the diaphragm line has been reached, massage the solar plexus for emotional stress. An indication for finding the solar plexis is an inverted 'V' at the centre point of this reflex.

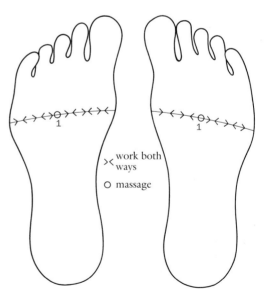

Hand position: the solar plexus and diaphragm, reflex point 1 (both feet). Working hand over supporting hand. Refer to Nervous, Respiratory and Digestive Systems.

Direction for working: the solar plexus and diaphragm, reflex point 1 (both feet).

123

CASE STUDY WITH POLYMYALGIA RHEUMATICA

Sally came for reflexology in desperation of finding help with polymyalgia rheumatica. Her story is told below.

I suffered from polio at the age of seven, very mildly but have felt unsure whether I ever had a full recovery, as I suffered muscle and ligament problems from the age of twelve. I also had bad back and cystitis problems, which went untreated during my teens and early twenties. After a difficult birth with my daughter, I suffered back problems. I went to my doctor and he suggested that I had an X-ray which showed that I had a 'slipped disc'. I received no medical treatment and finally found relief from chiropractic treatment in 1970. I have also suffered bladder and kidney problems and have had several minor operations on the bladder.

My back problems went away until 1981 when I resumed periodic chiropractic treatment and in 1988 I had an operation to remove calcium deposits from my kidney, which had practically ceased working. My back problems became worse from 1987 onwards, culminating in two frozen shoulders and severe pain in my upper arms. This went on for two years.

Finally, by 1995 I was in so much pain that I couldn't sit or lie down in bed for more than half-hour periods and I had to give up driving my car as I could not lift my arms above my chest. My doctor sent me for blood tests, which showed high ESR (erythrocyte sedimentation rate) and immediately put me on 30mg Prednisolone without telling me that this was a steroid. I was advised several days into the course by a friend that I was taking steroids and voiced my fears to my doctor who told me that they were completely safe and that the side-effects were nil, other than to put on weight. I was told that if I did not take these steroids I would probably go blind through temporal arteritis.

However, the steroids caused damage to both my eyes and I had to pay to have a new lens put in my right eye, and I now need an operation for the left eye. I had, and reported to my doctor, very severe side-effects from the steroids right from the beginning of the treatment, but my doctor ignored everything I said, even when I was losing my sight.

Finally I got myself off the steroids after two years and refused to take any medication offered by both my doctor and a specialist. In desperation, I sought help from a local complementary clinic and was told to consult a nutritionist and a reflexologist. I started treatment with Jenny and was, by this time, in terrible pain and mentally very frightened by my experiences. I have been having reflexology and Jenny has been able to highlight specific problems for me. The first problem being obviously that my whole system was in a mess! She pointed out that my liver was a big problem area and suggested that I ask my doctor for a cholesterol test. The test showed that my cholesterol had gone up from 5.7 before taking steroids to nearly 8 since taking the steroids. My doctor immediately wanted to give me tablets to lower my cholesterol but I refused and once again consulted the nutritionist. She felt sure that within six months or so, if I stayed on the diet the cholesterol would resolve itself.

My doctor reluctantly agreed but said that if my cholesterol was not down in twelve months he would again ask me to take the tablets. With Jenny's help and my diet, my cholesterol reduced to 5.7 in three months. My ESR is still high (52). This, the nutritionist feels, could well be down to my adrenal glands, which will probably not have recovered from taking steroids. Jenny has pointed out to me on several occasions that my adrenal glands are still a problem area, but my doctor does not agree on the subject of adrenal deficiency and advises me that he can see no valid reason to carry out an expensive test, so it looks as though I will have to pay to find out.

After not sleeping for ten years I am now sleeping well and can walk briskly for at least an hour each day. Whilst I was on steroids I could not even walk 100 yards without having palpitations and severe cramping. My general health, energy levels and my self esteem have rocketed since being helped by the nutritionist and Jenny. They have both given me faith in my own judgement. I feel that I am in charge and responsible for my health and I now know that there is great support and help to be found with a natural and complementary approach to health problems.

This client continues to improve in her overall health, so much so that she has since begun her own business! She has also remained on the diet given to her by the nutritionist and feels that this has stopped toxicity accumulating in her muscles and joints.

CHAPTER 14

The Cardio-Vascular System

Overview of the Cardio-Vascular System

Circulatory system
Major transport system ————————
|
Three divisions of the circulatory system
|

———— SYSTEMIC (GENERAL CIRCULATION) ————
heart
|
plasma – carries nutrients and waste products
|
erythrocytes (red cells) – carry oxygen and carbon dioxide
|
thrombocytes (platelets) – involved in blood clotting
|

———— PULMONARY CIRCULATION ————
heart/lungs – gaseous exchange
lungs – release carbon dioxide and absorb oxygen
|
superficial vessels carry oxygenated blood
(arteries, arterioles, capillaries)
|
deep vessels carry deoxygenated blood (veins, venules, capillaries)
|

———— PORTAL CIRCULATION ————
small intestine – absorption of nutrients
|
hepatic portal vein – transports nutrients to liver from small intestine
|
hepatic vein – transports nutrients and waste products to the
pulmonary and systemic circulation

breathing, muscular action, dilation and contraction
of blood vessels required to push venous blood and
lymph fluid up towards the heart

the left and right subclavian veins in the neck
drain lymph fluid into the pulmonary circulation

Lymphatic system
Provides immunity and
cleanses blood
|
spleen (major lymphatic
organ), thymus gland,
tonsils, appendix
|
leukocytes (white cells)
|
lymphocytes – move into
blood vessels if needed
|
antibodies
|
macrophages
|
capillaries – drain lymph
into vessels and plasma
|
nodes – filter lymph fluid
and store lymphocytes
|
left thoracic duct – drains
lymph from cisterna chyli
|
right lymphatic duct –
drains lymph from liver
area
|
lacteals present in
intestinal villi absorb fats
|
Kupffer cells –
(macrophages present in
the liver)

LINKED TO: all other systems.

CIRCULATORY CARDIO-VASCULAR SYSTEM

The cardio-vascular system is made up of the circulatory and lymphatic systems, together with the heart. The circulatory system is the most important system in the human body – it travels to every part carrying nutrients and oxygen, and is consequently the major transport system of the body.

Exchange of gases in the lungs takes place in blood capillaries, with inhaled oxygen (O_2) taken into the blood and carbon dioxide (CO_2) eliminated by exhalation. Blood changes its composition as it moves around the body as it gives up nutrients, oxygen, hormones and water to cells and takes away waste products for excretion.

Blood 'feeds' the body and is classified as a soft connective tissue, as it is solid in its molecular content. Blood cells represent the solid part of blood and float in plasma which is mostly made up of water and other substances. The composition of blood is 45 per cent blood cells and 55 per cent plasma. Plasma is a straw-coloured fluid and is composed of 90–92 per cent water in which waste products are sent to the kidneys for excretion. The functions of blood are given below.

- The nutrients that are digested from our food are taken to all the cells around the body.
- Oxygen is exchanged for carbon dioxide. Carbon dioxide is transported in the blood to the lungs for exhalation as oxygen is inhaled into the bloodstream. As we cannot survive without oxygen and too much carbon dioxide in our blood will poison the body, the lungs and brainstem maintain a constant balance to meet the body's needs.
- Waste products from the liver, in the form of urea, and waste products from cell metabolism and the lymphatic system are taken to the kidneys for excretion.
- Hormones are sent from the endocrine glands to 'target organs'.
- Heat is vital in maintaining an internal environmental balance (homeostasis). Heat is taken from the muscles and liver to cooler parts of the body.
- Blood transports antibodies around the body to fight micro-organisms and viruses.

Blood Cells

Erythrocytes

Erythrocytes (or red blood cells) carry oxygen to the cells of the body and carry away carbon dioxide. This process is called gaseous exchange. Red cells need a substance called haemoglobin for O_2 and CO_2 to attach to the cell. Red cells live for approximately 120 days and when they are 'tired' they are transported to the spleen and liver where they are broken down to release iron and bilirubin, which are necessary in the formation of new cells. These cells are biconcave, which means that they are discs that are concave on both sides. The main place of manufacture of red cells is red bone marrow, especially in the femur and vertebrae.

Red cells are formed in the liver and spleen between the first six and seven months of foetal life. Bone marrow becomes the main source of blood cells during childhood and adult life. At birth, the formation of red blood cells begins in the bone marrow of almost every bone in the body. As the child grows the marrow cavity starts to be replaced by fat so that the formation of cells in an adult occurs in the central skeleton and the ends of the long bones. The control of the formation of red blood cells is by the hormone erythropoietin, which is formed in the kidneys and the liver.

Leukocytes

Leukocytes (or white cells) do not contain haemoglobin and are therefore colourless. These cells are part of the immune system and form antibodies and lymphocytes. Lymphocytes are concerned with producing antibodies to kill off microbes and viruses that may enter the body. Lymphocytes and antibodies are formed in the spleen, which is the major lymphatic organ in the body. The function of lymphocytes is concerned with the formation and storage of antibodies.

Macrophages and Neutrophils

Specialized white cells called macrophages and neutrophils – *macro* means 'big' and *phage* means 'eat' and so another way of thinking of them is as 'big eater' – are produced in red bone marrow and their lifespan is variable. These cells are concerned with crushing, poisoning and strangling invaders (phagocytosis). These cells can remain in tissue or circulate in the blood and large numbers can be found in the spleen, lungs, liver and lymph nodes. Inflammation is the body's defence against irritants and produces pain, heat, redness and swelling. In injury, histamine is released from damaged cells, which causes blood vessels to dilate, thereby also causing redness, heat and swelling.

Thrombocytes

Thrombocytes (or platelets) are concerned with blood clotting and rush to the site of a wound to begin the repair. Platelets are fragments of cells and are very small compared with other cells in the blood. The place of manufacture of platelets is the bone marrow. Their lifespan is unknown and their function is to release enzymes that cause the blood to clot.

DIVISIONS OF THE CIRCULATORY SYSTEM

The circulatory system is divided into three major areas.

- **The pulmonary circulation**, which takes blood to the heart from the lungs and from the lungs to the heart.
- **The portal circulation** takes nutrients through the villi in the small intestines to the liver via the hepatic portal vein. Nutrients are either broken down or stored in the liver. Nutrients pass through the liver via the hepatic vein into the inferior vena cava, thence to the heart and into the main circulation.
- **The systemic or general circulation** is the rest of the route of blood around the body. This means that it goes everywhere else other than through the digestive processes, lungs and heart.

Blood Flow around the Body

Gravity is only useful for parts of the body above the heart. Breathing assists venous blood flow back to the heart from the lower extremities with movements of the rib cage and diaphragm encouraging blood to be sucked towards the heart.

Blood moves through vessels called arteries, which carry oxygenated blood, and veins, which carry deoxygenated blood. Each organ has an artery taking oxygen-rich blood to it and a vein taking deoxygenated blood away.

Arterial Circulation

Arteries and arterioles have three muscular layers. The outer layer consists of fibrous tissue, the middle layer consists of a smooth muscle and elastic tissue, and the inner lining

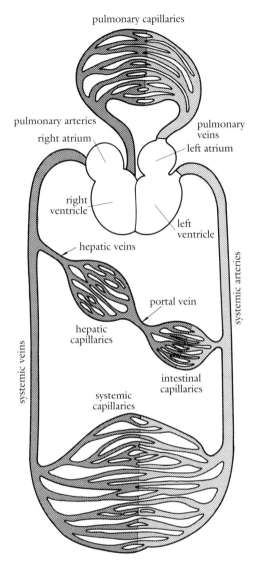

Fig 31. The circulation of the blood around the body.

The major arteries are:

- carotid artery;
- pulmonary artery;
- ovarian artery;
- aorta;
- hepatic artery;
- renal artery.

Arterioles are very fine and delicate vessels, which carry oxygenated blood to the finest structures called the capillaries. Eventually, at the very extremities of our bodies we have a capillary network covering the whole surface of our bodies, nearest to the external environment.

Blood in the arteries flows at a higher pressure than that in the veins as the heart acts as a pump in pushing the blood through the arteries to the capillary beds. When the blood is in the capillary network an exchange of oxygen and carbon dioxide takes place. Capillary walls are only one cell thick so waste can diffuse from cells into the tissue fluid and then into the capillary.

Venous Circulation

The walls of veins and venules are thinner than those of arteries but have the same three layers. Veins have less muscle and elastic tissue, so there is a larger space for blood to flow through. Some veins possess cup-shaped valves, which ensure that blood flows in one direction towards the heart as it moves against gravity.

Blood in the veins is under low pressure because it is a long way from the heart and it has lost fluid and pressure as it travelled through the capillary bed. Blood flow in veins is maintained by muscles that lie next to them and exert pressure on the venous walls and valves.

Venules are similar to arterioles except that they carry deoxygenated blood away from the capillaries. The major veins are:

consists of endothelium. As the walls of the arteries have a thick muscle and elastic layer, blood is forced into the artery, pressing against the artery walls, which stretch the elastic tissue. As this elastic muscle springs inwards blood is squeezed along the artery.

129

- jugular vein;
- superior vena cava; drains the head, neck, arms and upper part of the trunk;
- inferior vena cava; drains the lower part of the trunk, legs and pelvis;
- hepatic portal vein;
- common iliac vein;
- renal vein;
- ovarian vein.

Plasma

Plasma has many functions. It is mainly composed of 90–92 per cent water and carries waste products, such as urea and uric acid, and useful substances, such as salts, amino acids, glucose, hormones, nitrogen, oxygen, carbon dioxide, blood plasma proteins (necessary for blood clotting), nutrients, enzymes and antibodies.

Blood Groups

A blood-group system is based upon the presence or absence of antigens associated with the membranes of the red blood cells. There are four blood groups: A, B, AB and O. The type of antigen associated with the red blood cell gives the blood its group name:

- group A, type antigen A;
- group B, antigen B;
- group AB, antigen AB;
- group O, none.

A person who needs a blood transfusion must only be given blood of a certain type, that is, a person needing blood who has group A can take compatible blood of O and A; group B can take O and B; group AB can take O, A, B and AB; group O can only take O. From this we can see that a person with an AB group can receive blood of any group, and anyone can receive group O blood.

Blood Plasma Proteins

- **Albumen** is formed in the liver. It is the most abundant plasma protein and its main function is to maintain a normal level of plasma osmotic pressure.
- **Globulins** are formed in the liver and lymphoid tissue. They are concerned with the immune response to the presence of antigens (microbes, viruses, foreign bodies), the transportation of some hormones and mineral salts and the inhibition of some enzymes.
- **Clotting factors** are substances essential for the coagulation of blood.
- **Fibrinogen** is synthesized in the liver and is essential for blood coagulation.

Blood Clotting

Thromboplastin (an enzyme) is found in blood platelets and tissue cells, which when released at the site of a wound comes into contact with prothrombin and calcium in the blood. In the presence of prothrombin and calcium, thromboplastin is converted into thrombin, which interacts with fibrinogen, a protein always present in blood plasma, to form fibrin. Fibrin consists of needle-sharp crystals which, with the assistance of the blood platelets, forms a fine network in which the blood corpuscles become enmeshed and form a blood clot. Serum is plasma from which clotting factors have been removed and which remains after the formation of a fibrin clot in a wound.

Route of Blood through the Heart

The function of the heart is to provide a constant circulation. The heart is a muscular organ about 10cm (4in) long and is about the size of the owner's fist. It weighs about 225g (½lb) and is heavier in men.

Fig 32. Blood route
through the heart.

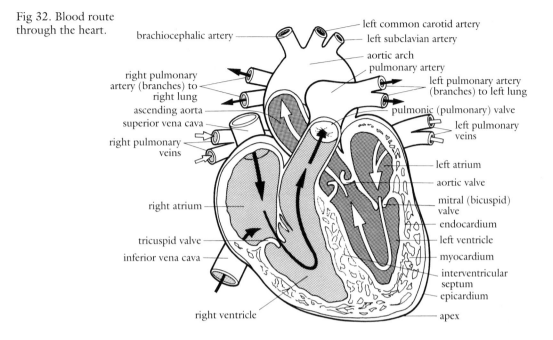

Blood enters the heart as deoxygenated blood and leaves as oxygenated blood. This occurs by the heart pumping blood into the lungs in the process of gaseous exchange of CO_2 for O_2. The part of the circulatory system that conveys blood between the heart and the lungs is the pulmonary circulation. The heart has four chambers: two on the right side and two on the left.

The right side of the heart fills with deoxygenated blood. The major veins that empty into the right side of the heart are called the superior and inferior vena cava, which empty into the top chamber of the heart called the right atrium; its function is to act as a collecting chamber for blood.

The blood is pushed through a one-way valve, called the tricuspid valve, into the right ventricle. 'Tri' means three so there are three flaps that act as a one-way valve to stop blood pumping backwards into the atrium once it has entered the right ventricle. Once the blood is in the ventricle, it is pumped under pressure through the pulmonic valve into the pulmonary artery and into the lungs. The pulmonary artery and the pulmonary vein are the only areas in the body where arteries and veins serve an opposite purpose. The pulmonary artery carries deoxygenated blood and the pulmonary vein carries oxygenated blood.

Blood re-enters the heart under pressure through the pulmonary vein into the left side of the heart and empties into the left atrium at the body's blood pressure. The valve between the atrium on the left side of the heart and the left ventricle is called the bicuspid valve ('bi' means two). The bicuspid valve therefore has two flaps, which stops blood moving backwards into the left atrium. Pressure increases dramatically in the ventricle once the bicuspid valve is closed, and as the ventricle relaxes the pressure drops.

The aortic valve closes as blood falls back due to lack of pressure from the left ventricle.

From this point, blood is pushed up through the aortic valve and in to the aortic arch and the main aorta, where it is pushed under pressure around the body.

The atria on the left and right sides of the heart fill with blood and contract at the same time. Both ventricles fill with blood when the atria contract, and both ventricles contract at the same time. At the end of this sequence the heart relaxes, while the atria fill with blood once more. The ventricle on the left side of the heart is much thicker than that on the right side because the left ventricle has the job of pumping blood with force through the aortic arch on its journey around the body.

Heart Rate

Each repeating sequence is a heart cycle or a heartbeat. The heart beats at about 76 times a minute. The number of beats per minute is the heart rate. The heart rate varies from person to person and increases during exercise, so that oxygenated blood and glucose can be carried to the tissues faster. The heart rate for a person depends on age, health and exercise taken and can be influenced by hormones, ions and drugs. The heart rate is determined by counting the pulse rate, which can be found either where an artery is close to the surface of the body, for example, the carotid artery in the neck, or where it crosses a bone, such as the radial artery in the wrist.

Cardiac Cycle

The name given to the pressure of blood during the relaxed phase of the cardiac cycle is 'diastolic', and the name given to the pressure of the blood during the contraction of the cardiac cycle is 'systolic'. Normal blood pressure is considered to be 120/80, the top figure representing systolic pressure when the heart is contracted and the lower figure diastolic pressure when the heart is relaxed. If blood pressure rises or falls below the norm, then blood pressure may be considered to be high or too low.

Muscle Layers of the Heart

There are three layers of muscle surrounding the heart. These are the endocardium (the innermost layer), the myocardium (the middle layer) and the pericardium (the outermost layer). The septum divides the left and right side of the heart. The endocardium is the only layer of the heart that comes into contact with blood in the chambers. The myocardium has its own blood vessels to supply it with oxygen and nutrients and to take away waste products. The heart muscle is supplied by blood from the left and right coronary arteries, from the first branches of the aorta, which begins above the aortic valve. The arteries fill with blood as the heart relaxes. Blood passes through the capillaries in the myocardium, then drains into the cardiac veins for return to the right atrium.

Conduction of the Heart

The chambers (atria) of the heart produce a hormone known as atria natriuretic peptide (ANP) as they fill with blood. This substance increases loss of salt by the kidneys and lowers blood pressure.

Specialized areas in the heart wall provide the conduction system of the cardiac cycle. Two areas are called nodes whilst the third is a group of fibres called the atrio-ventricular bundle. The sinatrial (SA) node, located in the upper wall of the right atrium, initiates the heart beat and is known as the pacemaker. The second node is located in the bottom of the right atrium and is called the atrio-ventricular (AV) node. Fibres from the top of the ventricular walls branch to all parts of the ventricular chambers. Impulses in the heart travel as follows:

- the SA node generates an electrical impulse that begins the heartbeat;
- contraction of the atria takes place as waves travel throughout the muscle;
- the AV node is stimulated; a slower conduction through this node allows time for the atria to completely fill with blood and contract;
- waves rapidly travel throughout the ventricular walls through the bundles of fibres;
- both left and right ventricles contract almost at the same time.

The volume of blood pumped through the ventricles of the heart each minute is approximately 5 litres (9 pints).

Heart murmur is due to a faulty action of heart valves when blood leaks back from the ventricle into the atrium. A narrowing of a valve opening is called stenosis.

Nerve Supply

The heart is independent in its nerve supply from the brain and is influenced from a part of the brain called the medulla oblongata, a part of the brain-stem. It can also be stimulated or depressed by hormones or nerve impulses.

SPECIAL INTEREST

The following reflexes will help to stimulate elimination of waste products, thereby reducing undue pressure on blood vessels and providing homeostatic balance within the endocrine system. Remember that heart referral pain may be found extending to the medial edge of the left foot and onto the ball of the right foot. It may also be found as puffiness on the top of the tho-racic area of the left foot. This is because heart problems affect the shoulders and arm on the left side of the body. Hard, impacted skin over the heart reflex point and surrounding area can indicate unexpressed feelings and emotions, both conscious and unconscious.

Coronary Heart Disease

The main cause of heart disease is an atheroma, which is formed by fatty deposits in the blood leading to blood clotting. Cigarette smoke contains two substances that affect the heart: nicotine encourages atheroma formation, and carbon monoxide reduces the amount of oxygen the blood can carry, meaning less oxygen reaches the tissues.

Cholesterol is a main ingredient of atheroma and nicotine indirectly increases its level in the blood by stimulating the release of adrenalin, which in turn raises cholesterol levels. Adrenalin is stimulated by the sympathetic part of the autonomic nervous system, and its presence triggers the release of fatty acids, which can be broken down to supply the body with energy. If physical exercise does not follow, the liver will convert the fatty acids to cholesterol.

Heart failure is associated with high blood pressure. The left side of the heart becomes thickened when blood pressure rises. Insufficient oxygen will then be supplied to the heart, causing breathlessness, and failure of the left and right sides of the heart may occur. Risk factors of heart failure include:

- **Gender**: more men than women suffer from coronary heart disease. Women are protected by hormones until after the menopause.
- **Heredity**: this can be alleviated by watching diet.
- **Diabetes**: obesity is linked to diabetes and high blood pressure.
- **Salt**: causes retention of water.

133

- **Soft water**: more people die of coronary heart disease in soft water areas than in hard water areas. The reasons are unclear.
- **Alcohol**: the heart may become enlarged or be poisoned.
- **Coffee**: creates abnormal heart rhythms.
- **Oral contraceptives**: slightly less risk than smoking, high blood pressure or high cholesterol levels. There exists a link between oral contraceptives and high blood pressure. The risk increases with the length of time a woman is on the pill and over the age of thirty-five years.

Reflex Points 2–6 & 6a – Thymus gland, Oesophagus, Heart, Lungs, Shoulder and Axillary Lymph Nodes

Begin working the thoracic cavity by working up the ball of the foot beneath the big toe for the thymus gland and anatomical oesopha-gus. Now work the rest of the thoracic cavity by holding the toes open with the supporting hand index finger so that the reflexes can be found between the metatarsal joints. Work medially to laterally across the foot using the medial edge of the thumb in an upward movement only. Then work laterally to medially back across to the edge of the foot. You may find it easier to change hands so that the hand nearest the lateral edge of the foot works the shoulder reflex (no. 6)

Remember to work over the whole pad under the little toe for the shoulder area and axillary lymph nodes. These reflexes can be worked horizontally, just over the pad. Also remember, work upwards only between the metatarsal joints, except when working on the 5th zone.

Refer to diagrams of reflex points in the colour section: 17, 18, 42, 43, 44, 46, 47, 49, 49a, 49b, 52, 53, 54, 54a, 55, 56.

The Circulatory System

System(s)	Associated Reflexes	Disorders
REFLEX POINTS 5 & 50: THE HEART		
Circulatory	Whole foot	Angina pectoris,
Digestive	Large colon, sigmoid flexure	angiomas, bruise,
	Ileo-caecal valve, liver	arrhythmias, stroke,
		coronary occlusion
Endocrine	Hypothalamus, pituitary,	
	thyroid/parathyroid glands,	
	adrenal glands	
Lymphatic	Lymphatic ducts and nodes	
Respiratory	Lungs	
Nervous	Solar plexus, spine, brain	
Muscular	Diaphragm	

Nerve Innervation: Heart 2nd Thoracic

See Chapter 26 for a description of disorders associated with the Circulatory System

---

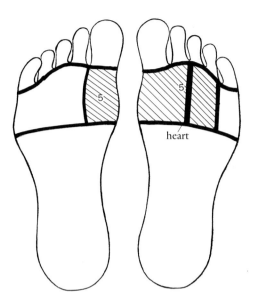

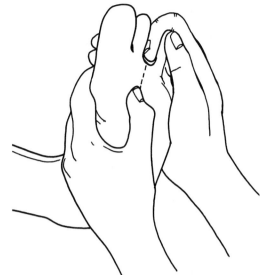

Heart supporter area on right foot, reflex point 5.

The heart, reflex point 5 (left foot only).

Hand position: the heart, reflex point 5 (left foot only). Working hand over supporting hand.

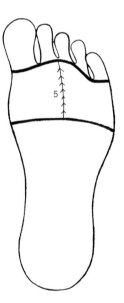

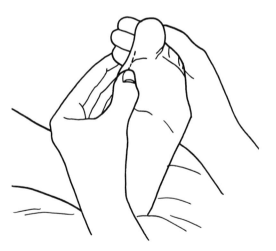

Direction for working: the heart reflex point 5 (left foot only).

Hand position: the thymus gland, reflex point 2 (both feet). Working hand over supporting hand.

135

Refer to the Lymphatic, Digestive, Endocrine, Respiratory and Skeletal Systems.

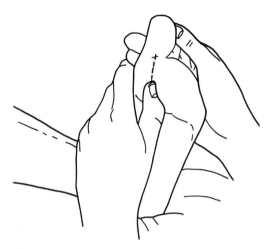

Hand position: anatomical oesophagus, reflex point 3 (both feet). Working hand over supporting hand.

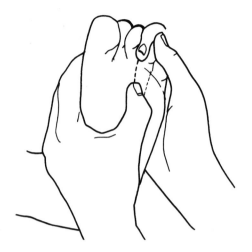

Hand position: the lung, reflex points 5, 5a and 5b (both feet). Working hand over supporting hand.

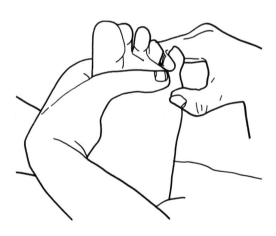

Hand position: the shoulder, reflex point 6 (both feet). Working hand over supporting hand.

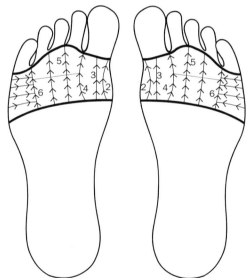

Directions for working: the thymus gland (2), anatomical oesophagus (3), thyroid gland supporter (4), heart (5), lungs (5) and shoulder (6). Refer to Endocrine/Lymphatic, Digestive, Respiratory and Skeletal Systems.

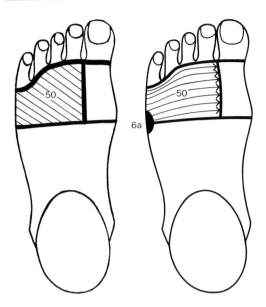

Heart supporter area on top of left foot. Refer to Respiratory and Skeletal Systems.

Directions for working: heart supporter on top of left foot and axillary lymph nodes.

CASE STUDIES WITH CARDIO-VASCULAR DISORDERS

Myocardial Infarction (Heart Attack)

Margaret came to see me having suffered from a heart attack and a bypass operation and was currently suffering from breathlessness, anxiety and bowel-related problems. It transpired that her husband had died of cancer a few years before she came to see me and, although her daughter was currently living with her, she felt stressed and unable to cope with everyday life due to breathlessness and low energy levels.

Within a short time, Margaret felt more able to cope with life and began to find more enjoyment – so much so that she sold her home and moved into a warden-secured luxury flat. She has currently made a new social life for herself and states that the major benefits she received from reflexology were relaxation, increased energy levels and an overall sense of well-being, which had been missing from her life since her heart attack and her husband's death.

Although still on high levels of medication, Margaret feels in charge of her life and has recognized a growing sense of independence. Her daughter has since trained in reflexology and continues to give her mother regular treatments.

Hypertension

David came for reflexology treatment some years ago, suffering from hypertension, chronic digestive problems and urinary problems. He was a businessman in his mid-fifties who did little exercise, drove constantly around the country, smoked and who entertained his business colleagues frequently. As often happens with men, he found the concept of reflexology hard to accept and he was defensive, sceptical and somewhat patronizing! However, he agreed to come for weekly treatments and was soon amazed at the general improvement with all his multi-various health problems.

I remember especially his urinary problem, which resembled cystitis and had left the urethra reflex extremely tender. He had avoided telling me about the problem in the consultation, but during the treatment the reflex point told me everything!

He was taking medication for high blood pressure, and after almost three months of reflexology treatments had a check-up with his doctor who said that his blood pressure had lowered to a point where medication could be reduced, much to his amazement!

With dietary advice, which David followed to a certain extent as he found that with his business entertainment it was difficult to keep to a strict diet, he found his digestive problems improved and he felt more like taking gentle exercise at weekends and felt a general sense of improved alertness and well-being.

CHAPTER 15
The Lymphatic System

INTRODUCTION

The lymphatic system provides protection from invaders and cleanses the blood. It is a separate system in its own right, although closely linked to the circulatory system and, with it, forms part of the cardio-vascular system (*see* overview in Chapter 14).

Cells that are part of our immune system, or lymphatic system, are responsible for killing invaders before they manage to get a grip on our body and destroy cells and tissues. Lymph fluid in the lymphatic vessels carries away the waste products from cell metabolism, carries fats from our digestive processes to the circulatory system, which are eventually stored under the skin if not required for heat and energy, and returns some protein to plasma. Lymph fluid has a milky white appearance because of the presence of fats. Lymphocytes can squeeze their way through lymph vessels and into blood vessels in the circulatory system, so that they can go wherever needed to fight infection in the body.

The lymph system does not have a heart, unlike the circulatory system. The force of gravity 'pulls' the fluid downwards to the lower extremities, for example, the legs and ankles. In addition to exercise and muscular movement in the lower limbs, lymph fluid is helped to travel up towards the subclavian veins by the act of breathing with the diaphragm muscle and contraction and dilation of blood vessels. Lymph vessels have cup-shaped valves, similar to veins, which stop back-flow of lymph.

The organs associated with the lymphatic system are:

- the spleen (the major organ) produces 'B' and 'T' lymphocytes and antibodies;
- the tonsils, which comprise lymphoid tissue present in the throat;
- the thymus gland, which also produces the hormone thymosin that is necessary in the manufacture of 'T' lymphocytes;
- lymph nodes, which filter lymph fluid and are composed of lymphoid tissue;
- lymph vessels and capillaries.

The ways in which white cells act to combat infection consist of:

- making chemicals that destroy the trapped bacteria;
- producing antibodies to combine with antigens to neutralize their effects;
- engulfing the bacteria;
- making antitoxins to counteract the effects of poisonous chemicals produced by some bacteria; and
- removing cell debris caused by bacterial attack.

Lymphocytes originate from stem cells in bone marrow and are manufactured in the lymph nodes and the spleen. Their lifespan is variable. They form almost half the body's circulating white cells. Circulating lymphocytes are larger than red cells. There are two main types:

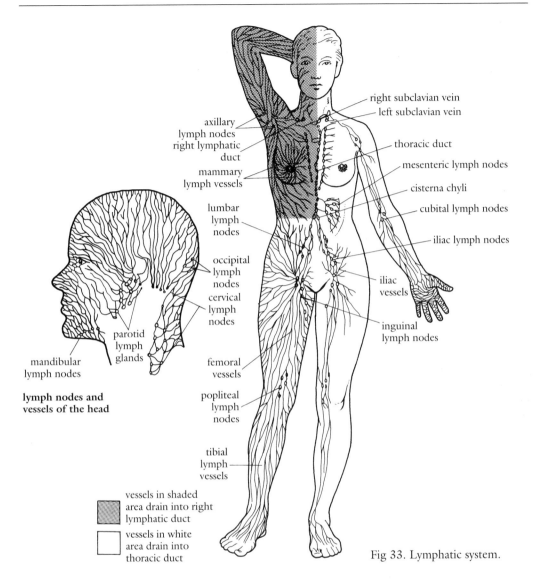

axillary
lymph nodes
right lymphatic
duct
mammary
lymph vessels

lumbar
lymph
nodes

occipital
lymph
nodes
cervical
lymph
nodes

parotid
lymph
glands

mandibular
lymph nodes

**lymph nodes and
vessels of the head**

femoral
vessels

popliteal
lymph
nodes

tibial
lymph
vessels

right subclavian vein
left subclavian vein

thoracic duct

mesenteric lymph nodes

cisterna chyli

cubital lymph nodes

iliac lymph nodes

iliac
vessels

inguinal
lymph nodes

vessels in shaded
area drain into right
lymphatic duct

vessels in white
area drain into
thoracic duct

Fig 33. Lymphatic system.

- 'T' lymphocytes, which are concerned with immunity within cells and form about 80 per cent of the circulating lymphocytes; lymphocytes enter the thymus gland before birth and are processed as T-lymphocytes and then stored in the lymph nodes.
- 'B' lymphocytes, which are concerned with immunity.

Macrophages are found in the lymphatic system. These cells, which can change their shape, are phagocytic as they crush, strangle or poison microbes and invaders in the body.

Lymph capillaries are blind-end tubes, where tissue fluid is exchanged through the sides of the capillary wall. Cell waste and water are excreted into lymph capillaries, then carried into lymph vessels and ducts.

139

ORGANS OF THE LYMPHATIC SYSTEM

Spleen

The spleen is the largest lymphoid organ in the body and is situated in the left side of the abdominal cavity behind the stomach. It is purplish in colour and varies in size in different individuals. It is about 12cm (5in) long, 7cm (3in) wide and 2.5cm (1in) thick, and it weighs about 200g (7oz). The spleen consists of red pulp, which contains sinuses lined by macrophages, and white pulp. The spleen provides about 25 per cent of the body's T-lymphocytes and 15 per cent of B-lymphocytes present in the spleen.

The spleen shares the function of producing antibodies and lymphocytes. Up to one-third of the platelets are stored in the spleen. It is in the spleen (and liver) that worn-out red blood cells are broken down, and iron and bilirubin released. Once released, iron is stored in the liver. The spleen is thought to be a reservoir for blood. Normal red cells, which are flexible, pass through the red pulp into the venous system without difficulty. Old or abnormal cells, which are damaged, are removed by phagocytosis (the function of macrophages).

Thymus Gland

The thymus gland weighs at birth 10–15g (½oz), is 6cm (2½in) long and continues to grow until the individual reaches puberty when it begins to shrink. Its maximum weight at puberty is between 30 and 40g (1–1½oz), and by middle-age it has returned to approximately its weight at birth. The location of the thymus gland is behind the sternum (breast bone).

The development of the thymus and other lymphoid tissue is stimulated by thymosin, a hormone secreted by the epithelial cells that form the framework of the thymus gland. As we grow older, the effectiveness of T-lymphocyte response to antigens decreases.

The functions of the thymus are to:

• destroy foreign cells;
• release substances that stimulate other lymphocytes and macrophages which destroy invaders; it is these 'T' helper cells that become infected and are destroyed by the AIDS virus;
• 'T' lymphocytes suppress the immune response in order to regulate it.

Lymph Nodes

The functions of the lymph nodes are to filter the lymph fluid, manufacture and store lymphocytes that fight infection, and form antibodies. Major groups of lymphatic nodes are found in the armpits (axillary), groin (inguinal), under the jaw (parotid and mandibular), behind the knee (popliteal), in the abdomen and in the neck (see Fig. 33).

Lymphatic Vessels

Some lymphatic vessels are superficial and some are deep. There are superficial lymphatic vessels in the face, neck and fingers. The superficial inguinal lymphatic glands are placed immediately beneath the skin in the groin.

The deep cervical glands form a chain along the carotid artery and internal jugular vein, lying by the side of the pharynx, oesophagus and trachea, and extend from the base of the skull to the thoracic cavity, where they communicate with the lymphatic glands. The deep lymphatic glands are subdivided into those in the arm and the axilla (armpit).

The popliteal glands surround the popliteal vessels embedded in the cellular tissue and fat of the popliteal space behind the knee. The deep inguinal glands are placed around the femoral artery and vein.

Lymphatic Ducts

The left thoracic duct and right lymphatic duct are the major areas where lymph is collected. The left thoracic duct collects lymph fluid at the second lumbar vertebrae by a group of muscular pouches called the cisterna chyli. These pouches collect lymph fluid from the lower extremities and pump (through the action described above) the lymph fluid upwards towards the subclavian veins. The left thoracic duct is the largest duct and drains two-thirds of the body's lymph fluid. The remaining third is drained by the right lymphatic duct, which begins at the level of the liver.

Waste Products

Once lymph fluid joins the circulation at the subclavian veins, waste products are carried with the waste products collected by the circulatory system to the kidneys for excretion by the urinary system.

IMMUNITY

Immunity is the body's protection against invasion by foreign substances. Examples of natural immunity are:

- tears containing enzymes that destroy bacteria with saliva;
- hairs and mucus in the nose that prevent the entry of dust and microbes;
- sneezing, which expels foreign material from the respiratory tract;
- white mucus and cilia in the respiratory and digestive tracts trap foreign particles;
- stomach acid destroys microbes;

- some beneficial bacteria in the intestines control harmful organisms;
- the vagina and urethra are protected by mucus and beneficial bacteria;
- sebaceous glands in the skin secrete chemicals, which are toxic to many bacteria;
- breastfeeding, which supplies antibodies from the mother to the newborn baby.

'T' cells provide a defence against viruses and bacteria, are involved in the rejection of tissue from transplanted organs, and help combat cancer cells. Macrophages and 'T' lymphocytes work together by macrophages carrying antigens on their surfaces which enable the 'T' cells to recognize the macrophages as 'self' and the antigen as an invader. The 'T' cells combine with the macrophages, which release substances called interleukins (meaning 'between white blood cells'). Interleukins stimulate growth of 'T' cells and are used in medicine to boost the immune system. The 'B' lymphocytes originate in bone marrow and mature in lymphoid tissue, such as the spleen or the liver in the growing foetus. Encounters with antigens stimulate 'B' cells to reproduce rapidly and to produce large numbers of plasma cells. These plasma cells produce specific antibodies that float in the blood, providing immunity.

Antibody response to an antigen involves the antibody creating the same shape as the antigen when it 'locks' itself onto the antigen. In this way it binds with the antigen and deactivates it.

Active immunity is where a disease is contracted and antibodies are manufactured in response to infected cells to act against the toxin or invasive substance. Each time a disease is contracted, an antibody is created that provides protection, usually for years or a lifetime.

The foetus can acquire immunity from the mother. Antibodies are transported from the mother to the foetus and because they have arrived from outside of the foetus, this kind of immunity is termed *passive immunity*.

Acquired immunity is when an automatic immunity is provided through exposure to disease. In cases where a disease can be potentially harmful to the quality of life, or life-threatening, vaccination with the disease in a reduced form can stimulate production of antibodies without causing serious illness.

Vaccines can be made from toxins, live organisms or with organisms killed by chemicals or heat. For example, cowpox is a live organism, but is non-virulent in humans and so can be administered for use as a form of immunization against smallpox. Vaccination works by introducing the dead or weakened organisms into the body by injection to produce an immune response. When the immune system is sensitized to recognize these, it destroys similar micro-organisms which later invade the body.

Autoimmunity refers to body cells reacting abnormally to the self. Under normal circumstances, the immune system learns before birth to ignore the body's own tissue by destroying or inactivating those lymphocytes that attack them. Loss of immune tolerance may cause diseases such as multiple sclerosis, lupus erythematosus, rheumatoid arthritis, glomerulonephritis, early-onset diabetes mellitus and Grave's disease.

Cancer cells vary slightly from healthy body cells and should be recognized by the immune system. Those suffering from immune deficiency disease appear to contract cancer at a higher rate than those with a healthy immune system. Under normal circumstances, cancerous cells are probably killed by the immune system, but as we grow older cellular immunity decreases and cancer is more likely to develop. A form of immunotherapy for cancer patients involves stimulating the body's natural immune system by activating 'T' cells with interleukins and then re-injecting the 'T' cells

into the patients. *See* Overview of the Lymphatic System, Chapter 14).

SPECIAL INTEREST

The thymus is a dual-functioning gland, belonging to both the endocrine system and the immune system, which is a main function of the lymphatic system. Remember to ask female patients if they suffer from tender axillary lymphatic nodes – if so, have they had them checked by their GP.

Milk the lymphatic ducts when massaging the feet at the end of the treatment and cream has been applied to the feet. This stops friction of fingers against any dry skin that may be present and encourages the flow of lymph upwards towards the subclavian veins. This reflex is also on the hands between the thumb and index finger. Stroke firmly, away from the body several times.

WORKING THE REFLEXES

Reflex Point 16 – The Lymph Nodes and Tonsils

Massage between the base of the toes for the lymph nodes in the neck and the tonsils. Work with either the index finger or little finger until you see the tip of the finger through the toes of the foot.

Remember to check for mushrooms growing between the toes before you begin, for example, athlete's foot! These reflexes should be worked when working the eyes and ears as they are closely related.

For reflex point 20 – the spleen – refer to the Digestive System. For reflex points 40 and 41 – the anatomical and supporter areas for the Fallopian tubes, vas deferens and inguinal lymph nodes – refer to the Reproductive System.

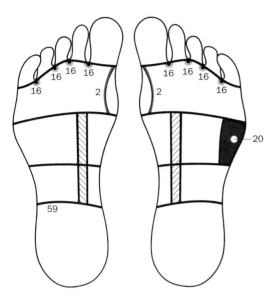

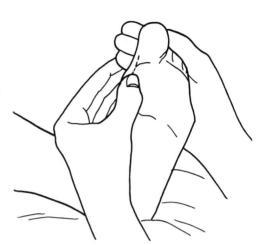

The lymphatic system, reflex points 2, 16, 20 and 59. Refer to endocrine, respiratory and skeletal systems.

Hand position: the thymus gland, reflex point 2 (both feet).

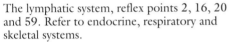

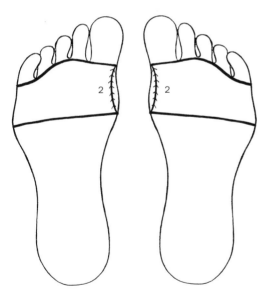

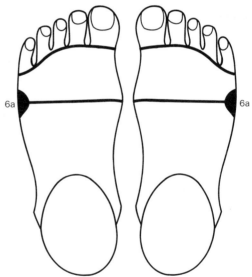

Directions for working: the thymus gland, reflex point 2.

Position for axillary lymph nodes (right foot). Make a special note when working the shoulder and spleen reflexes for sensitivity on the top and soles of the feet.

143

The Lymphatic System

System(s)	Associated Reflexes	Disorders
REFLEX POINT 2: THE THYMUS GLAND		
Endocrine	Hypothalamus, pituitary, thyroid, parathyroids, thymus, adrenal glands	HIV-AIDS, myasthenia gravis
Lymphatic	Lymph nodes in the neck, inguinal nodes (anatomical and supporter)	

Nerve Innervation: 3rd Thoracic

REFLEX POINT 6A: THE AXILLARY LYMPH NODES		
Cardio-vascular	Heart, lymph nodes, thymus gland	Cardio-vascular,
Urinary	Kidneys	lymphoedema
Digestive	Spleen, liver, gall-bladder, large colon, sigmoid flexure, ileo-caecal valve, small intestine	
Muscular	Diaphragm	
Nervous	Brain, spine, solar plexus	
Endocrine	Hypothalamus, pituitary	

Nerve Innervations: 2nd, 3rd Thoracic

REFLEX POINT 16: THE TONSILS AND LYMPH NODES IN THE NECK		
Lymphatic	Lymph nodes and ducts, spleen	Tonsillitis, pharyngitis,
Skeletal	Neck, spine	laryngitis, mumps
Special senses	Eyes, ears, nose, face	
Respiratory	Trachea	
Digestive	Ileo-caecal valve, small intestine	

Nerve Innervations: 5th, 6th Cervical

REFLEX POINT 20: THE SPLEEN		
Cardio-vascular	Lymph nodes and ducts, heart	Splenegomaly
Digestive	Liver, small intestine	

Nerve Innervations: 8th Thoracic

REFLEX POINTS 40 & 41: THE INGUINAL LYMPH NODES		
Reproductive	Ovaries, testes, uterus, prostate gland	Vasectomy, ectopic
Lymphatic	Lymph nodes and ducts	pregnancy, pelvic
Urinary	Kidneys, bladder, urethra, ureter	inflammatory disease
Endocrine	Hypothalamus, pituitary gland, adrenal glands	(PID), obstructed
Digestive	Large colon, intestines, sigmoid flexure, ileo-caecal valve, lymphatic ducts	Fallopian tubes, lymphatic oedema,
Nervous	Brain, spine	inguinal hernia, femoral hernia, constipation

Nerve Innervation: 3rd, 4th and 5th Lumbar

REFLEX POINT 60: MILKING THE LYMPHATIC DUCTS		
Cardio-vascular	Heart, lymph nodes, thymus gland	Cardio-vascular

Urinary	Kidneys	lymphoedema and
Digestive	Spleen, liver, gall-bladder, large colon, sigmoid flexure, ileo-caecal valve, small intestine	digestive disorders
Muscular	Diaphragm	
Nervous	Brain, spine, solar plexus	
Endocrine	Hypothalamus, pituitary	

Nerve Innervations: 12th Thoracic

See Chapter 26 for a description of disorders associated with the Lymphatic System

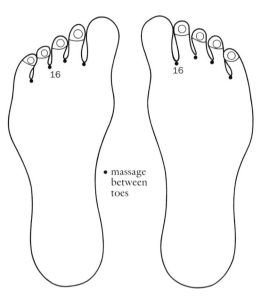

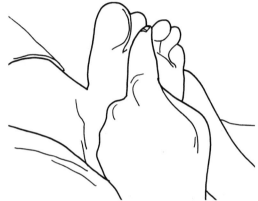

Hand position: massaging the tonsils/lymph nodes in the neck, reflex point 16 (both feet). Rest supporting hand on the top of the foot with the thumb supporting the sole of the foot.

Tonsil lymphatic nodes between each toe, reflex point 16.

Milking the Lymphatic Ducts and Solar Plexus Relaxation – Reflex Point 60 – Lymphatic System

This reflex point should be worked at the beginning of the foot massage at the end of the treatment when cream has been applied to the foot. Place your supporting hand thumb on the solar plexus and with the index and third finger of the working hand, stroke in an upward movement between the big toe and first toe on top of the foot, towards the base of the toes. Use the working hand thumb to support the

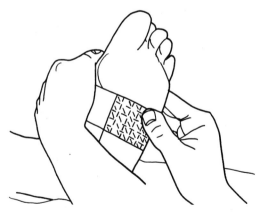

Hand position: the stomach, spleen and pancreas, reflex points 19, 20 and 24 (left foot only). Working hand on top of supporting hand. Refer to the Digestive System.

145

movement by placing it on the ball of the foot. The supporting hand should gently hold the medial edge of the foot. *See* reflex points 40 and 41 for how to work the inguinal lymph nodes and reflex point 20 for working the spleen (*see* Chapter 19, The Digestive System).

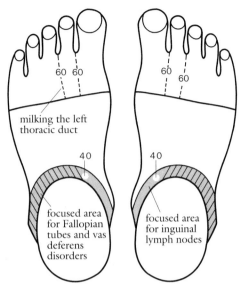

Anatomical inguinal lymph nodes and lymphatic ducts, reflex points 40 and 60 (both feet).

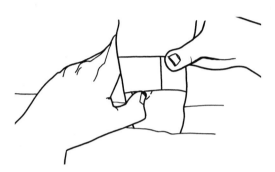

Hand position: hooking the ileo-caecal valve, reflex point 58 (right foot only). Working hand on top of supporting hand, or under heel. Refer to the Digestive System for directions for working the ileo-caecal valve.

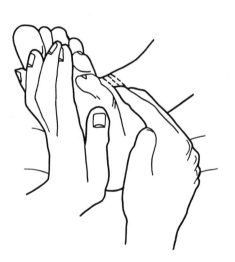

Hand position: the inguinal lymph nodes, reflex point 40 (both feet). Supporting hand pushes the foot into an upright position.

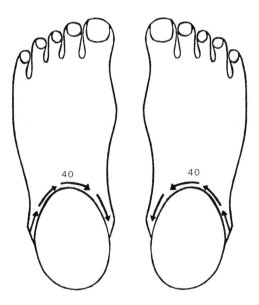

Directions for working: the anatomical inguinal lymph nodes, reflex point 40 (both feet).

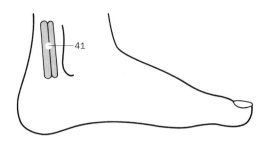

Inguinal lymph nodes supporter, reflex point 41 (both feet).

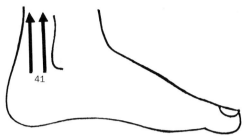

Directions for working: the inguinal lymph nodes supporter, reflex point 41 (both feet).

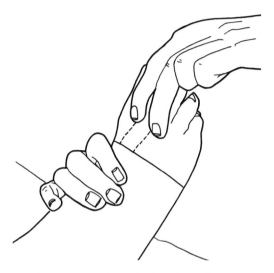

Hand position: milking the lymphatic ducts, reflex point 60 (*see* directions for working the reflexes). Thumb of supporting hand rests on the sole of the foot.

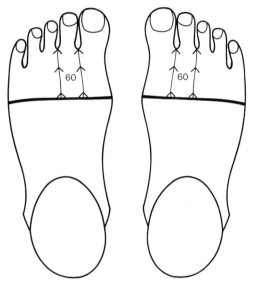

Directions for working: the left and right thoracic duct, reflex point 60.

CASE STUDY OF A DEBILITATED IMMUNE SYSTEM

Alison came for reflexology treatment having been to see her doctor who had encouraged her to seek treatment. Her story is given below.

During the birth of my son, his head got trapped for two hours, in such a position that he stopped my bladder from working as he'd trapped the nerves as he pressed down. The midwives did not notice anything was wrong until six days after the birth when I looked just about ready to deliver again, due to two litres of fluid trapped in my ever-expanding bladder. I had to be catheterized through the urethra and then had a supra pubic catheter inserted below the bikini line. During the nightmare month I had one infection after another and went in and out of hospital like a yoyo. At one point, I had a temperature of 105°F after suffering from infected stitches from my episiotomy, mastitis (from breast feeding) and a protozoan infection in my bladder. At the end of that month I was rushed into hospital to have an infected catheter tube removed. Thankfully, the new month brought with it new luck – my bladder started to function on its own and the infections began to clear up.

In the spring of the following year, I discovered that I had a suspected rectal abscess, probably caused by a difficult labour, and I went into hospital to have the abscess drained. Having returned to work after the statutory maternity leave, I intended returning after two weeks convalescence from the operation. However, only four days after surgery, I became very ill with a deep-seated chest infection caught from the general anaesthetic. I was prescribed antibiotics but nothing would shift the infection and although I saw every doctor in the practice, in the hope of effective treatment, they all said it would take time to get better because my immune system was so low after all the problems with the birth of my son. The various sick notes given to me to send into school gave different diagnoses because no-one was really sure what was happening to my body.

Eventually, I asked one of the doctors to treat me homeopathically as I was desperate to try anything. Around this time I decided to try reflexology and discussed it with my family and friends, thinking they would think I was mad! To my amazement, my aunt in North Wales was already undergoing treatment and two friends went for reflexology for stress and a debilitated immune system. Maybe it would work after all!?

In my first treatment with Jenny, I discovered that every part of my body was run down or not functioning properly, especially my clogged lungs. My feet were agonizingly painful, even with the slightest pressure. I wanted to believe this prodding and poking about on my feet would make me better but the scientific part of me kept saying 'take it with a pinch of salt'. I was absolutely amazed that by manipulating my feet it could make parts of my body better and I could not believe that Jenny could know I was feeling pain when she touched certain areas associated with my illness. I tried my best to fake her out by chatting and smiling but she still seemed to know that there was a sensation of pain.

When I got home I crudely poked my own feet, just to prove it was touch and not the act of reflexology that stimulated the feet but nothing I did had the same effect. At the start of reflexology treatments I had weekly treatments and my progress was very good, and by the spring term I was back at school, not quite as good as new but functioning.

I still can't say how or why reflexology works but I am a converted believer in complementary medicine! Maybe my recovery would have happened on its own given a little extra time, but I doubt it. I still go for reflexology treatments with Jenny every two weeks to maintain my immune system and help alleviate the stress build-up, due to my job as a teacher with responsibility of 240 children aged twelve and thirteen.

I have since recommended reflexology to other people who may be just under the weather, stressed or not getting relief from their conventional medical treatments. Even if you go for treatment for no other reason, one hour spent just for you can help you relax without interruption from the demands of your job or family and is well worth it.

When working on Alison's feet, I 'held' the reflexes on painful areas for a considerable time in the first few treatments. It was this method, I felt, that shifted her chest infection and speeded her immune system back to full strength.

CHAPTER 16
The Respiratory System

Overview of the Respiratory System

Gaseous exchange – oxygen (O_2) inhaled provides energy for cells as carbon dioxide (CO_2) is exhaled as a waste product of cell metabolism.

PULMONARY CIRCULATION

Structures	*Functions*
Heart	Conveys blood to and from the lungs
Pulmonary veins	Carry oxygenated blood
Pulmonary arteries	Carry deoxygenated blood

THE PROCESS OF BREATHING: INHALATION AND EXHALATION

Mucous membrane	Produces a sticky substance (mucus) that traps organisms harmful to the body
Nose	Allows inspiration and expiration; traps harmful organisms in hair cells; centre for smell (*see* The Special Senses)
Sinuses	Air passages give resonance to the voice and lighten the bones of the skull
Mouth and pharynx (forms the throat)	Divided into the nasal, oral and pharyngeal air passages
Larynx	The voice box
Bronchi and bronchioles	Air passages that end in the lungs
Lungs	Muscular sacs that through movement of the ribs and diaphragm expand, allowing air containing oxygen into the lungs, and contract, pushing air containing carbon dioxide out
Alveoli	The smallest units of the lungs where gaseous exchange takes place; they are balloon-like structures surrounded by blood capillaries that allow oxygen to enter the blood and carbon dioxide to diffuse out of the body
Dust cells	Specialized lymph cells, present in the mucous membranes of the respiratory passages, that destroy harmful organisms
Ribs	Protect the lungs and heart and give attachment to the intercostal muscles: external muscles contract and assist in lifting the rib cage upwards and outwards; internal muscles contract to push the rib cage in on the lungs to expel air during expiration
Diaphragm	Separates the abdominal cavity from the thoracic cavity; assists in breathing

LINKS TO: circulatory, muscular, endocrine, urinary and lymphatic systems.

INTRODUCTION

The respiratory system comprises the upper respiratory tract, which contains: the mouth, nostrils, larynx, pharynx, trachea and sinuses; and the lower respiratory tract, which contains: the bronchi, with one bronchus going to each lung, the bronchioles and smaller air passages, two lungs and their coverings called the pleura, and the muscles of respiration the intercostal muscles and the diaphragm.

The muscle that separates the thoracic cavity from the abdominal cavity is called the diaphragm. It is dome-shaped and aids in the expiration of air from the lungs by pushing upwards under the lungs as we breathe out. The diaphragm muscle is the main muscle involved in respiration and is attached to the spine, ribs and sternum (breastbone).

The functions of mucus are to protect the lining of the respiratory tract, moisten and lubricate the respiratory tract, and trap dust and harmful particles. The tear ducts and the Eustachian tubes open into the back of the nose.

UPPER RESPIRATORY TRACT

Nose and Mouth

The nose has a dual function: as the organ of the sense of smell (olfactory) and as a receptacle for air currents. There are nerve endings and fibres that detect smell, which are located in the roof of the nose, that are stimulated by smell. Olfactory nerve impulses are transmitted to the brain where the sensation of smell is received. Once olfactory nerves have become accustomed to a particular smell, the sensory part of the brain concerned with smell will no longer detect it.

The nose, which contains mucous membrane, is lined with hair cells. The nose is the first part of the respiratory passage through which incoming air passes. The functions of the nose are to begin the process of warming, moistening and filtering air; to expel large particles through sneezing; and to protect the lining of the respiratory tract. The nose also carries microbes in mucus to the throat to be swallowed. Ducts open into the back of the nose from the Eustachian tubes (forming part of the middle ear) and the lacrimal (tear) ducts.

The mouth provides inhalation and exhalation.

Pharynx

The pharynx is a tube 12–14cm (7–7½in) long and lies behind the nose, mouth and larynx.

The nasal part of the pharynx lies behind the nose, above the soft palate. On the outside walls are two openings, the auditory tubes, one leading to each middle ear, and the pharyngeal tonsil (adenoid), consisting of lymphoid tissue. The tonsil is most prominent in children up to about the age of seven years, after which it shrinks in size.

The oral part of the pharynx lies behind the mouth. The walls of the pharynx merge with the soft palate to form two folds on either side. Between each pair of folds there is a collection of lymphoid tissue, called the palatine tonsil.

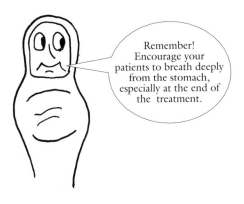

Remember! Encourage your patients to breath deeply from the stomach, especially at the end of the treatment.

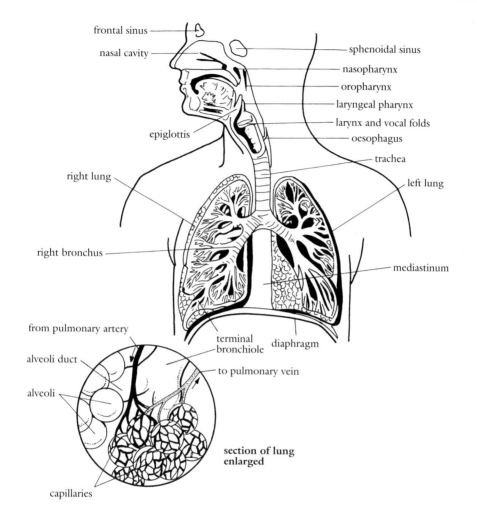

frontal sinus
nasal cavity
sphenoidal sinus
nasopharynx
oropharynx
laryngeal pharynx
larynx and vocal folds
epiglottis
oesophagus
trachea
right lung
left lung
right bronchus
mediastinum
from pulmonary artery
alveoli duct
alveoli
terminal bronchiole
diaphragm
to pulmonary vein
section of lung enlarged
capillaries

Fig 34. The respiratory system.

The lymphatic tissue of the pharyngeal and laryngeal tonsils produces antibodies in response to antigens.

Larynx

The larynx or voice-box extends from the root of the tongue into the trachea. The larynx provides a passageway for air between the pharynx and trachea. As air from the outside passes through, it is moistened, filtered and warmed. The vocal cords produce sounds of loudness and pitch. Until puberty, there is little difference in size of the larynx between the sexes. Thereafter it grows larger in the male, which explains the prominence of the 'Adam's apple' and the development of a deeper voice.

During swallowing, the larynx moves upwards, closing the opening into it from the pharynx. This ensures that food passes into the oesophagus and not into the respiratory passages. In the event of food entering the respiratory passage, a reflex action provokes choking, which regurgitates the food for entry into the oesophagus.

Trachea

The trachea, or windpipe, is a continuation of the larynx, and divides into the left and right bronchi, one bronchus going to each lung. The structure of the trachea is an elastic tube, held open by loops of cartilage, which lead from the larynx to the bronchi, and is approximately 10–11cm (4–4½in) long. It lies in front of the oesophagus.

The main functions of the trachea are: to trap inhaled particles in the mucous lining so that cilia (hair cells) can move the mucus up and out of the respiratory system; and to form a passageway to convey air to the lungs.

LOWER RESPIRATORY SYSTEM

Bronchi

The two bronchi are formed where the trachea divides. The right bronchus is a wider, shorter tube than the left bronchus and is approximately 2.5cm (1in) long. After entering the right lung, it divides into three branches, which then divide into smaller branches.

The left bronchus is about 5cm (2in) long and is narrower than the right bronchus; it divides into smaller tubes within the lung itself, becoming the bronchioles. The smallest bronchioles divide until they become the alveoli. In the alveoli interchange of gases takes place in the walls of the alveolar ducts and alveoli, and those of the pulmonary artery capillaries.

Lungs

The lungs are composed of the bronchi and smaller air passages, alveoli, blood vessels, lymph vessels and nerves. The two lungs lie one on each side of the mid-line of the thoracic cavity. The area between the lungs is occupied by the heart, blood vessels, trachea, the right and left bronchus, the oesophagus, lymph nodes, lymph vessels and nerves. The right lung is divided into three lobes, and the left lung is divided into two lobes comprising an upper and a lower lobe.

The right lung is larger and heavier than the left, and is broader. This is due to the position of the heart; it is shorter in consequence of the diaphragm rising higher on the right side to accommodate the liver.

Air breathed in moves through the air passages and is warmed or cooled to accommodate body temperature, and moistened and cleaned as particles of dust stick to the mucus which coats the lining membrane containing lymphatic macrophages called 'dust cells'.

Blood Supply

The pulmonary artery carries deoxygenated blood from the heart to the lungs. It divides in two, one branch reaching each lung. Each artery divides into many branches until it becomes a capillary network in the walls of the alveoli. As pulmonary capillaries converge, they become pulmonary veins. They leave the lungs and convey oxygenated blood to the left atrium of the heart.

Alveoli

Air sacs in the lungs are called alveoli, where CO_2 is exchanged for O_2. A capillary network surrounds the alveoli, which at this point is one cell in thickness, and is where blood is nearest to the external environment. The capillary network is where gaseous exchange takes place. Air moves in the lungs by diffusion.

Gaseous Exchange

Most of the energy required by cells can only take place in the presence of O_2. The waste product of chemical reactions is CO_2. The respiratory system can therefore be described as the route by which the supply of O_2 present in the atmospheric air gains entry into the body and provides a route for excretion of CO_2.

Pleura

The pleura is a thin, double-layered membrane, one layer of which is attached to the lung and the other lines the thoracic cavity. The pleural cavity is a space where the two layers of the pleura are separated by serous fluid. Fluid between the layers provides lubrication and stops friction between the rib cage and the lungs in the expiration and inspiration of air as the lungs expand and contract.

RESPIRATION

External Respiration

In external respiration, expansion and contraction of the lungs ensures that a regular exchange of gases takes place between the alveoli and the external air.

Internal Respiration

In internal respiration, gaseous exchange of CO_2 and O_2 takes place in the capillaries surrounding the alveoli.

Thoracic Cage

The thoracic cage consists of one sternum, twelve pairs of ribs and twelve thoracic vertebrae. The sternum is a flat bone and can be felt in the middle of the front of the chest. The first rib does not move during respiration. The spaces between the ribs are occupied by the intercostal muscles.

Intercostal Muscles

There are eleven pairs of intercostal muscles that occupy the spaces between the twelve pairs of ribs. These are arranged in two layers known as the external and internal intercostal muscles. The external intercostal muscles extend downwards and forwards when breathing in (inhalation). The internal intercostal extend downwards and backwards and are involved in breathing out (exhalation).

When we breathe in, the ribcage is lifted up and outwards, and as we exhale the ribcage is pushed in and downwards. In expiration, the diaphragm is relaxed and the abdominal contents rise up within the abdominal cavity and in inspiration the diaphragm is contracted and pushed down on the abdominal contents.

Functions of the Diaphragm

The diaphragm separates the thoracic cavity from the abdominal cavity, by forming the floor of the thoracic cavity and the roof of the abdominal cavity. The intercostal muscles and the diaphragm contract simultaneously, ensuring enlargement of the thoracic cavity.

The Respiratory Centre

The brain-stem, or medulla oblongata, regulates the respiratory nerve reaction. We need CO_2 as well as O_2 in the maintenance and balance of healthy cell metabolism.

SPECIAL INTEREST

All mucus-related problems can be exacerbated by excess intake of dairy produce. Recommend to your patient to cut out dairy produce altogether or to reduce consumption.

Chronic sinusitis and congestion reflexes can be found a little to the sides of the pads of the toes and towards the bottom of the toe pad.

The lungs and upper respiratory reflexes, found under the root of the toes, reflect coughs, sore throats, smoking or any other condition affecting the trachea and upper bronchial tubes.

The lower respiratory reflexes reflect conditions relating to the lower lobes of the lung; for example, asthma, bronchitis, emphysema. Check the lower ribs on top of the foot at the waistline for sensitivity, caused commonly by prolonged coughing and muscular strain.

WORKING THE REFLEXES

Refer to Chapter 17, The Special Senses, under Working the Reflexes for directions for working the ears and eyes and refer to the Circulatory, Lymphatic, Endocrine and Skeletal Systems for additional reflexes in the thoracic cavity.

Reflex Point 15 – The Sinuses

Massage the pads of the toes by keeping your working hand fingers vertically over the supporting hand and grip the whole pad of the toe with the thumb pad to find the sinus reflex.

CASE STUDY WITH ASTHMA

Peter, a young man, came for reflexology treatments some years ago complaining of asthma, which he had suffered from on and off since a child. He was on high levels of medication, which were increasingly ineffective when he felt stressed by his work. I suggested I saw him twice weekly to begin with to give an impact on the key reflex areas of the lungs, bronchial tubes and adrenal glands. Within six weeks, he found that he could reduce his ventolin inhaler for the first time in years and that his air volume had increased considerably. He also commented on his increased energy and renewed ability to cycle – a thing he hadn't been able to do for years without fear of an attack with possible hospitalization for oxygen.

Over a period of six months, Peter reduced treatments to weekly sessions and found – to

---

The Respiratory and Special Senses Systems

System(s)	Associated Reflexes	Disorders
REFLEX POINTS 5 & 50: THE HEART AND LUNGS		
Respiratory	Sinuses, trachea	Emphysema, asthma, croup,
Circulatory	Heart	pleurisy, pneumonia, silicosis,
Special senses	Nose, ears	tuberculosis, bronchitis, cough,
Muscular	Diaphragm	head cold, diaphragmatic fatigue
Nervous	Solar plexus, brain, spine	
Endocrine	Adrenal glands	
Skeletal	Ribs	

Nerve Innervation: 3rd Thoracic

The Respiratory and Special Senses Systems *continued*

The Special Senses Reflex Points 12, 13, 14, 15, 18

REFLEX POINT 12: THE EYES

Endocrine	Adrenal glands, hypothalamus, pituitary, pineal gland	Glaucoma, eyestrain, conjunctivitis, strabismus,
Special senses	Ears, nose, face	cataracts, diabetic retinopathy,
Urinary	Kidneys	retinal detachment
Nervous system	Brain, spine	
Respiratory	Sinuses	

Nerve Innervation: 2nd Cervical

REFLEX POINTS 13 & 14: THE EARS

Special senses	Eyes, nose, face	Tinnitus, vertigo, hypertension,
Cardio-vascular	Heart, lymph nodes and ducts (and for the eyes)	motion sickness, Meniere's disease, labyrinthitis, otitis, otalgia,
Respiratory	Lungs, sinuses, trachea,	(earache), glue ear, otomycosis,
Nervous system	Brain, spine, solar plexus	otosclerosis
Skeletal	Neck	

Nerve Innervation: 1st, 2nd, 3rd and 4th Cervical

REFLEX POINT 15: THE SINUSES

Respiratory	Lungs, trachea	Allergens, head cold, sinusitis,
Lymphatic	Neck, lymph nodes and ducts	snoring, hay fever
Special senses	Eyes, ears, nose, face	
Nervous	Brain, spine	
Endocrine	Pituitary, adrenal glands	
Digestive	Ileo-caecal valve, small intestine, large colon	
Skeletal	Spine, brain	

Nerve Innervations: 1st and 2nd Cervical

REFLEX POINT 18: THE NOSE AND FACE

Nervous	Brain, spine, solar plexus	Neuralgia, Bell's palsy, neuritis,
Muscular	Diaphragm	rhinitis, olfactory desensitization,
Special senses	Ears, eyes	skin disorders, head cold, sinusitis
Endocrine	Pituitary, hypothalamus and pineal glands	
Respiratory	Lungs, sinuses	
Skeletal	Spine	

Nerve Innervations: 1st, 2nd, 3rd, 4th Cervical

See Chapter 26 for a description of disorders related to the Respiratory System

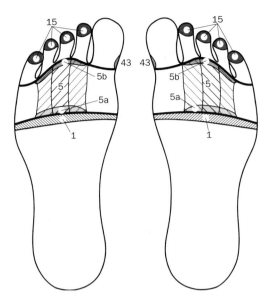

Respiratory tract and diaphragm, reflex points 1, 5, 5a, 5b, 15 and 43.

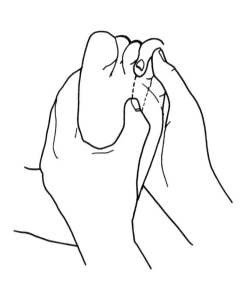

Hand position: the lung, reflex points 5, 5a, 5b (both feet). Working hand on top of supporting hand.

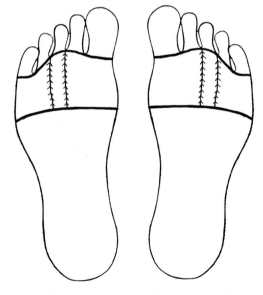

Directions for working: the lungs, reflex point 5.

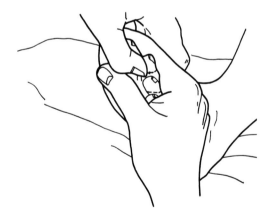

Hand position: massaging the sinus pads, reflex point 15 (both feet). Working hand held vertically over the supporting hand, which supports the toes from the tips.

156

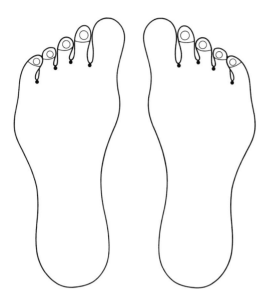

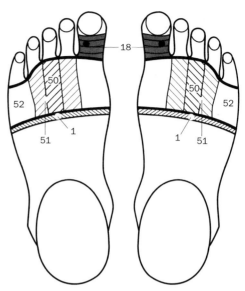

Directions for working: massaging the sinuses (both feet), reflex point 15.

The respiratory system (top of foot), reflex points 1, 18, 50, 51 and 52. Refer to the Special Senses, Muscular, Circulatory, Reproductive and Skeletal Systems (both feet).

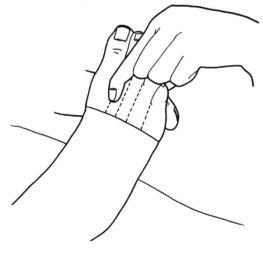

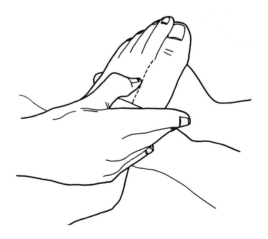

Hand position: working the whiplash lung and heart, breast and shoulder, reflex points 50, 51, 52 and 53. Supporting hand makes a fist on the ball of the foot.

Hand position: the whiplash, reflex point 53 (both feet). Supporting hand makes a fist on the ball of the foot.

157

his amazement – that he could live a 'normally' active life, which for him meant exercising without repercussions and increased medication, less wheezing, increased energy levels, mental alertness and improved confidence levels. He now attends reflexology sessions every four to six weeks and although still requiring medication occasionally, feels that he has an increased life quality for the first time in his life.

CASE STUDY WITH MUCUS-RELATED PROBLEMS

Dorothy had been suffering from mucus-related problems for many years and encountered reflexology by chance. She was on medication for ear-related problems, sinusitis, arthritis and diverticulitis but found little or no relief from symptoms. During a demonstration reflexology treatment, which I gave her whilst giving a talk to a group of ladies, I found all of her health problems, which she describes below.

I first met Jenny when she gave a talk on reflexology to our ladies group at our local Methodist Church. She invited one or two people to be demonstrated on and I volunteered. About one month before this I had been in hospital for an ear operation, for 'wet' ear and chronic sinusitis. I had also suffered from diverticulitis, which, again, I had suffered from for many years. I went to see my doctor and I was surprised to hear her say that she thought reflexology would help my problems and she was all for me having treatment.

When I began treatments with Jenny, she found the sinus reflex areas on my left foot, the spine, joints and the bowel reflexes especially painful. Over a period of eighteen months, although I have treatment fortnightly, I have found it has helped a lot, especially with the diverticulitis and I know that when I get home, I shall need to visit the bathroom! I feel it has been of great benefit and I look forward to my visits very much.

The health problem of arthritis in her feet made walking difficult and it also affected her fingers, spine and knees. Her doctor adjusted her medication for the arthritis and chronic sinusitis, and whilst she has received treatment, she has found that in conjunction with reflexology, she can walk more easily as the pain has lessened. Her sinusitis and ear problems have also decreased and she finds a marked improvement with the arthritis and a greater sense of well-being and feeling in control of her health problems.

Overall, her sense of well-being has improved dramatically. She has also felt more relaxed and calmer in herself since beginning reflexology treatments.

COLOUR SECTION

Suggested Sequence for Working the Reflexes

Reflexes are found on both feet, unless stated otherwise.

THORACIC CAVITY
1   Diaphragm and solar plexus
2   Thymus gland
3   Anatomical oesophagus
4   Thyroid supporter
5   Anatomical heart (left foot) and lungs
5a   Lower respiratory tract
5b   Upper respiratory tract
6   Shoulder
6a   Axillary lymph nodes

CRANIAL CAVITY
7   Cranial zones of energy
8   Brain
9   Hypothalamus and pineal gland
10   Pituitary gland
11   Anatomical thyroid and parathyroid glands
12   Eyes
13   Ears
14   Inner ear
15   Sinuses
16   Tonsils and lymph nodes in the neck
17   Neck and teeth
18   Face and nose

ABDOMINAL CAVITY
19   Stomach (left foot)
20   Spleen (left foot)
21   Pancreas supporter (left foot)
22   Duodenum (left foot)
23   Oesophagus supporter (left foot)
24   Anatomical pancreas (left foot)
25   Transverse colon
26   Descending colon (left foot)
27   Sigmoid flexure (left foot)
28   Pelvic extension
29   Sciatic nerve
30   Rectum and anus
31   Small intestine
31a Food allergy line

Suggested Sequence for Working the Reflexes *continued*

PELVIC CAVITY

32 Bladder
33 Urethra and penis
34 Ureter tubes
35 Adrenal glands
36 Kidney cortex
37 Kidney pelvis
38 Uterus/prostate
38b Cervix and vagina
39 Ovaries/testes
40 Anatomical Fallopian tubes, vas deferens and inguinal lymph nodes
41 Fallopian tubes, vas deferens and inguinal lymph node supporter area

REFLEXES RELATED TO ALL CAVITIES

42 Spinal vertebrae and spinal cord
43 Trachea
44 Innominate bone (pelvic bones)
45 Sciatic nerve
46 Shoulder supporter area
47 Hip, elbow, knee, lower back
48 Reinforcement of reflexes from the sole of the foot
49 All joints
49a Arm
49b Leg
50 Heart referral pain (left foot) and lungs
51 Breasts
52 Shoulder
53 Whiplash
54 Chronic neck
54a Chronic neck and shoulder supporter
55 Neck and teeth
56 Ribs

Working the right foot: all reflexes are the same and worked in the same way as the left foot, except for: the heart, stomach, spleen, pancreas, oesophagus supporter, duodenum, sigmoid flexure and descending colon which are found on the left side of the body and thus are on the left foot only.

Reflexes found on the right foot only

ABDOMINAL CAVITY

57 Liver
57a Gall-bladder

PELVIC CAVITY

58 Ileo-caecal valve (ICV)
59 Ascending colon

Reflex found on both feet

60 Milking the left thoracic duct and right lymphatic duct – work as part of a foot massage

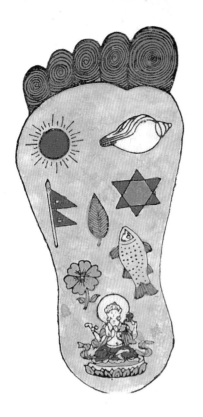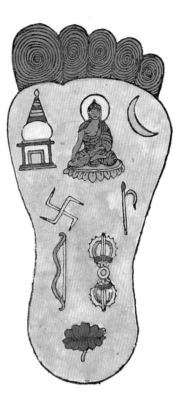

Hindu foot chart.

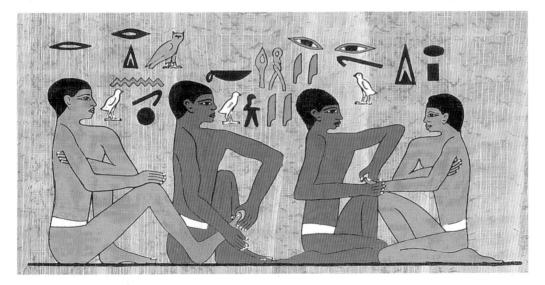

Egyptian reflexology treatment. Wall painting on the tomb of Ankhmahor (highest official after the king), early 6th dynasty, about 2330BC. The tomb at Saqqara is known as the Physician's Tomb. The translation reads: 'Don't hurt me.' The practitioner's replies: 'I shall act so you praise me.' Reproduced with permission from *Better Health with Foot Reflexology* by Dwight C. Byers, published by the International Institute of Reflexology.

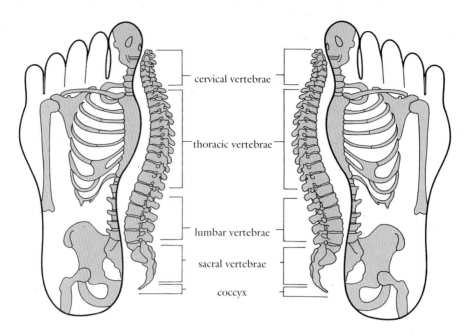

cervical vertebrae

thoracic vertebrae

lumbar vertebrae

sacral vertebrae

coccyx

The skeletal frame.

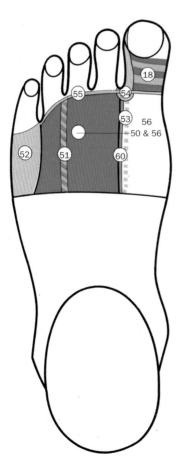
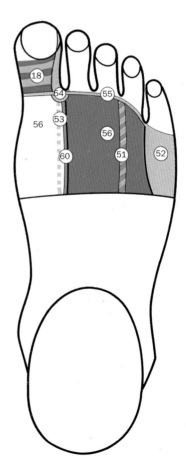

Reflex points on the tops of the feet.

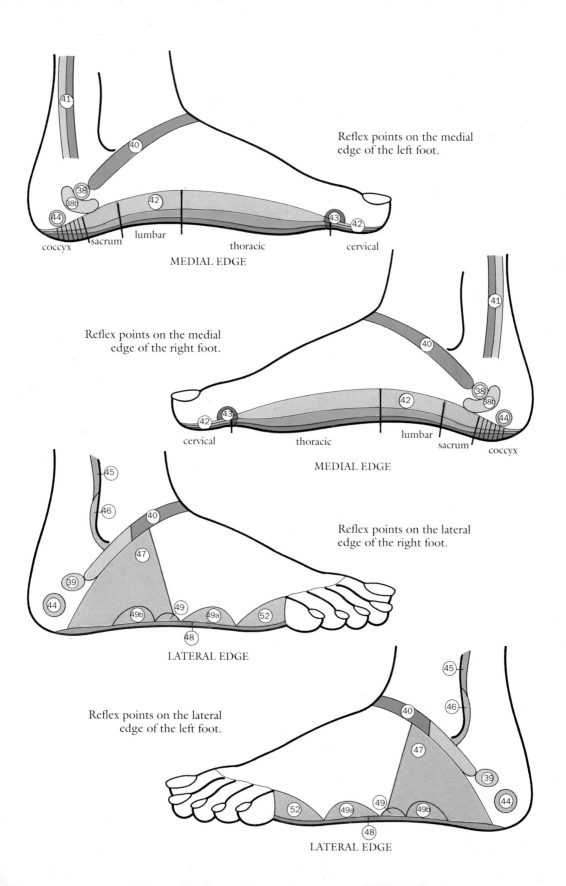

Reflex points on the medial edge of the left foot.

coccyx   sacrum   lumbar   thoracic   cervical
MEDIAL EDGE

Reflex points on the medial edge of the right foot.

cervical   thoracic   lumbar   sacrum   coccyx
MEDIAL EDGE

Reflex points on the lateral edge of the right foot.

LATERAL EDGE

Reflex points on the lateral edge of the left foot.

LATERAL EDGE

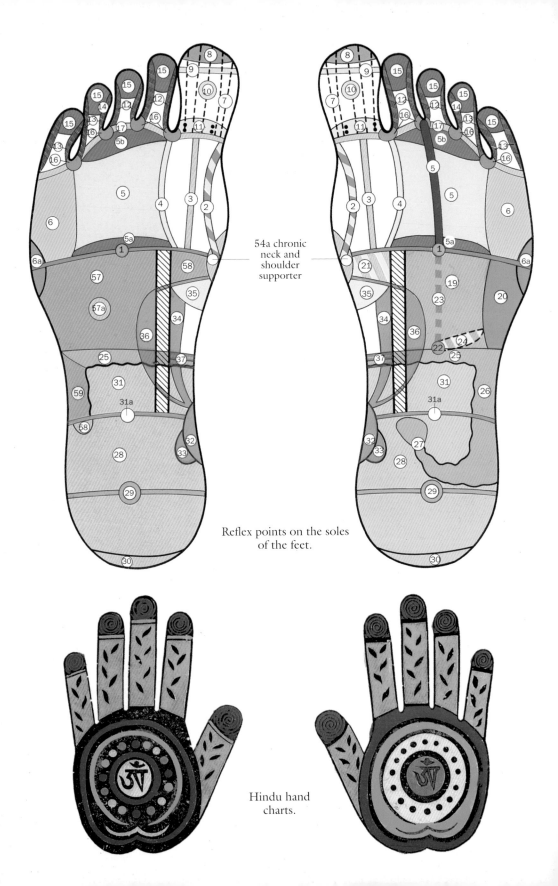

54a chronic
neck and
shoulder
supporter

Reflex points on the soles
of the feet.

Hindu hand
charts.

CHAPTER 17
The Special Senses

Overview of the Special Senses

Gives contact with the external environment, warns of danger, and
gives pleasure through touch, listening, sight and emotions

EARS	*Sections of the Ears*	*Function*	*Part of Brain*
Outer Ear	Pinna and auditory canal	Collect sound waves	Cerebellum and cerebrum
Middle Ear	Eustachian tubes	Equalize air pressure; amplify sound-waves 100 hundred times	
Inner Ear	Semi-circular canals and cochlea	Convert sound waves to water-borne waves; semi-circular canals give balance and coordination; cochlea provides volume of sound	
	Auditory nerve	Relays vibrations to the brain	
EYES	*Sections of the Eyes*	*Function*	*Part of Brain*
	Sclera – the white of the eye	Keeps the shape of the eyeball and gives attachment to muscles	Cerebellum and cerebrum
	Cornea	Refracts light waves and is a continuation of the sclera; it is a transparent membrane	
Choroid	Lines the back of the eye	Prevents incoming rays scattering and reflecting, and provides nutrients to the eye	

continued overleaf

Overview of the Special Senses *continued*

EYES	*Sections of the Eyes*	*Function*	
Ciliary body	Suspends the lens	Controls the thickness of the lens	
Iris	Consists of muscle fibres	Controls the amount of light entering eye	
Retina	The inner nervous layer, sensitive to light	Cells called rods and cones are sensitive to light and send nerve impulses to the brain	

Structures inside the eye-ball

Lens	A transparent and circular body	Refracts light waves onto the retina	
Aqueous humour	Has two fluid-filled chambers	Refracts light waves onto the retina	
Vitreous body	Contains a jelly-like substance	Stops the eye from collapsing by supporting the retina against the choroid process; refracts light waves onto the retina	

NOSE	*Features*	*Functions*	*Part of the Brain*
Olfactory nerves	Sense of smell affects appetite; nostrils assist in breathing	The sensory nerves of smell, which when stimulated relay the message to the nerve endings in the nose and the brain.	Cerebrum
	Sniffing concentrates particles and increases number of nerves stimulated	Air entering the nose is heated and convection carries inspired air to the roof of the nose	

TONGUE			
Taste buds	Found on the tongue, soft palate, pharynx and epiglottis	Enables taste; sweet and salty at the tip, sour at the sides and bitter at the back	Cerebrum

Smell and taste work together

LINKS TO: nervous, endocrine, muscular, skeletal, joints and respiratory systems.

INTRODUCTION

The special senses tell us about our external environment and the nature of our surroundings. The senses include sight, hearing, taste, smell and touch.

THE EYE

The eye is the organ of sense of sight and is situated in the orbital cavity. It is almost spherical in shape.

There are three layers of tissue in the walls of the eye, which are:

• the sclera and the cornea;
• the choroid, ciliary body and the iris;
• the inner nervous layer, which is called the retina.

The structures inside the eyeball are: the lens, the aqueous fluid (humour) and the vitreous body. These structures refract (bend) light waves.

Sclera

The sclera, or the white of the eye, forms the outermost layer of the eyeball, and is continuous with the transparent cornea. It consists of a firm fibrous membrane that maintains the shape of the eye, and provides attachment for muscles.

Cornea

At the front of the eye, the sclera continues as a clear transparent membrane and becomes the cornea. Light rays are refracted (bent) as they pass through the cornea.

Lens

The lens is an elastic, circular and transparent body, lying immediately behind the pupil. It is suspended from the ciliary body by the suspensory ligament. Light from distant objects needs least refraction, and as the object comes closer the amount of light needed increases.

The thickness of the lens is controlled by the ciliary muscles through the suspensory

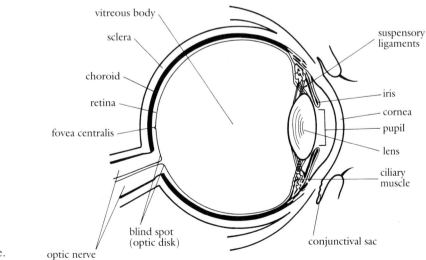

Fig 35. The eye.

ligament. The lens refractor bends light rays, reflected by objects in front of the eye, and it is the only structure in the eye that can vary its refractory power. When the ciliary muscle contracts, it moves forwards, releasing its pull on the lens, thereby increasing its thickness. In this way, the nearer the object, the thicker the lens becomes.

Ciliary Body and Suspensory Ligament

The ciliary body is at the front of the eye and is a continuation of the choroid, and consists of the ciliary muscle and secretory cells. It provides attachment for the suspensory ligament, which, at the other end, is attached to the capsule enclosing the lens. When the ciliary muscle relaxes, it slips backwards so that the pull on the suspensory ligament is increased making the lens thinner. Looking at near objects tires the eyes more quickly due to the continuous use of the ciliary muscle.

Light Waves

Light waves travel at a speed of about 299,250km/sec (186,000 miles/sec). White light is a combination of all of the colours of the rainbow and although the spectrum of light is broad, only a small part is visible to the human eye. In order to achieve clear vision, light reflected from objects is focused on to the retina of both eyes.

Light Refraction

The parts of the eye involved in refracting (bending) light waves onto the back of the eye are:

- the cornea;
- the aqueous humour;
- the vitreous ('glassy') humour;
- the lens.

Iris

The iris consists of two layers: one of circular and one of radiating muscle fibres. Contraction of the circular fibres constricts the pupil, and contraction of the radiating fibres dilates it. The iris extends from the front of the ciliary body and lies behind the cornea in front of the lens.

The iris divides the front section of the eye into the anterior (front) and posterior (back) chambers, which contain aqueous fluid secreted by the ciliary body. In the centre there is an aperture called the pupil. The colour of the iris depends on the number of pigment cells, for example, people with blue eyes have fewer than those with brown eyes.

Pupil

The pupil varies in size depending on the intensity of light. In bright light, the circular muscle fibres contract and constrict the pupil, while in dim light the radiating muscles contract, thereby dilating the pupil. If the pupils dilated in a bright light, too much light would enter the eye and damage the retina; conversely, in a dim light, if the pupils were constricted, insufficient light would enter the eye to stimulate the nerve endings in the retina.

Choroid Process

The choroid lines the back of the eye on the surface of the sclera. It is rich in blood vessels and is a deep chocolate brown in colour. The choroid prevents incoming rays from scattering and reflecting off the inner surface of the eye, and provides nutrients to the eye through minute blood vessels.

Retina

The retina is the size of a postage stamp, is the photosensitive part of the eye and is the innermost layer of the wall of the eye. It consists of an extremely delicate membrane and is especially adapted to be stimulated by light rays. It is composed of several layers of nerve cells and nerve fibres lying on layers of cells, which attach to the choroid process, called rods and cones. The retina lines about three-quarters of the eyeball and is thickest at the back; it thins out at the front to end just behind the ciliary body. Near the centre at the back of eye there is a little depression called the fovea, which consists of cone-shaped cells. Towards the front part of the retina, there are fewer cone and rod-shaped cells.

Rods and Cones

The retina contains rods and cones, which are receptors for the sense of vision. Cones are concerned with the colours, red, blue and green, and rods with black and white vision. The rods and cones contain photo-sensitive pigments, which are involved in the conversion of light rays into nerve impulses. Visual purple (rhodopsin) is a pigment in rod cells that is so sensitive it is bleached by dim light – vitamin A is essential for its synthesis.

The rods are more sensitive than the cones and are stimulated by low intensity or dim light, for example, by the dim light in a darkened room or at night. In a bright light, light rays are focused on to the fovea. Reading this page requires using cells in the fovea, which is a very sensitive area where most of the cones are clustered. Cones are fewer above and below the fovea and non-existent at the front of the retina, where only rod cells are found. The rods are more numerous above and below the fovea and extend to the front of the eye.

When moving from an area of bright light to one of dim light, it is difficult to see. This time lapse of readjustment from bright to dim light is called 'dark adaptation' and is dependent upon the reconstitution of the colour purple (rhodopsin).

Forming Images

The images from the two eyes are fused in the cerebrum of the brain, so that only one image is perceived. Binocular vision provides an accurate assessment of one object in relation to another, for example, distance, depth, height and width, which give us three-dimensional vision. Binocular vision has other advantages, as each eye sees a scene slightly differently; there is an overlap in the middle, with each eye seeing more on its own than can be seen by the other eye.

Aqueous Humour

In the spaces between the cornea and the lens, which are created by the iris, both chambers contain a clear aqueous fluid (humour) secreted into the back chamber of the eye by the ciliary glands. Fluid passes in front of the lens, through the pupil and into the anterior chamber and returns to the circulation through the angle between the cornea and the iris.

Vitreous Body

The vitreous humour is found behind the lens, filling the cavity of the eyeball. It is a soft colourless transparent jelly-like substance composed of about 99 per cent water, salts and protein. It maintains sufficient pressure to support the retina against the choroid process and prevents the walls of the eyeball from collapsing in on itself. The eye keeps its shape because of pressure exerted on to the surrounding structures by the vitreous body and the aqueous fluid.

Muscles of the Eye

The muscles of the eye are attached to the eyeball and are concerned with movement of the eyeball in the eye socket. They rotate the eyes so that they converge on the object in view and provide a clear image.

Optic Nerve

The fibres of the optic nerve originate in the retina of the eye. The small area of the retina where the optic nerve leaves the eye is the blind spot. There are no light sensitive cells at this point.

Protective Structures of the Eye

As the eye is a delicate organ, it needs to be protected by several structures. These are:

- the eyebrows, which protect the eye from sweat, dust and foreign bodies;
- the eyelids and eyelashes, which protect the eye from injury;
- the lacrimal ducts, which spread tears and secretions over the cornea, preventing the surface of the eye from drying in the action of blinking.

Conjunctiva

The conjunctiva is a fine transparent membrane that lines the eyelids and covers the front part of the sclera. The function of the conjunctiva is to protect the delicate structures of the cornea and the front of the eye. As the conjunctiva extends from the eyelid to the front of the eye, sacs are formed which enable tears formed by the lacrimal glands to keep the conjunctiva moist. These tears are spread over the surface of the eye by blinking. They wash away irritants such as dust, grit and foreign bodies and are carried into ducts near the nasal corner of the eye. An excess of tears causes a runny nose or overspill from the eyes, as when crying. The eyelid margins contain sebaceous glands with ducts opening into hair follicles of the eyelashes, with some between the hairs. They secrete an oily solution that is spread over the conjunctiva by blinking, which slows the evaporation of tears.

THE EAR

The ear is the organ of hearing. Sound waves are changed into nerve impulses for interpretation by the brain. The ear is divided into three parts.

- **The external ear** consists of the pinna, auditory canal, tympanum or eardrum, which becomes the entrance to the middle ear.
- **The pinna** is the expanded portion projecting from the side of the head and is composed of fibro-elastic cartilage covered with skin.
- **The auditory canal** is a slightly S-shaped tube and is about 2.5cm (1in) long, extending from the pinna to the tympanic membrane (eardrum). There are numerous sweat glands that secrete a waxy substance that is a sticky material containing lysozymes (an enzyme) and immunoglobulins. Foreign materials, such as dust, insects and microbes, are prevented from reaching the tympanic membrane by wax, hairs and the curve of the canal.

The Middle Ear

The middle ear separates the external ear from the inner ear. It consists of the eardrum (tympanum), three ossicles, the oval window and Eustachian tube. Sound waves cause the three ossicles to knock against each other, thereby magnifying sound waves by 22-fold.

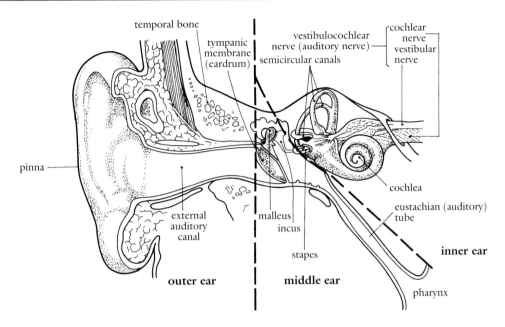

temporal bone

tympanic
membrane
(eardrum)

vestibulocochlear
nerve (auditory nerve)

semicircular canals

cochlear
nerve

vestibular
nerve

pinna

external
auditory
canal

malleus
incus

stapes

cochlea

eustachian (auditory)
tube

inner ear

outer ear

middle ear

pharynx

Fig 36. The ear.

The middle ear is an air-filled cavity and the presence of air at atmospheric pressure on both sides of the tympanic membrane enables it to vibrate when sound waves strike it. There are two openings: the oval window and the round window.

Ossicles

The auditory ossicles extend across the cavity of the middle ear, from the tympanic membrane to the oval window. These bones are the smallest in the body. They form a series of movable joints with each other. The bones are called the malleus, the incus and stapes. The malleus is a hammer-shaped bone and is in contact with the tympanic membrane. The head forms a movable joint with the incus, which is the middle, anvil-shaped bone. The body of the incus articulates with the hammer, and the long process of it with the stapes. The stapes is a stirrup-shaped bone, which articulates with the incus; its base fits into the oval window. The ossicles are held in place by fine ligaments.

Balance and Air Pressure

Air pressure on both sides of the eardrum is the same unless atmospheric pressure changes, as when going up in a plane, the air pressure drops. This causes air to push outwards on the eardrum and sound waves cannot be transmitted comfortably because pressure is different each side of the eardrum, resulting in a distortion of hearing. Swallowing, yawning and chewing, which introduce additional external air into the Eustachian tube, give a 'popping' sensation. Hearing returns to normal as pressure resumes balance on each side of the drum.

Descending in a plane causes the reverse to happen – pressure outside the eardrum pushes air inwards on to the drum. Chewing, swallowing or yawning again introduce additional air into the Eustachian tube in the middle ear, until the ears 'pop'.

167

The Inner Ear

The inner ear consists of the cochlea and semi-circular canals, the utricle, saccula and ampulla, which are fluid-filled with endolymph and perilymph. The inner ear contains the organs of hearing and balance and is generally described in two parts:

- the bony labyrinth, which consists of the vestibule (the expanded part nearest the middle ear, containing the oval and round windows);
- the cochlea, three semi-circular canals and the membranous labyrinth, which contains fluid called endolymph and perilymph.

Endolymph and perilymph surround the canals and change air-borne waves into water-borne waves. These waves cause movement of the membrane on which hair cells sit. Hairs are embedded in a jelly shelf and are pulled or crushed as cells rise or fall on the membrane. Movement of hair cells sends nerve impulses along the auditory nerve.

Due to the shape of the pinna, waves are concentrated and directed along the auditory canal, causing the tympanic membrane to vibrate. The tympanic membrane sends vibrations through the middle ear by the movement of the ossicles. The stapes rocks to and fro in the oval window, setting up fluid waves in the perilymph. These waves indent the membranous labyrinth with a wave-like motion in the endolymph.

Semi-Circular Canals

The semi-circular canals are three tubes arranged so that one represents each of the three planes of space. They have no auditory function, although they are closely associated with the cochlea. They provide information about the position of the head in space, and contribute to maintenance of equilibrium and balance.

The semi-circular canals, like the cochlea, are composed of an outer bony wall and inner membranous tubes. The membranous tubes contain endolymph and are separated from the bony wall by perilymph. Any change in the position of the head causes movement in the perilymph and endolymph, which stimulates the nerve endings and the hair cells in the utricle, saccule and ampullae. Impulses from these three sources are co-ordinated and efferent nerve impulses pass to the cerebrum, where position in space is perceived and, with the aid of motor nerve impulses to the muscles, posture and balance are maintained.

The utricle is a membranous sac, which is part of the vestibule, and the three membranous ducts, which open into it, are called the ampullae. Inside the ampulla (meaning a swelling in the semi-circular canals) are hair cells capped with jelly which move like a swing-door. The saccule is a part of the vestibule and communicates with the utricle.

Cochlea

The cochlea resembles a snail's shell and the principle part is called the organ of Corti, which is concerned with the volume of sound and is the organ of hearing.

SENSES OF SMELL AND TASTE

Smell

Olfactory nerves provide the sense of smell. They originate in special cells in the mucous membrane in the roof of the nose. When we inhale, chemical particles that have a 'smell' are carried into the nose and stimulate nerve cells when they hit the mucous membrane. In 'sniffing', the density of the smell concentrates particles on the roof of the nose, which in turn stimulates nerve cells in a greater quantity. When we are continuously exposed to an odour, the sense of smell decreases and eventually ceases. This sensory loss only affects specific odours.

The air entering the nose is heated and currents carry inspired air to the roof of the nose. The sense of smell may affect the appetite, and if the odours are pleasant, the appetite may improve and vice versa. Inflammation of the nasal mucosa prevents odorous substances from reaching the olfactory area of the nose, causing loss of the sense of smell and possibly appetite. When we have a cold in the head, our sense of smell is diminished because mucus prevents smells hitting the olfactory part of the nose. This can also happen to our taste buds when we have a cold.

Taste

Taste buds are found in the tongue and the soft palate, the pharynx and the epiglottis. Some tastes consistently stimulate taste buds in specific parts of the tongue: sweet and salty at the tip, sour at the sides and bitter at the back. Smell and taste work together.

THE SPATIAL MAP

It is with the maintenance of balance that we draw a spatial map of where we are in time and space and the external environment generally. Proprioceptors located in muscles, tendons and joints, joint capsules and the inner ear relay impulses and aid in judging position and changes in the locations of body parts in respect to each other and the external environment. They also inform the brain of the amount of muscle contraction and tendon tension. These rather widespread end organs

are aided in their function by the semi-circular canals and related internal ear structures. Information received by these receptors is needed for the co-ordination of muscles and is important in such activities as walking, running, complicated skills, such as playing a musical instrument, and other activities concerned with manual dexterity. These receptors also have an important role in maintaining muscle tone and good posture, as well as allowing for the adjustment of the muscles for the particular kind of work to be done.

The nerve fibres that carry impulses from these receptors enter the spinal cord and are sent to the brain. The cerebellum is a main co-ordinating centre for these impulses.

SPECIAL INTEREST

As the Special Senses imply, we gain sensory pleasure and pain from outside of ourselves or from internal sensations and feelings. Stress can affect our eyesight, hearing and facial muscles. Blotting out sights and sounds which are unpleasant to us or that we wish to avoid can eventually lead to impairment of these vital senses. Our facial muscles reveal our emotional and thinking selves – looking sad, happy, in pain or when concentrating with the mind can give the facial muscles a set expression. Laughing, listening to music, looking at beautiful things and facial exercises are good ways of maintaining flexibility with these expressive muscles. The relaxation enjoyed through reflexology will help to relax them as well!

Enjoyment of food and drink not only physically exercises the jaw muscles when chewing but also gives sensory pleasure and is thought to alter moods – as anyone who is a 'choc-o-holic' will testify! Smell can also give us sensory pleasure and bring back memories, such as the smell of flowers or perfume. Sadly, touch, unless accepted by those we know or in a professional capacity, has become unacceptable to a large extent in our society today, because of the fear of sexual connotations. Although this is understandable, it does mean that the humanness of touch to give comfort or show affection becomes inhibited. From my experience as a reflexologist, the elderly or those living alone may have no-one to give them this precious comfort. Reflexology offers touch in an acceptable way with those we do not know personally and is very much a part of the patient's healing process. For many, their time with you may be the only physical contact they have in their week.

Always ask permission before touching your patient, apart from working the feet or hands, as it could feel like an invasion of their personal space if you just assume that they want comforting with a hug. Very often I have found that if the patient wants comforting, it can allow a greater release of pent-up feelings and enhance the healing process.

There are two main types of hearing loss: conduction (reduction of sound waves) deafness and nerve deafness. Conduction deafness is due to interference with the passage of sound waves from the outside to the inner ear. In this condition there may be obstruction of the external canal by wax or a foreign body. Nerve deafness is due to a sensory disorder affecting the cochlea, the auditory nerve or the brain areas concerned with hearing. It may result from prolonged exposure to loud noises, to the prolonged use of drugs or to exposure to infections or toxins.

The fourth toe (little toe) can reflect deafness and the third toe, inner ear problems.

Magnetic wrist bands, which apply pressure to the pulse, are an aid in the prevention of motion sickness. Focusing on a static object whilst movement is present also reduces the symptoms of motion sickness.

WORKING THE REFLEXES

Refer to Chapter 17, the Respiratory System, for Special Senses systems, associated reflexes and disorders.

Eyes and Ears – Reflex Points 12, 13 and 14 – the Special Senses and Respiratory System

When working the eyes and ears you may find it easier to work with the index finger on curly toes and with the thumb on broad or straight toes. When working the toes with the index finger, it is important to hook the fingers not being used underneath the palm of the hand. This way the index finger can move freely and the hands are kept tidy. If you wish to work with the thumb, make sure that the working hand fingers are over the supporting hand.

When working the toes, remember to support from the tips of the toes at all times with the supporting hand to stop them wobbling

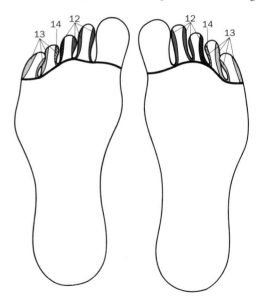

The ears and eyes, reflex points 12, 13 and 14 (both feet). Refer to the Respiratory System.

about, and use the thumb of the supporting hand to support the toe firmly. Work the centre of the toes then the medial side, continue across to the little toe then swap hands and work the centre and then the lateral side back towards the big toe. Hold the little toe firmly by using a 'scissor' movement with the third and index fingers by holding the toe firmly between them. Once worked, revert to sup-porting the tips of all toes with the support-ing hand.

Work the neck and teeth by pulling the pad of the thoracic cavity downwards so that the roots of the toes are exposed. Work with the thumb or index finger with ripple movements from the lateral edge to the medial edge of the foot. You can continue to work the face and nose by changing hands so that the working

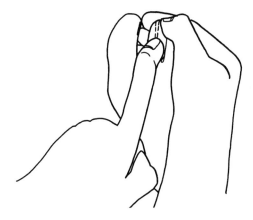

Hand position (1): the eyes, working the centre of the toes, reflex point 12 (both feet). Supporting hand supports the toes from the tips, using the thumb to lightly support the toe.

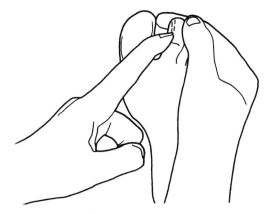

Hand position (2): the eyes, working the sides of the toes, reflex point 12 (both feet). Supporting hand position as before.

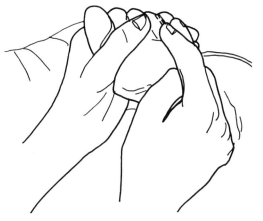

Hand position: the inner ear, working the sides of the toes, reflex point 14 (both feet). Supporting hand position as before.

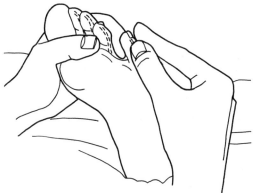

Hand position (1): the ear, reflex point 13 (both feet). The 'scissor' hand support.

171

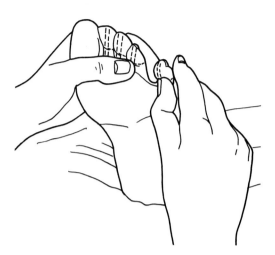

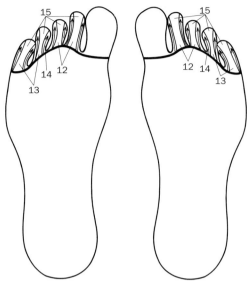

Hand position (2): the ear, using the 'scissor' hand support, reflex point 13 (both feet).

Directions for working: the ears and eyes, reflex points 12, 13 and 14.

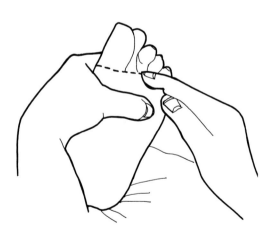

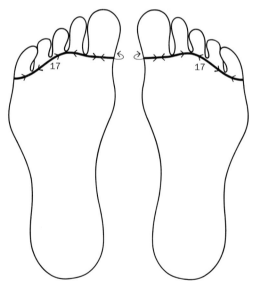

Hand position: neck and teeth, reflex point 17 (both feet). Supporting hand fingers on top of the foot, thumb on the sole of the foot.

Directions for working: the neck and teeth, reflex point 17, leading to the face and nose.

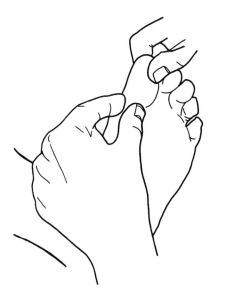

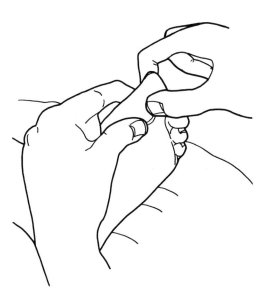

Hand position (1): the face and nose, reflex point 18 (both feet). Supporting the big toe with the thumb and index finger and supporting behind the big toe with the working hand.

Hand position (2): the face and nose, reflex point 18 (both feet). Supporting the big toe with the thumb and index finger and supporting behind the big toe with the working hand.

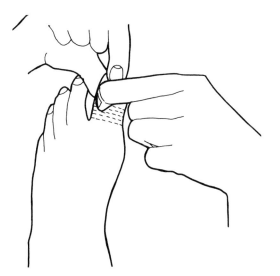

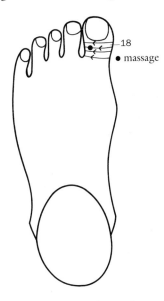

Hand position: the face and nose, reflex point 18 (both feet). Supporting hand position as before.

Directions for working: face and nose (both feet), reflex point 18.

hand becomes the supporting hand and the supporting hand becomes the working hand. To hold the big toe steady whilst you work around the front of the big toe, for the face and nose reflex, use your index finger to hold the toe from the nail bed on the front of the toe and the thumb on the pad of the toe. Remember to hold the supporting hand fingers under the palm of the hand – this enables you to see the front of the toe clearly. It also gives a tidy appearance. From the medial side of the toe, work with the index finger and support the back of the toe with the working hand thumb, this way your pressure will remain constant. Work to the inside of the lateral edge of the big toe for neck reflexes. Repeat this movement in tiny pathways towards the nail bed, massaging the indentation on the lateral side of the toe joint for the nose reflex point. Once completed go back to the neck and teeth and work medially to laterally as before.

CASE STUDY: EAR INFECTIONS AND DEAFNESS

Eileen had been suffering from ear infections, deafness and sinusitis for a number of years before coming for reflexology treatments. Her story is given below.

> After experiencing recurring spells of sinusitis, ear infections and deafness, which courses

of antibiotics only seemed to subdue, it was suggested by my daughter, who also has reflexology with Jenny, and my sister, who has ongoing reflexology treatments, that reflexology would help me.

I went for my first consultation with the vague knowledge that 'hands on' treatment on my feet would find the weak spots in my body. As weeks have passed I have discovered the true depth of reflexology.

As a patient, I have experienced all the skills of reflexology interacting during my treatments resulting in an improvement in my sinusitis. My ear infections have now cleared and my hearing is much improved. But more than this, I have found I have sustained a physical stamina to cope with my long strenuous days as a senior citizen looking after a boisterous toddler full-time. I have a more patient attitude when dealing with my chronically sick husband, a keener mental alertness and a calmer sleep pattern.

Reflexology has left me with an all-round feeling of physical and mental well-being, with stimulating mental and physical activity, providing restful relaxation. Importantly, I feel the essence of reflexology is the healing hands.

In addition to the benefits described, this client feels calmer and more able to cope emotionally with the demands she has on her.

CHAPTER 18
The Endocrine System

Overview of the Endocrine System

Hormones are sent as chemical messengers to target organs.

Structures	*Functions*
BRAIN	
Hypothalamus	Produces: oxytocin, which causes uterine and mammary gland contractions in childbirth and lactation respectively; vasopressin, which becomes the anti-diuretic hormone (ADH) in the posterior lobe of the pituitary gland
Pituitary gland	Produces a range of hormones as outlined below

POSTERIOR LOBE OF THE PITUITARY

Hormones	*Functions*
Oxytocin	*See* above
Antidiuretic hormone (ADH)	Inhibits the kidneys from excreting excess water

ANTERIOR LOBE OF THE PITUITARY

ACTH (Adrenocorticotropic hormone) (sent to the adrenal glands)	Stimulates production of three groups of hormones in adrenal cortex: *glucocorticoids:* major hormone is cortisol, which stimulates the pancreas to secrete insulin and glucagon *mineralocorticoids:* major hormone is aldosterone, which regulates excretion of potassium and reabsorption of salt from kidney tubules *androgens:* promote sexual development in the male
TSH (thyroid-stimulating hormone) (sent to thyroid gland)	Controls metabolism and regulation of blood calcium levels (together with parathormone released by the parathyroid glands)
GH (growth hormone) (released into blood, bone and thyroid gland)	Involved in growth and repair of body tissue and wound healing. Increases blood sugar levels

continued overleaf

Overview of the Endocrine System *continued*

FSH (follicle-stimulating hormone) (sent to ovaries and testes)	Stimulates ripening of ova (egg) and production of oestrogen levels in the ovarian follicles of the female, and production of sperm cells in the male; responsible for secondary sexual characteristics in the female
LH (luteinizing hormone) (sent to ovaries and testes)	Leads to production of progesterone, which stimulates ovulation in the female and is required in maintenance of pregnancy; known as ICSH (interstitial cell-stimulating hormone) in the male, where it stimulates interstitial cells in the testes in production of testosterone
PRL (prolactin)	Stimulates production of milk in lactation (breast-feeding)

Negative feedback: regulation of the secretion of hormones is controlled by nerve impulses transmitted to the brain from the stimulated target organs.

LINKS TO: nervous, digestive, special senses, reproductive, skeletal, circulatory, muscular and urinary systems.

INTRODUCTION

The endocrine system is the hormonal messenger system in the body. The word 'hormone' comes from the Greek word '*hormon*', meaning 'to set in motion'. The word endocrine means 'secreting within', meaning that the glands secrete their contents directly into the bloodstream. Some hormones can be manufactured in synthetic form or produced by genetic engineering. Hormones attach to receptors on the surface of specific types of tissue. Some hormones are long lasting, for example the thyroid hormone, which lasts for approximately two weeks; others are renewed rapidly. Hormones are composed of protein, compounds which are made up of amino acids. The endocrine glands are as follows:

- 1 hypothalamus;
- 1 pituitary gland;
- 1 pineal;
- 1 thyroid gland;
- 4 parathyroid glands (two embedded in each of the thyroid glands);
- 2 adrenal glands, which sit on the top of each kidney;
- the islets of Langerhans, found in the pancreas;
- 2 ovaries;
- 2 testes.

A hormone is a chemical substance which stimulates a 'target' organ at a distance from its point of release. They have three major functions in the body:

- **Growth** is under the influence of the growth hormone and two hormones secreted by the thyroid gland which regulate metabolism.

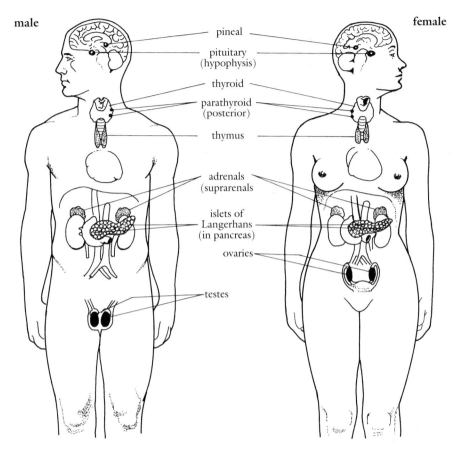

male

female

pineal

pituitary
(hypophysis)

thyroid

parathyroid
(posterior)

thymus

adrenals
(suprarenals

islets of
Langerhans
(in pancreas)

ovaries

testes

Fig 37. The main endocrine glands.

- **Activity** is under the influence of two hormones secreted by the adrenal glands in response to stress.
- **Nutrition** is regulated under the influence of three groups of major hormones secreted by the adrenal glands and the pancreas.

The release of many hormones is controlled by the central nervous system and the stimulating and inhibiting functions of the hypothalamus.

ENDOCRINE GLANDS

Hypothalamus

The hypothalamus is now considered to be the master hormonal gland as it computes nerve messages received by the brain, which are relayed to the pituitary gland, which turns on or off several major hormones. The hypothalamus is also responsible for our sleep patterns, metabolism of fat, carbohydrate, water balance, body temperature, genital functions, hunger, thirst and provides a nerve centre for our physical and emotional behaviour.

The hypothalamus produces two hormones called oxytocin and vasopressin, which are transported to the posterior lobe of the pituitary gland. Oxytocin stimulates uterine contractions in labour and the mammary glands during lactation, while vasopressin is an antidiuretic hormone. Release of these two hormones is under the control of nerve impulses, which travel between the hypothalamus and the posterior lobe of the pituitary gland.

Once in the pituitary gland, vasopressin is called the antidiuretic hormone (ADH). Excessive amounts of this hormone cause contraction in the walls of blood vessels and raise blood pressure. Inadequate amounts of ADH cause excessive loss of water, resulting in a disorder called diabetes insipidus. This condition should not be confused with diabetes mellitus, which occurs due to inadequate amounts of insulin.

The hypothalamus also triggers release of adrenocorticotropic hormone (ACTH) from the anterior lobe of the pituitary gland. The hormones released from the adrenal cortex (outside edge) as a result of stimulation by ACTH, raise blood sugar levels, inhibit inflammation, decrease immune response and inhibit the release of histamine.

The Pituitary Gland

The pituitary gland is often described as the conductor of the orchestra, meaning that it controls the release of hormones from the endocrine glands lying beneath it. The pituitary and hypothalamus act as a unit.

The pituitary gland lies in the sphenoid bone in the base of the skull, below the hypothalamus, to which it is attached by a stalk. It consists of two parts that originate from different types of cells, known as the anterior and posterior lobes. Blood supply to the pituitary gland is supplied directly by the carotid artery. Hormones are released from both lobes into the venous blood supply leaving the gland. Some of the hormones secreted by the anterior lobe of the pituitary stimulate or inhibit secretions by other endocrine glands (target organs), while others have a direct effect on target tissues.

Hormones produced in the anterior lobe of the pituitary gland are not released until chemical messengers, known as releasing hormones, are received from the hypothalamus via the portal system.

Hormones can act at the cell surface or within the cell membrane. Many hormones attach to cell surfaces where they trigger internal messengers. Some hormones, especially steroids, enter most of the cells of the body where they may be transmitted into the nucleus of a cell to interact with DNA.

Hormone secretions may be continuous, spasmodic or released at regular intervals. For example, the adrenal cortex follows a twenty-four-hour cycle related to sleep patterns, decreasing activity at bedtime and increasing it before waking. Thus hormones are released at regular intervals occurring over twenty-four hours of the day/night cycle. The menstrual cycle is the best example of a long biological rhythm, where certain hormones are released at different times of the month.

Negative Feedback

The control of hormones present in the blood is controlled by a negative-feedback mechanism, that is, when there is a low level of hormone in the

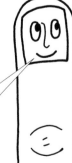

Hint! Find the pituitary by looking for the whorl on the puffy toe pad.

blood supplying the hypothalamus, it produces the appropriate releasing hormone, which in turn stimulates release of a hormone by the pituitary gland. This in turn stimulates the target gland to produce and release its hormones. As the blood level of that hormone rises, it inhibits the secretion of the releasing factor by the hypothalamus. Once a hormone has completed its task, it is deactivated by target cells or transported to the liver, where it is excreted or used to form new hormones.

Pineal Gland

The pineal (means shaped like a pine-cone) gland is thought to aid in the development of the ovaries and testes by influencing release of the gonadotrophic hormones (FSH and LH) from the anterior lobe of the pituitary gland. It also produces the hormone called melatonin, required for skin pigmentation. It is involved in sleep patterns as it is affected by light. The pineal gland is also thought to play a part in hormonal release and rhythms. Melatonin is also thought to delay the onset of puberty. Melanin is a dark pigment found in the skin, hair, some parts of the brain and parts of the eye.

Thyroid Gland

The thyroid gland is located in the neck, in front of the larynx and trachea. The lobes are roughly cone-shaped and are about 5cm (2in) long and 3cm (1¼in) wide. The thyroid gland produces the hormone thyroxine, a crystalline substance containing iodine, known as 'T4', which controls the rate at which we burn up our food, known as metabolic activity. Triiodothyronine (T3) increases the metabolic rate and influences physical and mental activity. Triiodothyronine is a substance which stimulates action of the thyroid hormone and is formed in the cells of the body by the de-iodination of thyroxine. It is

three times stronger than thyroxine and is produced synthetically for the treatment of hypothyroidism. The thyroid gland also produces the hormone calcitonin, which inhibits release of calcium into the blood.

Parathyroids

The parathyroids provide maintenance of phosphorous/calcium balance in the blood and bone structure, through the release of the hormone parathormone. A lack of parathormone leads to tetany (muscle spasm). Calcitonin causes a reduction in calcium levels in the blood and parathormone promotes the release of calcium from bone, thus increasing the amount of calcium circulating in the blood.

Thymus Gland

The thymus gland is composed of lymphoid tissue that lies in the upper part of the chest above the heart and behind the sternum. This gland is important in the development of immunity. It produces a hormone called thymosin, which assists in the maturation of white cells, called T-lymphocytes. After lymphocytes have left the thymus gland they are stored in lymph nodes throughout the body.

Adrenal Glands

The adrenal glands are situated on the top of each kidney and are about 4cm (1½in) long and 3cm (1¼in) thick.

Cortex

The cortex of the adrenal glands secrete three groups of hormones called the androgens, glucocorticoids and mineralocorticoids. All three groups of hormones are essential to life. **The androgens** are crucial in sex organ development and in development of secondary sexual characteristics, such as growth of pubic hair and deepening of the voice in the male, growth of the breasts and changes in the female pelvis to accommodate the growing foetus. Androgens include the hormone testosterone which is used in chronic illness to aid tissue repair and healing.

The glucocorticoids are a group of steroids, which include the growth hormone (GH), cortisone and cortisol, that affect fat, protein and carbohydrate metabolism. These hormones trigger the pancreas to release glucagon, and maintain the carbohydrate reserve by regulating the conversion of amino acids into sugar instead of protein. In times of stress, large amounts of this hormone are released, thus aiding the body. They have the ability to suppress inflammation and are thought to be involved in wound healing. The major hormone in this group is cortisol, also called hydrocortisone; 95 per cent of the glucocorticoids are composed of cortisol.

The mineralocorticoids function is to regulate the electrolyte balance (water and salts) in the body and help to control blood pressure. The hormone responsible for governing this function in the kidneys is aldosterone which controls the reabsorption of sodium (salt) and the secretion of potassium by the kidney tubules; 95 per cent of mineralocorticoids are composed of this hormone.

Medulla

The hormones secreted by the medulla of the adrenal glands are: adrenaline and noradrenaline. The 'fight or flight' response is caused by adrenaline action. The medulla (middle) of the adrenal glands is an extension of tissue from the autonomic part of the nervous system with functions connected to the sympathetic nervous system. We can survive without the medulla of the adrenal glands but the hormones secreted by the cortex of the adrenal glands are essential in the maintenance of life. **Adrenaline** raises blood pressure by vasoconstriction of smaller blood vessels and increases blood sugar levels by the release of glycogen into glucose from the liver.

Noradrenaline maintains blood pressure by causing vasoconstriction of blood vessels.

Stress and Hormone Levels

Stress has a direct effect on the hormones secreted in the body. For example, injury, disease and emotional response involves the nervous system and endocrine system as a unit. The response of 'fight or flight' is governed by parts of the brain, especially the hypothalamus, and by the autonomic nervous system.

Pancreas

The pancreas weighs about 60g (2oz) and is about 12–15cm (5–6in) long. The pancreas is attached to the spleen at its tail and is encased in the duodenum at its head. Distributed throughout the pancreas are little collections of different types of cells, called the islets of Langerhans, which secrete the hormones insulin and glucagon. The main function of insulin is to maintain the homeostatic balance of blood sugar levels within the liver. Specialized cells in the islets of Langerhans secrete beta cells, which produce insulin, and alpha cells, which produce glucagon. Together insulin and glucagon control the level of glucose in the blood in conjunction with the liver. Glucagon stimulates the amount of glucose released into the blood from the liver and insulin inhibits the release of glucose into the blood.

Ovaries and Testicles

The hormonal functions of these glands are described in Chapter 21, The Reproductive System.

MOOD AND HORMONE LEVELS

Changing hormone levels affect mood, for example: falling hormone levels before menstruation and high female hormone levels midway in the menstrual cycle, which give a sense of well-being; changes in the ovaries at the menopause, which cause hot flushes; and withdrawal of oestrogen and progesterone, which can lead to depression. A lack of sunlight can cause the pineal gland to secrete melatonin during daylight hours, which leads on to depression and Seasonal Affective Disorder (SAD).

See also Chapter 22, The Nervous System, for further information on the endocrine system.

SPECIAL INTEREST

Computerized axial tomography (CAT) and magnetic resonance imaging (MRI) scans are used to diagnose pituitary abnormalities. Remember that the controlling hormones secreted by the hypothalamus and the pituitary gland are interlinked with the hormones secreted by the other endocrine glands situated throughout the body. The pituitary gland reflex point is a deeply imbedded indentation in the feet and needs to be searched for. As an indicator, look for the puffiest part of the big toe, or where the whorl print is seen. Remember that the way we walk can push the flesh of the toe pad to one side so be prepared to look for this reflex towards the side of the toe.

Stress and tiredness will affect the thyroid gland and so foods rich in iodine, such as spinach and green vegetables, are a good source. Seaweed, sold as kelp tablets, is helpful in increasing thyroid efficiency as it has a high iodine content. There are many symptoms of an under-active thyroid gland (*see* table above) and an enormous number of

---

Symptoms and Signs of Hypothyroidism (Under-Active Thyroid Gland)

Dry skin and coarse skin
Lethargy and weakness
Slow speech and movements
Oedema (swelling) of eyelids, feet and face
Decreased sweating
Cold skin and general pallor
Thick tongue
Coarseness and loss of hair
Heart problems
Impaired memory
Constipation
Weight gain
Laboured or difficult breathing
Hoarseness
Loss of appetite
Nervousness
Excessive menstruation
Painful menstruation
Deafness
Poor vision
Loss of weight
Emotional instability
Fineness of hair
Cyanosis (bluish discoloration of skin)
Brittle nails
Depression
Muscle pain
Joint pain
Burning or tingling sensations
Slowing of mental activity and movements

---

people suffer from the lethargy and tiredness that accompany even a mild imbalance of the gland. If you suffer from any of the symptoms in the table, it is possible that your metabolic rate is too low. However, an under-active thyroid gland is hard to diagnose from a clinical blood test unless very low in activity. Studying what underlying reasons may be present to account for sluggishness and lethargy may be a route to help this important gland back to maximum efficiency.

Hormones have a direct effect on our personality and how we feel about ourselves. All endocrine glands should be worked extensively for depression, premenstrual tension and menopausal problems.

When working the pancreas supporter, make a special note of sensitivity as this can be an indication of refined sugar consumption – even a chocolate bar consumed before treatment! Refined sugar has been linked to aggression and instability, and is addictive when taken in excessive amounts. Most pre-prepared food products contain sugar as a preservative, and unless we eat a diet of fresh fruit and vegetables only, intake of refined sugar is unavoidable. It is worth noting that hyperglycaemia (high blood glucose levels) and hypoglycaemia (low blood glucose levels) can exist without diabetes mellitus being present. 'Choc-o-holism' or a diet with an excessive intake of refined sugar can lead to fluctuations of energy with resultant cravings for products high in sugar. Symptoms of low blood sugar can result in feeling faint, nauseas, with low energy whilst high intakes of sugar can lead to hyperactivity followed by lethargy as blood sugar levels drop. Over the years of practising reflexology, I have found that the following symptoms appear to coincide with low blood sugar levels:

- weakness
- tremors
- yawning
- hunger
- abdominal discomfort
- restless sleep
- convulsions
- coma
- lethargy
- sight related problems
- fatigue
- dizziness
- anxiety
- personality change
- headache
- sleepiness
- pallor
- mental confusion
- sweating
- palpitations
- cool skin
- bad dreams
- behaviour problems

- lack of drive and motivation

Those who 'crash' diet are especially vulnerable to hypoglycaemia as carbohydrate intake is usually low, and advising a balanced diet including carbohydrates is advisable. Withdrawal symptoms from refined sugar products, including honey, can leave the patient feeling worse, as with any addictive substance. Recommend that patients restrict their diets with milk, bread, cereals and fresh fruit and that they consult a nutritionist and inform their GP if they wish to reassess their diet. Encourage patients to eat as often as they like, providing the diet is balanced. Hair-mineral analysis can be useful in finding which supplements need to be increased and decreased. The pituitary gland secretes growth hormone (GH) and adrenocorticotropic hormones (ACTH), both of which have a blood-sugar elevating effect. The glucocorticoid hormone (one of the three major ACTH hormones) is responsible for increasing blood glucose levels. If there is a deficiency of the ACTH glucocorticoid hormone and the growth hormone, it is possible that low blood sugar (hypoglycaemia) can result. A lack of glucagon, released from the pancreas, results in low blood sugar as insulin levels rise. In contrast, high levels of glucagon resulting in high blood glucose levels and low levels of insulin can produce diabetes mellitus. As exercise increases the secretion of glucagon, it is possible that lack of exercise produces an imbalance of glucagon secretion, giving insulin a predominating influence in creating low blood sugar levels. When a low blood sugar level is present, adrenalin compensates in elevating blood sugar levels. When placed under stress, adrenalin output may become deficient. Adrenal deficiency is not widely accepted as a medical condition; however, I have treated individuals who present symptoms which describe this condition as listed below:

- excessive tiredness
- red and sore eyes
- mood swings
- demotivation and reduced sex drive
- psychological problems
- mental confusion
- kidney sensitivity
- depression
- lethargy
- caffeine addiction
- confusion

From these symptoms it becomes clear that some symptoms are similar to hypoglycaemia and may be connected with an imbalance of blood glucose levels, and other symptoms are related to the adrenocorticotropic group of hormones (ACTH) and hormones released by the pancreas.

Working the five energy zones stimulates all of the reflexes in the head and in the body as all ten zonal pathways converge at the neck.

WORKING THE REFLEXES

Reflex Points 7–11 – Nervous and Endocrine Systems; Energy zones – Brain, Hypothalamus, Pineal Gland, Pituitary, Thyroid/Parathyroids

Support the toes horizontally from behind, with the supporting hand, to stop them wobbling. Your index finger should be parallel with the tips of the toes. To work the five energy zones from the base of the great toe to the tip: with the thumb pointing in an upward direction, work with the ripple movement from the base of the great toe to the tip. Repeat this movement across the width of the toe.

To work the brain, support the big toe from the tip, and 'rock' the brain medially to laterally with the index finger held sideways with the nail facing towards the lateral edge of the foot.

Keeping the toes supported from the tips with the supporting hand, work the hypothalamus

---

The Endocrine System

System(s)	Associated Reflexes	Disorders
REFLEX POINTS 9 & 10: THE HYPOTHALAMUS, PINEAL AND PITUITARY GLAND		
Endocrine	All glands	Simmond's disease, insomnia
Nervous	Brain, spine, solar plexus	psychogenic factors, diabetes
Digestive	Pancreas, small intestine	insipidus, acromegaly, obesity
Urinary	Kidneys	

(For hormones secreted by the ovaries and testes, *see* Chapter 21.)

Nerve Innervation: 1st Cervical

REFLEX POINT 2: THE THYMUS GLAND		
Endocrine	Hypothalamus, pituitary, thyroid, parathyroids, thymus, adrenal glands	HIV–AIDS, myasthenia gravis
Lymphatic	Lymph nodes in the neck, inguinal nodes and supporter, spleen	

Nerve Innervation: 3rd Thoracic

continued overleaf

The Endocrine System *continued*

REFLEX POINTS 4 & 11: THE THYROID AND PARATHYROID GLANDS

Endocrine	Hypothalamus, pituitary gland, adrenal glands	Hyperthyroidism includes goitres, Grave's disease and myxoedema; renal colic, osteoporosis
Reproductive	Ovaries, testes	
Digestive	Stomach, pancreas, large colon, small intestine, liver/gall-bladder	
Urinary	Kidneys	

Nerve Innervation: 7th Cervical

REFLEX POINTS 21 AND 24: THE PANCREAS

Endocrine	All glands	Diabetes mellitus, diabetes insipidus, pancreatitis, cystic fibrosis, renal failure, gangrene weight loss
Digestive	Oesophagus, stomach, duodenum, liver/gall-bladder	
Urinary	Kidneys	
Nervous	Spine	
Special senses	Eyes	
Skeletal	Joints	

Nerve Innervation: 7th Thoracic

REFLEX POINT 35: THE ADRENAL GLANDS

Endocrine	Pituitary, hypothalamus, thyroid/parathyroids	Addison's disease, Conn's Syndrome, Cushing's Syndrome
Digestive	Pancreas, liver	
Urinary	All reflexes	
Reproductive	Gonads (ovaries and testicles)	
Nervous	Spine, brain	
Muscular	Diaphragm	

Nerve Innervation: 9th Thoracic

REFLEX POINT 7 – CRANIAL ENERGY ZONES

Nervous	Spine, solar plexus	Meningitis
Special senses	Ears, eyes, nose, face	Stroke
Muscular	Diaphragm	Fainting
Respiratory	Lungs, nose, sinuses	Shingles
Cardio-vascular	Lymph nodes, heart	Parkinson's disease
Endocrine	Adrenal glands, hypothalamus, pituitary, pineal gland	

Nerve innervations: 1st, 2nd, 3rd, 4th, 5th Cervical

See Chapter 26 for a description of disorders related to the Endocrine System. For hormones secreted by the ovaries and testes, *see* reflex point 39: Chapter 21, the Reproductive System.

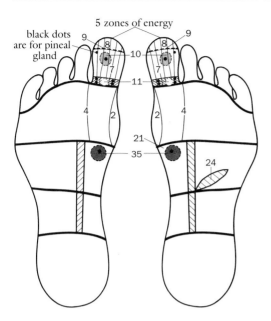

The endocrine system (both feet), reflex points 2, 4, 9, 10, 11, 21, 24 and 35. Refer to the Nervous System for brain reflex point.

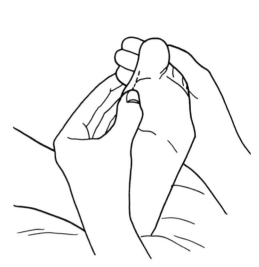

Hand position: the thymus gland, reflex point 2. Working hand over supporting hand. Refer to the Circulatory System.

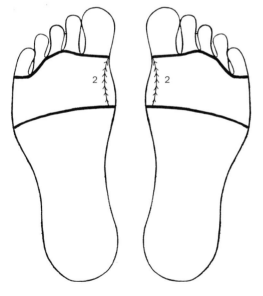

Directions for working: the thymus gland, reflex point 2 (both feet). Refer to the Circulatory System.

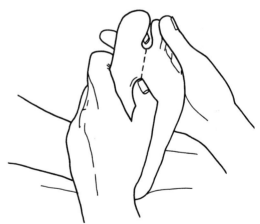

Hand position: for thyroid supporter gland, reflex point 4 (both feet). Working hand over supporting hand.

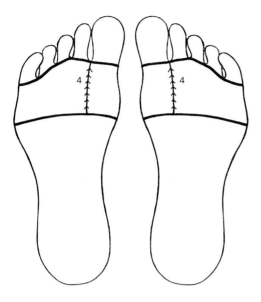

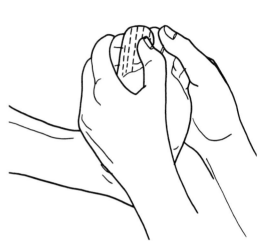

Directions for working: the thyroid supporter, reflex point 4 (both feet).

Hand position: zones of energy, reflex point 7 (both feet). Working hand over supporting hand.

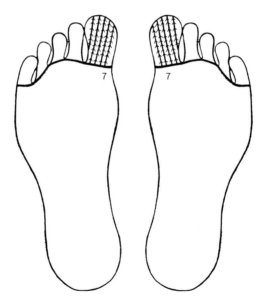

Directions for working: cranial zones of energy, reflex point 7 (both feet).

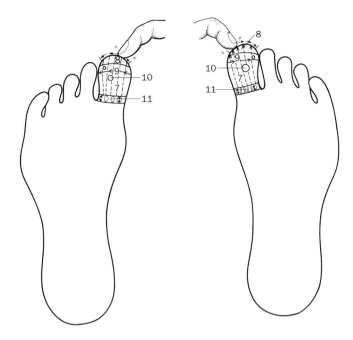

Directions for working: the brain, hypothalamus, pineal gland, pituitary gland, thyroid and parathyroids (both feet), reflex points 8, 9, 10 and 11. Refer to the Nervous System.

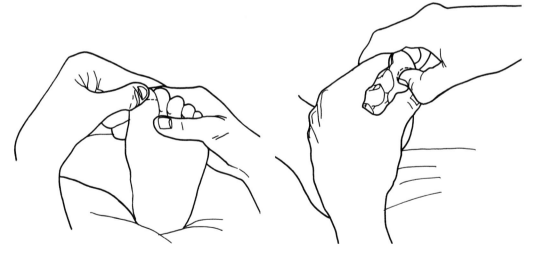

Hand position: the hypothalamus and pineal gland, reflex point 9 (both feet). Working hand over supporting hand.

Hand position: the pituitary gland, reflex point 10 (both feet). Working hand over supporting hand.

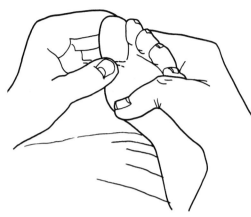

Hand position: the anatomical thyroid/ parathyroids, reflex point 11 (both feet). Working hand over supporting hand.

Hand position: the pancreas supporter, reflex point 21 (left foot only). Working hand over supporting hand.

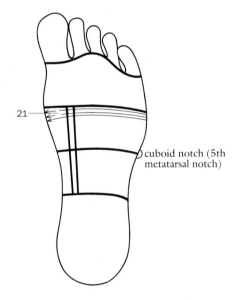

21

cuboid notch (5th metatarsal notch)

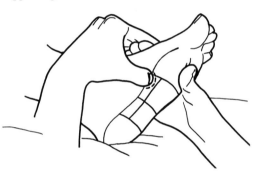

Hand position: massaging the adrenal gland, reflex point 35 (both feet). Working hand over supporting hand. Refer to the Urinary System.

Directions for working: the pancreas supporter, reflex point 21 (left foot only).

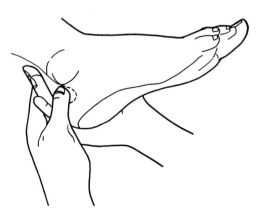

(Right) Hand position: the ovaries/testes, reflex point 39 (both feet). Working hand under supporting hand. Refer to the Reproductive System.

and pineal gland horizontally across the big toe, underneath the brain, with the thumb. Use the left hand when working the left foot and right hand when working the right foot.

Work the pituitary gland by holding your working hand fingers vertically over the supporting hand and use the hooking movement to work the puffy area of the big toe. Hook upwards and in towards the medial side of the body about eight to ten times. The left hand hooks the left foot and the right hand hooks the right foot. Alternatively, massage if this reflex is very tender.

Work the anatomical thyroid/parathyroid glands by massaging in rotating movements across the base of the big toe, from the lateral to the medial edge. Refer to the Urinary and Reproductive Systems for working the adrenal glands and ovaries and testes, and the Digestive System for working the pancreas and thymus gland.

CASE STUDIES WITH HORMONE IMBALANCE

Diabetes Mellitus

Some years ago, Jacky came for reflexology treatment because of diabetes mellitus. In classic style, she had developed the condition at the age of twelve years (early onset) and had been injecting insulin twice daily, which had embarrassed her as a teenager and interfered with her social and working life. At the age of twenty-four she decided to try complementary therapies as a way to improving her quality of life and she contacted me whilst I had a clinic at the local doctor's group practice.

I am always very nervous when beginning to treat a diabetic patient as the slightest overworking can cause hypoglycaemic symptoms when the pancreas knocks into action and begins to produce its own insulin. However,

no matter how gentle a treatment may be, even working on the hands as a substitute, Jacky still had several bouts of hypoglycaemic reaction after treatment. She always travelled prepared for an attack, carrying sweets, fruit and sweet drinks and we got into a routine of placing everything round her in case of a reaction during treatment! After several treatments, her symptoms began to decrease and by three months of weekly treatments, she proudly told me that her doctor had managed to reduce her insulin injections to one a day. We were both delighted at the news!

We continued weekly treatments, which were increasingly successful in stabilizing her, for a further three months until Jacky moved out of the area. I suggested she continued with her reflexology treatments and I hope that she has managed to stabilize and rely less on artificial amounts of insulin.

Word of warning: work extremely carefully with clients who suffer from diabetes mellitus, even if on oral medication. Reflexology is extremely powerful, especially when worked on the feet, and a diabetic patient's sugar levels are finely balanced and controlled by their insulin in-take. In the event of a continuous contraindication to treatment, work the hands or suggest an alternative complementary therapy which is less stimulating to the organs of the body.

Depression

Pam was a young girl in her late twenties who had suffered severe mood swings and depression, eventually experiencing the, literally, shocking form of treatment for severe depression called electroconvulsive therapy (ECT). This treatment had only succeeded in making her worse and she contacted me on recommendation by her twin sister.

It transpired throughout the consultation and first treatment that Pam was the second twin to be born and had always remained the 'weaker', mentally, emotionally and physically. When working her feet, which showed no pain at all in the first treatment session, I decided that most of her problems were psychological – her twin sister lived a stone's throw away from her and seemed to be a dominating influence. From the lack of sensitivity in her feet after receiving electric shock treatment, I began to build a picture of how Pam had felt 'un-alive', functioning but with no separate personality, mind or feelings of her own and how her feet accurately reflected how she felt, but was unaware of how she felt.

In the second treatment, Pam's feet were extremely sensitive and within minutes of working on her feet she began to sob uncontrollably. I held her feet, without working the reflexes to allow her time to release the pent-up feelings and emotions, which appeared to have been stored for years concerning her childhood and feeling in the shadow of her sister. Eventually she calmed herself and said that it was the first time she could remember when she had cried and released feelings she didn't know were there! I have found this a common experience when working the feet, that something happens through the feet which contacts the heart and feeling part of the person's psyche. Once in touch with these feelings, the wound can begin to heal.

I had also found every endocrine gland painful on Pam's feet and as the weeks went by the pain lessened, and after two months she laughed spontaneously for the first time. Up until then, it was as though she was stunned – not living and participating but on automatic pilot where nothing touched her.

Shortly after the two-month period, she went into counselling at my suggestion and made a 'new' relationship with her sister. Pam was convinced that her personality and perception of life events changed through stimulating the endocrine glands with reflexology, which encouraged her to begin a life for herself and not see herself in the shadow of her twin sister.

CHAPTER 19
The Digestive System

Overview of the Digestive System

Absorption of nutrients, production of heat and energy, and excretion of waste products.

Structures	*Functions*
THE ALIMENTARY CANAL	
Mouth and teeth	Teeth masticate and break down food; saliva begins breakdown of starch with the enzyme amylase
Pharynx (throat)	Assists in pushing masticated food (bolus) into the oesophagus
Epiglottis	Stops food entering the trachea (windpipe)
Oesophagus	Muscular tube that propels food towards the stomach
Stomach	Hormone gastrin stimulates pepsin, which breaks down protein with enzyme action; gastric juice contains hydrochloric acid which kills microbes, acidifies food, stops enzyme action and provides an acid environment for digestion
Small intestine	Intestinal juice completes breakdown of protein, fats and carbohydrates; protects against harmful organisms with lymphatic tissue; absorbs nutrients for transportation to the liver and fats into the lymphatic system
Portal circulation	Transports nutrients to the liver
Large colon	Produces vitamin K; reabsorbs water through the bowel wall, together with mineral salts and some drugs; manufactures healthy bacteria that synthesize folic acid; excretes waste products (faeces) from metabolic activity
ACCESSORY ORGANS	
Salivary glands	Produce the enzyme amylase that begins the breakdown of starch in the mouth; contains immunoglobulins that destroy harmful organisms
Liver	Processes nutrients for use in metabolic activities; stores useful substances; breaks down toxins and waste products; reorganizes useful substances; manufactures bile
Gall-bladder	Stores bile
Pancreas	Pancreatic juice contains the enzymes: trypsin (breaks down protein into amino acids); amylase (breaks down starch into sugar); lipase (breaks down lipids into glycerol and fatty acids)

LINKS TO: urinary, cardio-vascular, endocrine, nervous, muscular, skeletal/joints and integumentary systems.

INTRODUCTION

The function of the digestive system is to absorb nutrients from the external environment. Nutrients are needed for repair, growth, heat and energy. The respiratory system provides oxygen, which is a main source of energy needed for cell metabolism. The digestive system is divided into the alimentary canal and the accessory organs which aid in digestion without food passing through them. Digestion takes place in the gastro-intestinal tract (GI) which is a long tube capable of secretion, digestion, involuntary muscular action and movement (peristalsis), absorption, elimination and production of nutrients under the control of nerves, hormones and hormone-like compounds.

The process of digestion can be described as follows:

- **Mechanical digestion** involves breaking down of food by chewing, peristalsis and churning substances secreted in the digestive process. These reactions may alter the shape or composition of a given food.

- **Enzyme action** is the release of chemicals called enzymes, which are activated throughout the GI tract in the presence of food and which are involved in the breakdown of proteins, fats and carbohydrates into smaller chemical compounds.

Remember! Keep the thumb flexed or joint bent when working the reflexes, especially when massaging or hooking.

- **Chemical digestion** is the breakdown of food particles through the action of enzymes, acids and various substances secreted in the digestive process. These reactions may alter the shape or composition of a given food.

ALIMENTARY CANAL

The alimentary canal is approximately 10m (33ft) long and consists of:

- the mouth;
- the pharynx and epiglottis;
- the oesophagus;
- the stomach;
- the small intestine;
- the large colon, rectum and anus.

The alimentary canal is a long tube through which our food passes. It begins at the mouth and terminates at the anus, with the various parts given separate names although they are similar in structure. Various secretions are poured into the alimentary canal. Some secretions are made in the lining membrane of the organs, for example, gastric juice by the lining of the stomach, and some by glands situated outside the tract.

The organs of digestion and their secretions pass through ducts to enter the alimentary canal. The accessory organs consist of three pairs of salivary glands, the pancreas, the liver and the gall-bladder.

Process of Digestion Through The Alimentary Canal

Teeth and Mouth

When we eat food, we use our teeth and tongue. A child has twenty teeth (milk-teeth),

Fig 38. The digestive system.

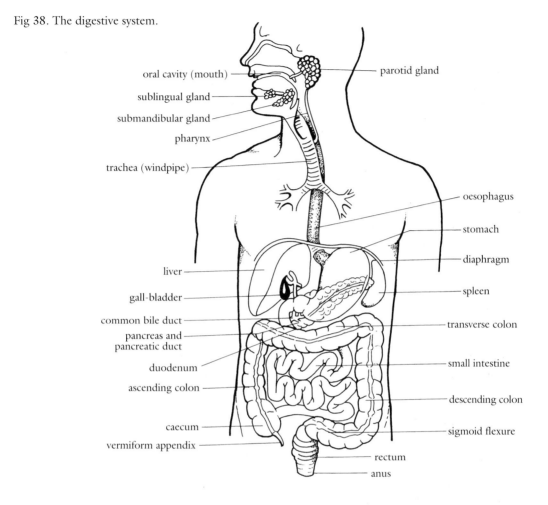

oral cavity (mouth)
sublingual gland
submandibular gland
pharynx
trachea (windpipe)

parotid gland

oesophagus
stomach
diaphragm

liver
gall-bladder
common bile duct
pancreas and
pancreatic duct
duodenum
ascending colon
caecum
vermiform appendix

spleen
transverse colon
small intestine
descending colon
sigmoid flexure
rectum
anus

and an adult has thirty-two. The incisors are for biting and the canines for biting harder, tougher food, and for tearing. The molars and premolars are for crushing and grinding. Tooth enamel is a very hard substance but can be broken if biting with undue pressure or by acid produced in the mouth as a result of bacterial action, which destroys the enamel, caused by food left between the teeth. These bacteria are very small organisms that live on the surface of teeth and in the crevices between them. Tooth decay can easily lead to gum disease.

After the food is chewed and broken down by the teeth, the tongue moves the food around to mix with saliva. This increases the size of the food, making it easier for enzyme action. Mucus in saliva sticks particles together and this reduces the food in size, making it easier to swallow. The pH (acid/alkaline balance) of the mouth is neutral to slightly alkaline.

The enzyme amylase in the saliva speeds up the breakdown of cooked starch to maltose. Water in the saliva softens the food so that amylase can flow around the food particles.

Saliva stimulates the taste buds on the tongue. Nerve impulses are sent to the stomach so that cells may start to produce digestive juices, in preparation of the digestive processes.

Food is pushed into a lump, called a bolus, and as the tongue quickly pushes it to the back of the mouth against the soft palate a swallowing action follows, pushing the bolus into the oesophagus.

Pharynx

The pharynx is a muscular tube that has several openings: the larynx, oesophagus, mouth, the nostrils and Eustachian tubes from the middle ear. These parts are involved in swallowing. Food passes from the mouth to the pharynx then to the oesophagus. When food reaches the pharynx, swallowing is no longer under voluntary control and food is conveyed into the oesophagus under peristalsis.

Epiglottis

The epiglottis automatically covers the entrance to the trachea (windpipe) when food is being swallowed. This action prevents food going into the trachea and produces a reflex action with choking if food enters the trachea whilst eating.

Oesophagus

The oesophagus is about 25cm (10in) long and about 2cm (⅞in) in diameter. Once food is swallowed, it enters the oesophagus and passes to the stomach. Alternate contraction and relaxation set up wave-like movements along the oesophagus, which pushes food downwards towards the stomach. This action is called peristalsis (muscular wave-like movements) and is found elsewhere in the body, for example, in the large bowel and small intestine.

Stomach

Once food has reached the end of the oesophagus it enters the stomach through the cardiac sphincter muscle. The functions of the stomach are to store food, to prepare it for absorption in the small intestine and to kill microbes. While the food is in the stomach its consistency is changed. A quantity of fluid in the form of gastric juice is secreted by churning movements of the muscular walls, which converts the mixture of food into a runny paste called chyme.

The wall of the stomach secretes highly acid (pH2) gastric juice. Food is mixed with the gastric juice and the process of digestion begins. Gastric juice contains mucus, rennin, which clots milk proteins, and pepsin. A hormone called gastrin stimulates the production of the gastric juice. Mucus is produced by special cells in the stomach lining called goblet cells, which allow easy movement of food and prevent enzymes and acid from damaging the stomach wall. The presence of hydrochloric acid stops the production of salivary amylase and stimulates the production of pepsin, an enzyme that breaks down protein and kills bacteria present in food. The only food digested in the stomach is protein, which is broken down into polypeptides and peptides. Chyme is pushed through the pyloric sphincter into the beginning part of the small intestine, called the duodenum. The hormone serotonin inhibits gastric secretion and stimulates involuntary muscle in the walls of the small intestine.

Small Intestine

The main function of the small intestine is to absorb nutrients into the bloodstream and lymphatic system. It is approximately 3–5m (10–16ft) in length and is longer than the large intestine, which is 1.2–1.5m (4–5ft) long. The small intestine is found mainly in the abdominal cavity, with the lower loops found in the pelvic cavity. Compared with the large colon, it is smaller in diameter. It begins at the pyloric sphincter, which leads from the stomach, and continues into the first section of the small intestine called the duodenum. The duodenum is about 25cm (10in) long and curves around the head of the pancreas. The jejunum is the middle part and is about 2m (6½ft) long. The final section is the ileum, which is about 3m (10ft) long and ends at the ileo-caecal valve. This valve controls the flow of waste from the ileum to the large intestine and prevents regurgitation (back flow) of waste into the small intestine.

Absorption of Nutrients After chyme has been released into the small intestine from the stomach, the absorption of nutrients takes place. The superior mesenteric artery feeds the small intestine, with the superior mesenteric vein joining other veins to form the large vein called the hepatic portal vein, which takes nutrient-rich blood to the liver. Finger-like processes called villi, present in the small intestine, are tiny antenna-like projections of about 0.5–1mm long. These villi absorb nutrients such as simple sugars, amino acids, some simple fatty acids and water. Intestinal juice consists of water, mucus and digestive enzymes, which work on proteins, reducing them to amino acids, and starch-reducing enzymes, which form simple sugars. Intestinal glands, which are tube-like structures found below the surface of the villi complete the digestion of carbohydrates, protein and fat.

Absorption of Fats Most fats are absorbed into the lymphatic system through the middle part of the villi in the small intestine, called a lacteal. Once in the lymphatic system, these substances are transported to the cisterna chyli where they are emptied into the left thoracic duct; they are then transported into the subclavian veins either side of the neck. At this point they enter the main circulation. Lymph fluid becomes milky white in appearance, due to the presence of fats. Once in the main circulation they are transported to the liver where the fats are processed.

Lymph Nodes There are numerous lymph nodes in the mucous membrane, which are scattered at irregular intervals throughout the length of the small intestine. The smaller nodes are known as solitary lymphatic follicles. The larger nodes are situated towards the further end of the ileum, and are known as Peyer's patches. Protection against infection by microbes that have survived the action of hydrochloric acid in the stomach are mostly destroyed by the lymphatic follicles in the small intestine.

Large Colon

The large intestine is about 1.5m (5ft) long, beginning at the caecum on the right side of the body and terminating at the rectum and anal canal. When waste matter enters the first part of the large intestine it contains mucus, dead cells from the lining of the gut, bile pigments and a large amount of water. Even though the absorption of water takes place in the large intestine, it still makes up about 60–70 per cent of the weight of the faeces, which provides a semi-solid consistency to ease its passage through the colon and anus. As the waste is pushed along the colon by peristaltic action, most of the water is reabsorbed into the bloodstream. The body would become dehydrated very quickly if this reabsorption did not take place.

Roughage is important because it helps the intestine to move the contents along and absorbs water, keeping the faeces soft and bulky. If the diet is low in fibre, constipation may become a problem causing the wall of the intestine to thicken. After a period of time little pockets called diverticula, which cover the surface of the intestine, begin to bulge at the weak areas.

Although enzymes are not produced in the colon, there are many bacteria, that feed on undigested material, which are thought to be responsible for releasing vitamin K (essential for the production of the blood protein involved in blood clotting, called prothrombin) and some B vitamins. The bacteria living in the colon do not harm the body but help to keep us healthy.

In the presence of dead and living microbes, epithelial cells from the walls of the tract, fatty acids, an adequate amount of roughage, and water and mucus secreted by the mucosa, lubrication of the faeces takes place. With a combination of peristaltic action and bulk, the contents of the colon can be stimulated to defecate.

As well as vitamin K, microbes synthesize folic acid, mineral salts and some drugs, which are absorbed into the blood capillaries. The red cell pigment broken down from erythrocytes gives the faeces a brown colour.

The caecum is the broadest part of the large intestine and becomes the ascending colon until it reaches the base of the liver at the hepatic flexure (or bend), where it becomes the transverse colon. It crosses the waistline where it turns sharply left under the spleen (called the splenic flexure or bend) becoming the descending colon. The sigmoid flexure, or colon, is where most constipation and bowel problems begin and which resembles the 'U-bend' under the kitchen sink, where waste accumulates. The sigmoid flexure leads to the rectum and anal canal. Once the rectum is distended a nerve impulse produces the urge to defecate.

Accessory Organs

Salivary Glands

There are three pairs of salivary glands, which secrete their contents into the mouth. There are two parotid, two submandibular and two sublingual. The parotid glands are situated one on each side of the face, just below the ear. The submandibular glands lie on each side of the face, under the jaw. These ducts open onto the floor of the mouth, one on each side of the tongue. The sublingual glands lie under the mucous membrane on the floor of the mouth in front of the submandibular glands. They have numerous small ducts on the floor of the mouth.

Functions of Saliva Secretions from the salivary glands are poured into the ducts by secretory cells, which join up to form larger ducts that lead into the mouth. Saliva consists of water, mineral salts, enzymes (salivary amylase), ptyalin and mucus. The functions of saliva are to:

- provide enzymes that will act on cooked starches;
- lubricate food;
- cleanse and lubricate the mouth;
- stimulate taste buds by particles of food, which are dissolved in water.

Pancreas

The pancreas weighs about 60g (2½oz) and is about 12–15cm (5–6in) long. Like the spleen, it lies behind the stomach. The pancreas is attached to the spleen at its tail and is encased in the duodenum at its head. The structure of the pancreas consists of a large number of lobules made up of small alveoli, which consist of secretory cells. Each lobule is drained by a tiny duct and these unite to form the pancreatic duct, which extends the whole length of the

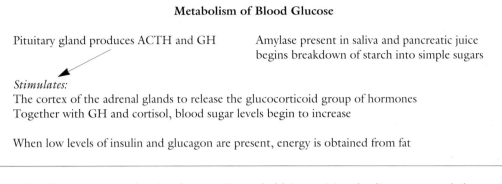

gland and opens into the duodenum. Just before entering the duodenum, the pancreatic duct joins the common bile duct.

Pancreatic juice is an alkali, composed of bicarbonate, water and mineral salts, which neutralizes the highly acidic chyme secreted by the stomach into the duodenum. Pancreatic juice is stimulated by hormones secreted by the cells in the intestinal wall. The pancreas is a dual functioning organ and gland:

- It releases hormones insulin and glucagon as an endocrine gland (*see* Chapter 18 for function of hormones).
- It provides pancreatic juice which contains enzymes, which digest carbohydrates, proteins and fats as an exocrine organ.

The action of enzymes released in pancreatic juice and released through the pancreatic duct into the duodenum have the following functions:

- **trypsin** breaks down proteins into peptides;
- **lipase** breaks down fatty lipids to fatty acids;
- **glycerol** and **amylase** break down starch to maltose.

Liver

The liver is the largest organ in the body, weighing between 1 and 2.3kg (2–5lb). It is held in position by ligaments and the pressure of organs in the abdominal cavity. It has four lobes, the two most obvious are the large right lobe and the smaller left lobe. The hepatic portal vein enters the liver carrying blood from the stomach, spleen, pancreas and small and large intestines and is fed by a blood supply from the hepatic artery. Approximately 1.7 litres (3 pints) of blood enter the liver every minute. The liver is an extremely important organ and some of its functions are listed below.

- It stores glucose as glycogen by action of the hormone insulin and converts glycogen to glucose by activation of the hormone glucagon.
- It breaks down (deaminates) amino acids by removing the nitrogenous portion forming urea, and it breaks down the worn-out cells of the body to form uric acid, both of which are excreted in urine.
- The liver requires a considerable amount of energy and, as a result of a high metabolic rate, it produces a great deal of heat and is the main heat producing organ of the body.
- It desaturates fats, for example, it converts stored fats into a form that can be used to provide energy.
- It manufactures bile. The liver cells synthesize the constituents of bile from the mixed

arterial and venous blood. These constituents include bile salts, bile pigments, water and cholesterol, which together provide an alkaline substance required in the duodenum with which to neutralize the high acid content of chyme and begin the breakdown of fats.

- It synthesizes vitamin A from carotene, which is found in carrots and green leaf vegetables.
- It detoxifies drugs and alcohol by removing ethanol.
- It stores vitamin B12, and the fat-soluble vitamins A, D, E and K
- It stores iron.
- It produces plasma proteins, which are mostly concerned with blood-clotting factors.
- It deactivates hormones, including insulin, glucagon, cortisol, aldosterone, thyroxine and the sex hormones.
- It produces red blood cells in foetal life (along with the spleen).

Gall-Bladder

The common bile duct is about 7.5cm (3in) long. The gall-bladder is a pear-shaped sac attached to the surface of the liver by connective tissue. The function of the gall-bladder is to act as a reservoir for bile, formed in the liver. The lining membrane adds mucus to bile and absorbs water, which makes bile more concentrated. When the muscular walls of the gall-bladder contract, bile is squeezed out and passed through the bile duct into the duodenum. Along with the acidity and fats present in the chyme hormones secreted by the duodenum stimulate the gall-bladder to contract. Bile flow is approximately 1 litre (1.8 pints) per day. Contraction of the gall-bladder in the presence of fat is under the influence of the hormone cholecystokinin (CCK).

Fats are broken down into small droplets in the presence of bile so that they can be absorbed through the intestinal wall more easily. Humans can live without a gall-bladder. The liver compensates for the storage of bile by continually producing and transporting it to the duodenal area. The amount of bile produced is dependent on the amount of fat eaten. Those who have the gall-bladder removed are usually put onto low-fat diets in order to reduce the amount of contraction by the gall-bladder prior to removal. The liver is allowed to rest after removal of the gall-bladder by encouraging patients to watch the amount of fat in the diet.

The bile pigment, called bilirubin, is the breakdown product of red blood cells (erythrocytes). It is yellow in colour, giving a yellow tint to bile and urine. If the body produces too much bilirubin the patient appears yellow, or jaundiced, in colour. As it becomes altered by microbes in the small intestine, some urobilin is reabsorbed and secreted in urine and the remainder, called stercobilin, is excreted in the faeces. The red pigment in stercobilin gives the dark colour normally associated with faeces.

As well as absorption of digested fats in the small intestine, the presence of bile is needed for absorption of vitamin K. Bile also deodorizes and colours faeces.

NUTRITION

Needs of Cells

The cells of the body require energy to carry out their metabolic processes including:

- multiplication of cells for replacement of worn-out cells;
- contraction of muscle fibres;
- synthesis of secretions produced by the cells of glands;

- oxidation of carbohydrate and fats, which provide most of the energy required by the body.

Some energy can be provided by glucose in the absence of any oxygen. This is known as an anaerobic process, where energy from the glucose molecule is not released immediately. This can only be maintained for a limited period, such as when participating in some sports where a sudden spurt of activity can be sustained over just a very short period of time. The end-products of fat metabolism are energy, heat, carbon dioxide and water.

The body requires the essential nutrients of protein, carbohydrate, fats, water, fibre, vitamins, minerals and oxygen in order to remain healthy and to provide heat and energy. Functions of vitamins, minerals, fibre, proteins, carbohydrates and fats are described as follows (for the functions of oxygen *see* Chapter 16, The Respiratory System, and for the functions of water, *see* Chapter 20, The Urinary System).

Minerals

Minerals are required in cell metabolism. Their functions are:

- cell formation;
- contraction of muscles;
- transmission of nerve impulses;
- formation of secretions;
- maintenance of balance between acid and alkaline.

A detailed breakdown of the essential minerals and their functions is given in the table overleaf. Trace elements are needed in very small amounts and include zinc, copper, fluorine and iron.

Vitamins

Vitamins enable certain chemical reactions to take place more quickly. There are two broad bands of vitamins: the fat-soluble vitamins A, D, E and K, which are found in lipids and can be stored in the liver; and the water-soluble vitamins B and C which need to be replaced each day. The functions of vitamins are:

- production of antibodies;
- formation of red blood cells;
- development and maintenance of bone;
- maintenance of blood capillary walls.

A detailed breakdown of vitamins and their functions is given in the table overleaf.

Carbohydrates

- Provide heat and energy.
- Converted into fat if eaten in excess.
- Saves depletion of protein as an energy source.

Protein

Proteins are broken down into essential and non-essential amino acids (*see* below). Their functions are as follows:

- Growth and repair of body cells and tissues;
- Provide energy as a secondary function when carbohydrate and fat stores are depleted;
- Required in the synthesis of enzymes, plasma proteins, antibodies and hormones.

Amino Acids

Proteins are made from small units of amino acids and contain carbon, hydrogen, nitrogen, and oxygen. There are twenty different types of amino acids: eight essential amino

Minerals: Their Source and Functions

Mineral	Source	Function
Calcium	Milk, cheese, eggs, dark green vegetables, soya beans, sesame seeds, fish, meat, blackstrap molasses	Needed for good bone and teeth structure, muscle contraction and blood clotting
Chlorine	Salt, cheese, eggs, meat, milk, butter, margarine	Contained in gastric juice and tissue fluids, including blood
Cobalt	Animal produce	Part of vitamin B12; involved in blood cell production and in synthesis of insulin; deficiency causes pernicious anaemia
Copper	Nuts, pulses, liver, fish, oysters	Formation of haemoglobin; absorption and oxidation of vitamin C and iron; deficiency causes anaemia
Fluorine	Added to some drinking water	Needed for strong enamel on teeth, aids the deposition of calcium in bone
Iodine	Water, iodized salt, wide range of foods	Forms part of thyroxine (a hormone which controls metabolic rate)
Iron	Eggs, meat, spinach, dark green vegetables, chick peas, black beans, soya beans, wheat-germ, oatmeal, potatoes	Forms part of haemoglobin (molecule which combines with oxygen and transports it around the body)
Magnesium	Green vegetables, grains	Enzyme reaction and carbohydrate metabolism; deficiency causes vaso-dilation, arrhythmia and spasticity
Manganese	Green leafy vegetables, nuts, pulses, cereals	Action involved in phosphorus and calcium; deficiency causes reproductive disorders
Phosphorus	Milk, peas, meat, fish, eggs, cottage cheese, almonds, wheat-germ, soya beans, pinto and black beans	Needed for good bone and teeth structure, and for muscle contraction
Potassium	Spinach, butter beans, raisins, prunes, oranges, milk, peas, brussel sprouts	Takes part in transmission of nervous impulses, and in chemical reactions inside cells
Sodium	As for chlorine	Part of tissue fluids, including blood; takes part in kidney functioning and transmission of nerve impulses
Zinc	A variety of foods	Present in enzymes; needed for transport of carbon dioxide and energy metabolism; it is thought to be involved in diabetes and alopecia

Vitamins: Their Source, Function and Effect of Deficiency

Vitamin	Source	Function	Deficiency
A	Milk, butter, egg yolk, fish-liver oils, liver, carrots, fresh green vegetables	Allows vision in dim light, maintains healthy skin	Poor vision in dim light, skin and cornea of eyes become dry, increased susceptibility to disease
B complex	Whole cereal grains, wholemeal bread, yeast, liver, egg yolk, peas, beans, fresh green vegetables, milk, nuts, cheese	Helps to release energy from food, and chemical reactions in cells	Functioning of the nervous system and digestive system is disrupted, skin and mucous membranes are affected
B12	Only found in animal products and in yeast extract	Involved in the development of red blood cells	Pernicious anaemia
C	Citrus fruits, tomatoes, potatoes, fresh green vegetables, rosehips	Involved in making connective tissue, also involved in respiration and pigment metabolism	Scurvy, bleeding under the skin and in the joints, bleeding gums, poor healing of wounds, irritability, loss of appetite and weight
D	Milk, eggs, butter, fish-liver oils, sitting in the sun	Enables calcium to be absorbed and promotes its deposition in bones and teeth	Rickets (softening and deformation of bones)
E	Seeds and green leaves, peanuts, lettuce, egg yolk, wheat-germ, whole cereal, milk, butter	Normally present in vegetable oils; its function is uncertain in humans	Occurs in severe malnutrition; may cause anaemia and failure to reproduce, muscle wasting or miscarriage
K	Foods containing lipids (bacteria in the bowel can make this vitamin)	Involved in the formation of prothrombin in the liver (prothrombin is involved in the clotting of the blood)	Bleeding under the skin; blood will not clot
Pantothenic acid	Eggs, liver, yeast	Essential for normal growth	Poor wound healing; lack of coordination; insomnia

acids, which must be ingested through food, and twelve non-essential amino acids, which can be synthesized in the body. The functions of amino acids are to:

- synthesize hormones, enzymes, plasma proteins and antibodies (immunoglobulins);
- synthesize new cells;
- provide growth and repair of body tissue and cells;
- provide energy if insufficient carbohydrate is present and fat stores depleted.

Excess amino acids cannot be stored in the body and are broken down in the liver by a process called deamination. Nitrogen is released and secreted as urea, a constituent of urine. The remainder is converted to fat for storage under the skin and used to provide energy and heat. Amino acids present in the liver form albumin, globulin, prothrombin, thrombin and fibrinogen.

Enzymes

Enzymes are proteins and are essential in aiding cells to break down (catabolism) and build up activities (anabolism) in the cell. Enzymes are unique shapes – like one key for one lock – and are produced by living cells. Some function outside the cell (extracellular), as in the digestive system, but most function within the cell (intracellular). Enzymes speed up the rate of a reaction but are not used up during the process. Enzymes require water in order to function and they work within a narrow range of acidity or alkalinity, dependent on where they are in the body.

Function of Fibre

- Provide bulk in faeces, easing defecation and lessening the risk of bowel disorders.

Lipids

Lipids (fats) are used as a source of energy and heat and are stored as adipose tissue (fat) under the skin and around organs. Lipids are involved in providing a surface membrane for cells. Fat cells release a hormone called leptin which travels to the hypothalamus (a part of the brain) to act as an appetite suppressant. A lack of this hormone can result in obesity as a dysfunction of appetite control.

Fats are divided into two groups: animal and vegetable. Animal fat contains mainly saturated fatty acids and glycerol; it is found in eggs, butter, cheese, milk, meat and oily fish. Vegetable fats contain unsaturated fatty acids and glycerol and are found in vegetable oils and margarine. Their functions are as follows:

- provide heat and energy;
- stored in fat depots when eaten in excess;
- transport fat-soluble vitamins A, D, E, and K;
- support and protect some organs in the body, for example, the kidneys and eyes;
- present in nerve sheaths and secretions of sebaceous glands found in the skin;
- required in the formation of steroids (hormones) and cholesterol.

Appetite, Hunger and Taste

Appetite is stimulated by social company and the sight, smell, colour, texture and presentation of food. The special senses are therefore involved in how we perceive food. A part of the brain called the hypothalamus controls appetite and the metabolism of food. They are influenced by the hormone leptin which is released by fat cells. It is transported to the hypothalamus where it acts as a tap by turning off the desire for food when we feel satiated. A lack of leptin has been found to lead to uncontrollable hunger and obesity and is thought to reduce blood sugar levels in diabetes mellitus. Other hormones linked to satiety include insulin and glucagon, released by the pancreas following a meal, and cholecystokinin (CCK), bombesin and somatostatin, which are released by the small intestine. Numerous neurotransmitters (substances which transmit the action of a nerve to cells), such as CCK, opioids, serotonin and adrenocorticotrophic releasing hormone (ACTH) also influence the feeling of satiation after eating a meal.

The sense of taste is perceived by receptors in the tongue and carried by nerves to the brain. Substances tasted in solution stimulate taste buds; hence eating an hors-d'oeuvre stimulates taste buds and the desire for more food. Different tastes can stimulate the feeling of hunger and the desire for a variety of foods. When we have a head cold, our sense of smell and taste are diminished and we lose our appetite. There are four basic taste buds, which are located on the tongue as follows:

- Sweet – at the tip of the tongue;
- Sour – at the sides of the tongue;
- Salty – towards the front sides of the tongue;
- Bitter – the back part of the tongue.

SPECIAL INTEREST

Teeth Sensitivity

I have found that the molars and pre-molars are sensitive at the base between the 2nd, 3rd and 4th toes, with the wisdom teeth found under the little toe (back of the jaw) and the incisors and front teeth found towards the medial edge of the neck/teeth reflexes. This is logical if we relate the lateral edge of the foot to the back of the jaw and the medial side of the foot to the middle of the body. Sensi-

tivity along these reflexes can also relate to ulcers in the mouth and throat.

Enteric Fevers

Meat may be contaminated at any stage between slaughter and the consumer. Outbreaks of food poisoning are associated with large-scale cooking. If food is not adequately reheated the microbes that have multiplied will not have been killed. After being eaten, the microbes that remain vegetative die and release endotoxins that cause gastroenteritis.

Acid Formation and the Stress Triangle

As most of us have experienced at some time in our lives, stress can affect our appetite and digestive processes. When tension is present in the solar plexus ganglia of nerves, the digestive organs are affected by constriction of the stomach, oesophagus, pancreatic duct and duodenum. The stomach produces excessive amounts of acid (hydrochloric acid) and with

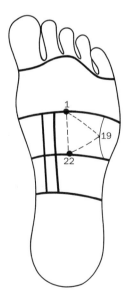

Fig 39. The stress triangle.

the constriction surrounding the pancreatic duct, which diminishes the amount of alkalinizing pancreatic juice, indigestion and the more serious problem of gastric and duodenal ulcers can develop. Specific attention can be given to this area, which begins at the solar plexus reflex point with tension, and which should be worked frequently throughout the treatment.

As the stomach becomes affected by tension and releases high levels of hydrochloric acid the stomach should be the next reflex to be worked frequently throughout the treatment.

The next reflex to be worked is the duodenum (on the waistline) and then the oesophagus supporter, both of which should be worked frequently throughout the treatment.

Thus, a triangle is formed – a vicious circle, which can increase in severity until either gastric (in the stomach) or duodenal ulcers form.

I have found that patients who suffer from a hiatus hernia present a painful anatomical oesophageal reflex point in addition to the above reflexes, and heart-burn and indigestion sufferers present sensitivity towards the top of the oesophagus supporter reflex. Those patients suffering from gastric or duodenal ulcers have presented extreme sensitivity around the duodenal reflex, lower stomach reflexes (towards the waistline and in close proximity to the duodenal reflex) and the lower oesophagus supporter area. To check for acid formation in joints, work all of the above reflexes, and the cuboid notch reflex point, for 'all joints', which can indicate acid present in the joints anywhere in the body.

Eating patterns and habits affect the digestive processes and can be exacerbated by:

- eating whilst unrelaxed, as in standing, driving or walking;
- rushed and irregular meals;
- an excess of rich food;
- an excess of alcohol whilst eating;

- eating too fast or too frequently;
- not chewing food adequately;
- strenuous activity too soon after eating;
- eating late at night, especially with increasing age;
- eating too much;
- drinking too much liquid whilst eating.

A balanced diet consisting of plenty of fresh fruit and vegetables provides vitamin C to strengthen the immune system and aids in the defence against heart disease, cancer and infections and provides a source of fibre in the large bowel.

Organically grown food stuffs do not undergo unnatural processes and are therefore preferable to include in the diet. Irradiation, intensive farming, genetic engineering, precooking, lengthy storage, refining, additives, hormones, artificial colourings and sweeteners, waxing and unnatural animal feed deplete food of essential nutrients and may cause physical symptoms in the body as a result of consumption over a period of time.

In our modern-day living, refined foods are the easy answer to preparing meals. Unfortunately, they are also high in additives, colourings and preservatives, such as sugar and salt, which can have the following effects:

- high calorie intake with low nutritional value;
- a deficiency in vitamin and minerals and those stored in the body as they are used to process refined foods;
- lack of high fibre necessary for the passage of faeces through the large colon;
- refined, processed and dairy produce create excess mucus, which coats the bowel with a hard covering leading to constipation and other bowel disorders;
- stress on the body to process foods that have lost their natural nutritional value;
- excessive amounts of sugar can lead to

hyper/hypoglycaemia and eventually to diabetes mellitus;

• tooth decay from excess sugar.

Candida albicans can be exacerbated by eating refined foods that contain preservatives, sugar and salt, which may be precursors to digestive and related conditions as important nutrients are lost in processing. Research has shown that sugar can cause or contribute to the following symptoms and conditions:

• contribute to diabetes;
• cause arthritis;
• cause asthma;
• cause candidiasis (yeast infection);
• cause ischaemic heart disease;
• cause appendicitis;
• lead to periodontal disease;
• promote tooth decay;
• cause increased acid in the stomach;
• raise adrenalin levels in children;
• suppress the immune system;
• upset the body's mineral balance;
• cause hyperactivity, anxiety, concentration difficulties, decreased interest and activity, aggression and mood swings in children, all of which affect learning;
• contribute to a weakened defence against bacterial infection;
• cause kidney damage and lead to the formation of kidney stones;
• reduce helpful high-density lipoproteins (HDLs);
• promote an elevation of harmful low-density lipoproteins (LDLs);
• may lead to chromium deficiency;
• cause copper deficiency;
• interfere with absorption of calcium and magnesium;
• may lead to cancer of the breast, ovaries, prostate and rectum;
• cause colon cancer, with an increased risk in women;

• be a factor in gall-bladder cancer;
• increase fasting levels of glucose;
• affect eyesight;
• raises the level of a neurotransmitter called serotonin, which can narrow blood vessels;
• cause hypoglycaemia;
• malabsorption is common in those with functional bowel disease;
• speed up the ageing process, causing wrinkles and grey hair;
• contribute to weight gain and obesity;
• high intake increases the risk of Crohn's disease and ulcerative cells;
• cause a raw inflamed intestinal tract in those with gastric or duodenal ulcers;
• lead to the formation of gallstones;
• exacerbate the symptoms of multiple sclerosis;
• indirectly cause haemorrhoids;
• cause varicose veins;
• elevate glucose and insulin responses in oral contraception users;
• contribute to osteoporosis;
• contributes to saliva acidity;
• cause a decrease in insulin sensitivity;
• leads to a decreased glucose tolerance;
• decrease growth hormone;
• increase cholesterol levels in the blood;
• increase systolic blood pressure;
• change the structure of protein, causing interference with protein absorption;
• cause food allergies.

Arthritis can be aggravated by phosphates, such as in soda pop, which interferes with the absorption of calcium, thus promoting arthritis and osteoporosis. Magnesium and vitamin C have been found to aid arthritis.

Transverse Colon, Descending Colon, Sigmoid Flexure and Rectal Area

Stress can affect the colon in different ways, depending on heredity factors and our emotional response to life events. Due to the sedentary life-styles most of us lead with driving cars instead of walking, bowel problems and spinal problems are only too common for the reflexologist. Working these reflexes as thoroughly as possible on constipated patients aids good evacuation of the bowel, lessens pressure on the spinal innervations and vertebrae and lightens the mood! However, caution should be applied when working with the reverse problem as your patient may find that they have more of a problem than before treatment!

Remember that the sigmoid flexure is a deeply embedded indentation and will need to be searched for. The descending and ascending colon are the widest parts of the large colon and to ensure that all of the possibilities of a distended bowel have been worked, we work the three pathways thoroughly into the middle of the foot.

Conditions such as diverticulitis distend the bowel and bloat the stomach by retaining water that would normally be reabsorbed back through the bowel wall into the bloodstream. I have found a faulty ileo-caecal valve with this condition and, in extreme cases, have found the diverticula to be affected on the ascending colon reflexes on the right foot and thus the right side of the body.

The splenic flexure (which means the bend under the spleen into the descending colon) on the left foot can indicate irritable bowel syndrome (IBS) or a 'nervy tummy', which may be upset through emotional tension, causing loose and watery stool movements of the bowel. Generally, I have found that if sensitivity persists into the descending colon then an irritable bowel is the most likely problem, which the patient will verify if that is the case. Sensitivity of the reflexes can continue into the sigmoid flexure and rectal and anal area, due to alternating periods of constipation and diarrhoea-like symptoms. Encourage patients who suffer from this condition to eat – sitting down

– regular meals and to learn how to relax and deal with their stress levels effectively.

With some bowel problems, there will be deeply held unconscious insecurities that have become locked into the sacral area. With chronic conditions, encourage your patients to try body therapies such as biodynamic massage, body psychotherapy or rolfing to release the memories of the origins of insecurities.

The sigmoid flexure is like the U-bend under the sink – it can get blocked easily and so is a common site for constipation. We finish working down all three pathways on the descending colon so that faeces move with the direction of gravity – expelling waste out of the body towards the ground. On the right foot and ascending colon we work in an upwards direction only as we aim to assist the movement of waste against gravity and across the transverse colon on the waistline. The hepatic flexure (pertaining to the liver) is the bend from the ascending colon into the transverse colon on the right foot.

The rectal area will show conditions associated with the rectum, such as haemorrhoids, fissures and polyps. There are no secrets with reflexology! Elderly patients may show embarrassment when discussing personal problems of this nature and so be diplomatic and sensitive to how you phrase your questions to check if they are conscious of any past or present problems in that area. The Achilles tendon up the back of the ankle is a supportive area to the rectal reflex and should be worked when giving a massage with cream on the foot by stroking from the calf towards the base of the heel.

Pelvic Extension

We can understand that people's bodies are not text-book-shaped by simply observing individual variations in height and width; thus, organs and glands vary in position with each person. When there is undue pressure from the digestive organs onto the intestine and large colon, through lack of exercise or invalidism where it is impossible for the patient to exercise the abdominal muscles, the muscle tone becomes lax in the pelvic cavity, resulting in a spastic colon and chronic bowel conditions such as constipation and diverticulitis. This results in the large colon dropping down into the top of the thigh. The natural position for the sigmoid colon is just below the bikini line on the legs – think where the anus is and draw an imaginary line round the buttocks onto the leg to see where the lower part of the colon sits in the body. With this in mind, we can work the heel area as a possible extension of the large colon.

Ileo-Caecal Valve (ICV)

This important valve is the origin of all bowel disorders. A faulty valve that becomes 'stuck', either closed or open, can create chronic constipation when closed or infective conditions when waste from the last part of the small intestine moves backwards and forwards between the valve and caecum (beginning of the large colon). Appendicitis is commonly caused by a build-up of faeces in the blind-end tube of the appendix caused by a faulty ICV. It is also connected with mucus build-up in the body and so all lymphatic and mucus-related organs should be worked in conjunction with the ICV. This reflex is a deeply embedded indentation and in some cases considerable pressure may need to be applied to find the reflex.

The Small Intestine and Common Food Allergies

If more serious conditions exist, such as Crohn's disease, work the reflexes diagonally from the heel line to the waistline, from the medial edge of the foot and the lateral. The food allergy line across the heel can indicate allergies to certain foods, including colourings and additives. The small intestine becomes inflamed when a food allergy is present and so it is probably no coincidence that tenderness across the lower part of this area reflects this problem. The best way of finding out what you may be allergic to is to have an allergy test and then to be guided by a nutritionist in eliminating the sensitivity from the digestive tract.

Work these reflexes deeply and recommend that your patient has an allergy test and advice from a nutritionist, with, possibly, hair analysis for mineral imbalances. The most common cause of mucus build-up in the body is an allergy to dairy produce. The ICV is a key reflex to work for all mucus-related conditions and abstinence from the intake of dairy produce altogether is highly recommended. Without the irritation to the mucous membranes and regular reflexology treatments, patients should find good relief from symptoms within a month of beginning the treatments. More chronic conditions may take longer to have an effect.

If your patient will not give up dairy produce altogether, recommend that they change to soya milk and milk products, or sheep's yoghurt (the nearest to human milk) or goat's milk. Allergies to gluten, found in wheat and yeast, are also common and recommendations are for gluten- and yeast-free products, such as soda and rye bread.

Working the Pancreas and Diabetes Mellitus

Care must be taken when working the pancreas supporter and anatomical reflex point with those who are hypoglycaemic or insulin or non-insulin dependent diabetics. Over-stimulation of the reflexes could result in a hypoglycaemic coma. Work these reflexes lightly with those who have these disorders, and have sweet drinks or sweets available if symptoms of low blood sugar become apparent.

Remember that the presence of hypo- and hyperglycaemia do not necessarily mean that diabetes is present. Both conditions can be present when a person starves themselves of either carbohydrate, fats or protein, thus creating hypoglycaemia. Cravings for refined sugar products heightens the blood glucose levels for a short while, creating hyperglycaemia, but then plummet a few hours later and the cycle begins over again. Excessive amounts of sugar are required to keep energy levels constant until, in the end, the pancreas may give up trying to keep pace with the insulin levels required and diabetes mellitus develops. Remember, chocolate is addictive as it contains caffeine (present in cocoa) and sensitivity to milk products may produce excessive amounts of mucus in the body.

Eventually, fainting and coma are the ultimate consequences of becoming a sugar addict. Suggest to the patient that they replace all refined sugar products with fresh fruit and vegetables and if they must have sweeteners in their drinks and food to use fructose, which is found in sweet fruits. Diabetes mellitus can be connected to high blood cholesterol levels (see below). Refined sugar is highly acidic and is thought to be connected with the development of joint-related problems, such as rheumatoid arthritis, as well general acid-related disorders.

Caffeine is a toxic substance and can have immunosuppressive effects on the lymphatic system. When taken orally it can cause the following symptoms and exacerbate existing disorders:

- adverse effects on digestive, urinary, circulatory and pancreatic processes;
- anxiety, nervousness and irritability;
- disturbed sleep patterns;
- as a diuretic, it can irritate the bladder and become a precursor to cystitis through the sympathetic nervous system, if taken in excess;
- excess stimulation to the nervous system can lead to fatigue;
- coffee can rob vital vitamins and minerals in the body, such as vitamin B1, and cause excess excretion of calcium and increase the risk of degenerative bone diseases, such as osteoporosis;
- coffee can increase cholesterol levels;
- an increased risk of precancerous breast disease, bladder and kidney cancers;
- an increase in the metabolic rate, which creates increased stress levels;
- inflammatory conditions may become exacerbated;
- it is a major migraine trigger;
- caffeine is addictive and can cause withdrawal symptoms.

Addiction to crisps, caffeine, chocolate and some varieties of soft drinks, which are high in caffeine and which give the effects of living on a 'high', if eaten without an adequately balanced diet, can result in immune-related disorders such as glandular fever, which is common in adolescents.

Refer to Chapter 18, The Endocrine System, for information on sugar-related problems.

The Liver and Cholesterol Levels

The liver manufactures cholesterol, which is naturally present in the blood and has several functions. Cholesterol is a waxy substance derived from animal and vegetable tissue and which resembles the steroid group of hormones. It is needed in the manufacture of the sex hormones, the hormones of the adrenal cortex and the repair of membranes and bile acids. It is found throughout the body, especially in the brain, nervous tissue, adrenal glands and skin. Blood cholesterol levels are considered to be high if over 6mmol/l of blood as there appears to be a correlation between high blood cholesterol and atheroma (fatty deposits) in the blood vessels and heart. There is a link with diabetes mellitus and myxoedema (under-active thyroid gland), where there is a high blood cholesterol present. This gives rise to arterial degenerative diseases, including coronary thrombosis and high blood pressure. It has been found that saturated fatty acids raise blood cholesterol levels, and unsaturated fatty acids lower it. Saturated fats include animal fats and unsaturated include vegetable oils, such as olive oil, corn oil and sunflower oil. If your patient has a diet rich in saturated fats, recommend to him or her that they change to unsaturated fats.

When working the feet, sensitivity on the liver and adrenal gland reflexes can indicate blood cholesterol levels that may be too high or on the low side. Secondary sensitivity may appear with all endocrine gland reflexes, which may also be connected with atheroma formation. Remember, never tell your patient that they have such-and-such a problem, just gently suggest that it may be a good idea to have a cholesterol check as your findings on the feet indicate a possible imbalance in that area. Remember that the gall-bladder is an indentation and will need to be searched for and worked gently if digestive problems exist.

WORKING THE REFLEXES

Oesophagus, Stomach, Spleen, Pancreas – Reflex Points 3, 19, 20, 21 & 24 – Digestive, Lymphatic and Endocrine Systems

Find the top of the cuboid bone, or 5th metatarsal notch, for the waistline and draw an imaginary line across the foot to the medial edge of the foot. Find the lateral edge of the plantar tendon and in the square formed by the tendon line, waistline and up to the diaphragm line, work the stomach, spleen and anatomical pancreas. Work horizontally, vertically and diagonally over this area.

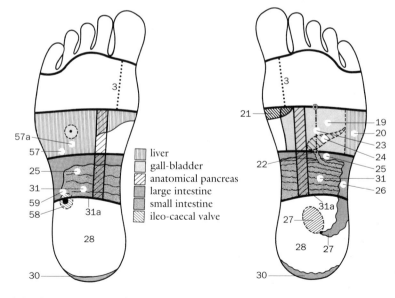

The digestive tract, reflex points 3, 19–28, 30, 31 and 31a.

209

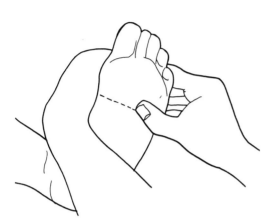

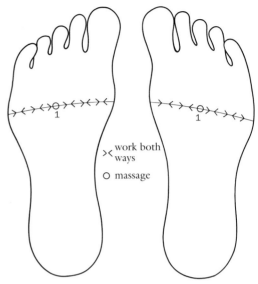

The solar plexus and diaphragm, reflex point 1 (both feet). Working hand over supporting hand. Refer to the Nervous, Respiratory and Muscular Systems.

Directional working: the solar plexus and diaphragm, reflex point 1 (both feet).

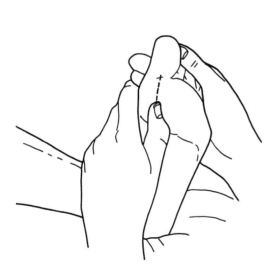

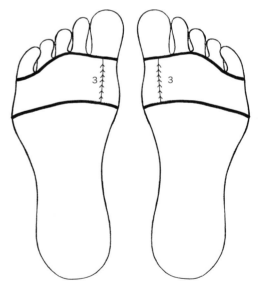

Hand position: the oesophagus, reflex point 3 (both feet). Working hand over supporting hand.

Direction for working: the anatomical oesophagus, reflex point 3 (both feet).

The Digestive System

System(s)	Associated Reflexes	Disorders
REFLEX POINTS 3 & 23: THE OESOPHAGUS		
Digestive	Stomach, pancreas, duodenum, large colon, small intestine, liver/gall-bladder	Cardiospasm, peptic reflux, oesophagitis, hiatus hernia
Muscular	Diaphragm	
Nervous	Solar plexus, spine, brain	
Endocrine	Pituitary, hypothalamus, thyroid, parathyroids, adrenal glands	

Nerve Innervations: 1st Thoracic, 5th Thoracic and 6th Thoracic

REFLEX POINT 19: THE STOMACH		
Digestive	Oesophagus, pancreas, duodenum, small intestine, large colon, pituitary gland	Oesophageal varices, peptic reflex, oesophagitis, thrush, peptic/gastric ulcers, cystic fibrosis
Endocrine	Hypothalamus, pituitary, adrenal glands, thyroid, parathyroids	
Muscular	Diaphragm	
Nervous	Solar plexus, spine, brain	

Nerve Innervation: 6th Thoracic

REFLEX POINTS 21 & 24: THE PANCREAS		
Endocrine	Hypothalamus, pituitary, thyroid, parathyroids, adrenal glands	Diabetes mellitus, hypo-/hyperglycaemia, pancreatitis
Digestive	Stomach, duodenum	
Urinary	Kidneys	
Lymphatic	Lymph nodes and ducts	
Special senses	Eyes	
Nervous	Spine, brain	

Nerve Innervation: 7th Thoracic

REFLEX POINT 22: THE DUODENUM		
Digestive	Stomach, pancreas, liver, gall-bladder, small intestine	Peptic ulcers
Endocrine	Hypothalamus, pituitary, thyroid, parathyroids, adrenal glands	
Nervous	Spine, brain, solar plexus	
Muscular	Diaphragm	

Nerve Innervations: 6th, 7th Thoracic

The Digestive System *continued*

System(s)	Associated Reflexes	Disorders

REFLEX POINTS 25, 26, 27, 28 AND 30: THE TRANSVERSE COLON, DESCENDING COLON, SIGMOID FLEXURE, PELVIC EXTENSION, RECTAL AREA. REFLEX POINTS 58, 59: ILEO-CAECAL VALVE AND ASCENDING COLON

System(s)	Associated Reflexes	Disorders
Digestive	Stomach, small intestine, sigmoid flexure, ileo-caecal valve, liver, gall-bladder	Food intolerance, appendicitis, enteric fevers, Crohn's disease, ulcerative colitis, physical and
Muscular	Diaphragm	emotional tension, constipation,
Nervous	Solar plexus, brain, spine	diarrhoea, irritable bowel
Cardio-vascular	Heart, lymph nodes and ducts	syndrome, psychogenic factors,
Endocrine	Hypothalamus, pituitary, adrenal glands	haemorrhoids, *Candida albicans*, rectal polyps, poor
Urinary	Kidneys	peristalsis, diverticulitis,
Skeletal/joints	Innominate bones, legs, all joints	sciatica, spinal misalignments

Nerve Innervations: Reflex Point 25: 1st, 2nd Lumbar; Reflex Point 26: 1st, 2nd Lumbar; Reflex Point 27: 1st, 2nd Lumbar, Coccyx; Reflex Point 28: 1st, 2nd Lumbar; Reflex Point 30: 1st, 2nd Lumbar, Coccyx; Reflex Point 59: 12th Thoracic: 1st and 2nd Lumbar; Reflex Point 60: 12th Thoracic, 1st, 2nd Lumbar

REFLEX POINTS 31 AND 31A: THE SMALL INTESTINE AND FOOD ALLERGY LINE

System(s)	Associated Reflexes	Disorders
Digestive	Stomach, pancreas, duodenum Oesophagus, liver, gall-bladder	Crohn's disease, food poisoning, poor peristalsis, food intolerance,
Muscular	Diaphragm	enteric fevers
Endocrine	Hypothalamus, pituitary, adrenal glands, thyroid, parathyroids	
Cardio-vascular	Lymph nodes and ducts, heart	

Nerve Innervation: 12th Thoracic

REFLEX POINT 57 AND 57A: THE LIVER AND GALL-BLADDER

System(s)	Associated Reflexes	Disorders
Digestive	Stomach, pancreas	Hepatitis A, B, C, D, E,
Endocrine	Thyroid, parathyroids, adrenal glands	gall-stones, cirrhosis, jaundice
Cardio-vascular	Lymph nodes and ducts, spleen, heart	
Urinary	Kidneys	

Nerve Innervations: 4th, 5th Thoracic

See Chapter 26 for a description of disorders relating to the Digestive System

---

Pancreas Supporter – Reflex Point 21 – Digestive and Endocrine Systems

Work the pancreas supporter by working three pathways just under the diaphragm line, laterally to medially only. The main area for sugar-related disorders is found on the medial side of the plantar tendon.

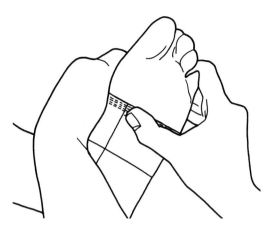

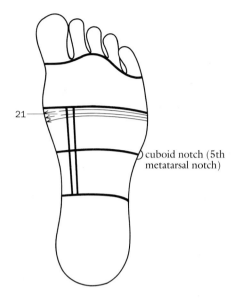

Hand position: the pancreas supporter, reflex point 21 (left foot only). Working hand over supporting hand.

Duodenum, Oesophagus Supporter and Solar Plexus – Reflex Points 1, 22 & 23 – Digestive System and Nervous System

Work the duodenum by massaging the reflex which is to be found on the lateral side of the plantar tendon on the waistline. Work upwards from this point towards the solar plexus for the helper oesophagus in the centre of the diaphragm and massage the solar plexus. Then

Directions for working: the pancreas supporter, reflex point 21 (left foot only).

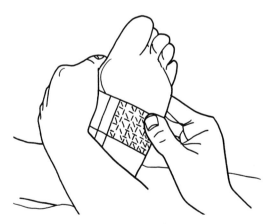

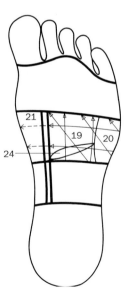

Hand position: the stomach, spleen and pancreas, reflex points 19, 20 and 24 (left foot only). Working hand over supporting hand.

Directions for working: the stomach, spleen, anatomical pancreas and pancreas supporter (left foot only), reflex points 19, 20, 21 and 24. Refer to the Lymphatic and Circulatory Systems for the spleen, and the Endocrine System for the pancreas.

213

work across the whole abdominal cavity between the diaphragm and the waistline, laterally to medially to include any reflexes missed and to reinforce the anatomical pancreas.

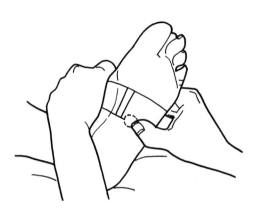

Hand position: the duodenum, reflex point 22 (left foot only). Working hand over supporting hand.

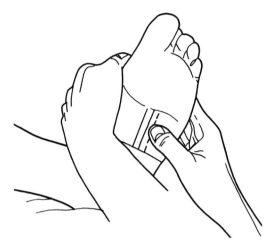

Hand position (1): the oesophagus supporter, reflex point 23 (left foot only). Working hand over supporting hand.

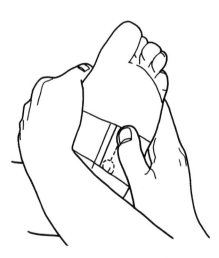

Hand position (2): the oesophagus supporter, reflex point 23 (left foot only). Working hand over supporting hand.

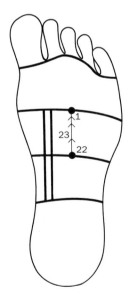

Directions for working: the duodenum, oesophagus supporter and solar plexus, reflex points 1, 22 and 23 (left foot only).

214

Transverse Colon, Descending Colon, Sigmoid Flexure – Reflex Points 25, 26 & 27 – Digestive System

1. Work the transverse colon lateral to medial then medial to lateral on the left foot. On the waistline of the lateral edge of the foot (top of the cuboid notch) turn the thumb downwards and work the descending colon into the sigmoid flexure.

2. With your right thumb held sideways, hook the sigmoid flexure towards the lateral edge of the foot. Turning the thumb into a diagonal position towards the medial edge of the foot, continue to work the sigmoid colon towards the top of the heel line in the shape of a fan. Repeat the hooking movement on the sigmoid flexure and,

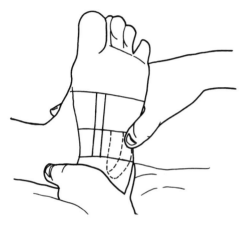

Hand position: the descending colon, reflex point 26 (left foot only). Supporting hand under the heel.

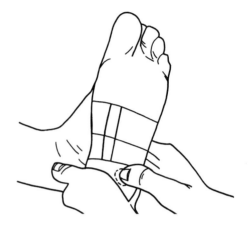

Hand position: the sigmoid flexure, reflex point 27 (left foot only) Supporting hand under the heel.

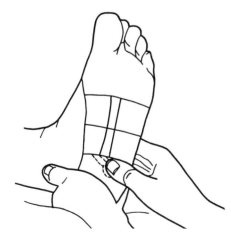

Hand position: the sigmoid flexure, reflex point 27 (left foot only). As above hand position.

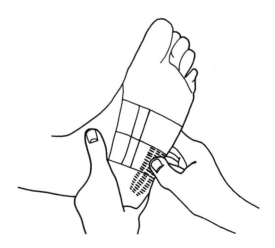

Hand position: the descending colon, reflex point 26 (left foot only). As above hand position.

215

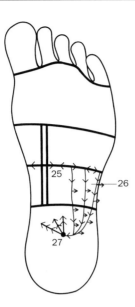

Directions for working: the transverse colon, descending colon, sigmoid flexure and rectal area (left foot only), reflex points 25, 26 and 27.

keeping the thumb in a sideways position, work back up to the waistline on the same pathway you worked down.

3. Work into the transverse colon on the waistline a little further (towards the middle of the foot) and repeat the movement of working down the descending colon into the sigmoid flexure. Repeat working the sigmoid flexure and colon as on the first pathway. Work up on the second pathway as before and once on the waistline work to the medial side of the foot for a third time so that your thumb is now in the middle of the sole of the foot, but still on the lateral side of the plantar tendon. Repeat steps 1–3 for the third pathway.

4. Once back on the waistline, turn the thumb down and work downwards only on each pathway. Hook the sigmoid flexure each time and take the thumb off the foot and then repeat working down on the two pathways previously worked. In this

way, we work with gravity by assisting passage of the faeces towards the rectum.

Pelvic Extension – Reflex Point 28 – Digestive System

Work the pelvic extension from the heel to the base of the heel line. You can work horizontally in either direction but upwards only from the base of the heel.

Rectal/Anus Area – Reflex Point 30 – Digestive System

Work the rectal area by supporting the heel of the foot and leg on the pads of your working fingers. The supporting hand gently holds the side of the foot without taking any of the weight. Thus, the weight of the leg and foot aids in finding reflexes as you work in a forward motion, with three fingers around the heel, from the centre, about 1.5 inches. Swap hands and repeat the process, moving from the centre of the heel in a forward movement.

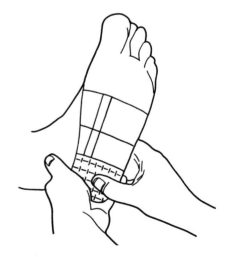

Hand position: the pelvic extension, reflex points 28 and 29 (including the sciatic nerve; both feet) and sigmoid flexure (left foot only). Supporting hand under the heel.

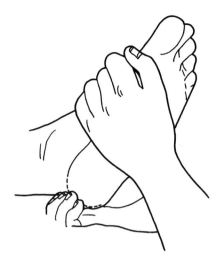

Hand position: the rectum and anus, reflex point 30 (both feet). Supporting hand lightly held on medial edge of the foot.

Small Intestine – Reflex Point 31 – Digestive System

Working from the top of the heel line with the thumb in an upward position, work vertically up to the waistline making tiny pathways across the whole width of the foot. Then work horizontally across the width of the foot between the waistline and the top of the heel. When working the last pathway at the top of the heel, work deeply to find the food allergy reflex which extends across the whole width of the foot.

Food Allergy Line – Reflex Point 31a – Digestive System

As you move to the food allergy line, at the top of the heel line, remember to keep your supporting hand on the top of the foot, with the working hand over the top of the sup-porting hand. Work lateral/medial, using as much pressure as possible to find sensitivity in this area.

Directions for working: the pelvic extension, rectum and anus, reflex points 28 and 30 (both feet).

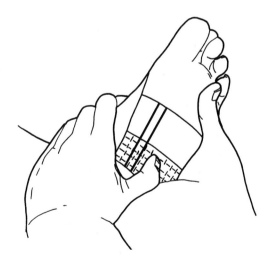

Hand position: the small intestine and food allergy line, reflex points 31 and 31a (both feet). Working hand over supporting hand.

217

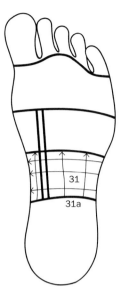

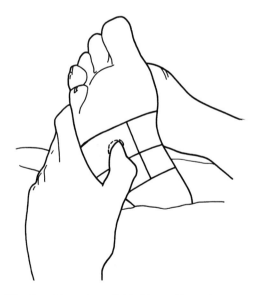

Directions for working: the small intestine, reflex points 31 and 31a (both feet).

Liver and Gall-Bladder (Right Foot Only) – Reflex Points 57 & 57a – Digestive System

The liver (right foot) should be worked in the same way as the stomach, spleen and pancreas on the left foot – horizontally, vertically and diagonally – in the same area: in the square formed by the lateral edge of the plantar tendon, the waistline and diaphragm line. The gall-bladder is worked by massaging with the left thumb towards the lateral edge of the foot at approximately the centre of the liver reflex. Look for a difference in skin tone, colour and puffiness to help you find the gall-bladder reflex.

Ileo-Caecal Valve/Ascending Colon (Right Foot Only) – Reflex Points 58 & 59 – Digestive System

The ileo-caecal valve is found either on, or just beneath, the thick part of the heel line,

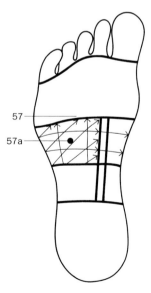

Hand position: the gall-bladder, reflex point 57a (right foot only). Working hand over supporting hand.

Directions for working: the liver and gall-bladder, reflex point 57 (right foot only).

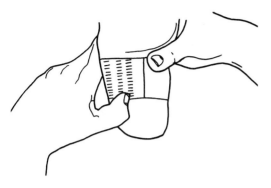

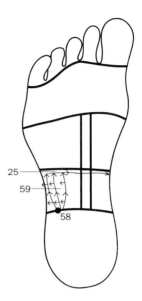

Hand position: the ileo-caecal valve and ascending colon, reflex points 58 and 59 (right foot only). Working hand over supporting hand on top of the foot.

towards the lateral edge of the right foot. Hook this deep indentation sideways with the thumb towards the lateral edge of the foot. To work the ascending colon as on the left foot and descending colon reflexes, you will need to work into the centre of the sole of the foot on three pathways. Work with the thumb sideways up the first pathway of the ascending colon to the waistline. Then work laterally to medially across the transverse colon. Take the

Directions for working: the ileo-caecal valve, ascending colon and transverse colon, reflex points 58, 59 and 25 (right foot only).

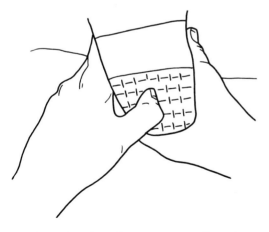

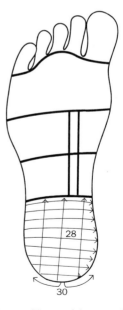

Hand position: the pelvic extension, reflex points 28 and 29, including the sciatic nerve supporter (both feet). Supporting hand under the heel.

Directions for working: pelvic extension, rectum and anus, reflex points 28 and 30 (both feet).

219

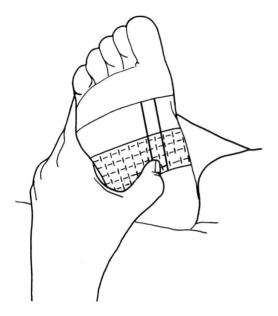

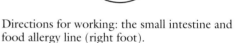

Hand position: the small intestine, reflex point 31, and food allergy line, reflex point 31a (both feet).

Directions for working: the small intestine and food allergy line (right foot).

thumb away from the foot and return to the ileo-caecal valve, with each ascending colon pathway move in towards the centre of the foot, by repeating the previous movements. Do not work down the ascending colon, as waste must be pushed upwards and across the transverse colon on its journey towards the rectum.

The small intestine can be worked on this foot before the ileo-caecal valve and ascending colon, if you wish, as nutrients are absorbed through the small intestinal walls before reaching the ileo-caecal valve, and the large colon and small intestine are joined by the ICV.

Reinforcement of Lateral Reflexes

Overlapping reflexes from the digestive cavities extend from the soles of the feet on to the tops of the feet. Work up the outside of each, from the heel, with the thumb, to the base of

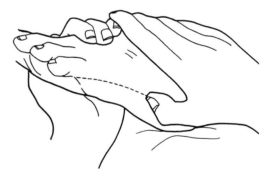

Hand position: reinforcement of lateral reflexes in the pelvic, abdominal and thoracic cavities, reflex point 48, and massaging the cuboid notch for 'all joints', reflex point 49 (both feet). Working hand on top of supporting hand.

the little toe to ensure all reflexes have been worked. Refer to Chapter 23, The Skeletal System, for working 'all joints' reflex point 49 on the cuboid bone.

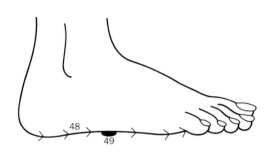

Directions for working: reinforcement of lateral reflexes in the pelvic, abdominal and thoracic cavities, reflex point 48 (both feet), and massaging the cuboid notch for 'all joints', reflex point 49 (both feet).

CASE STUDIES WITH DIGESTIVE PROBLEMS

Diverticulitis

Lyn came to see me for reflexology treatments, complaining of diverticulitis and sinusitis. I also found acid build-up in the duodenum, which Lyn confirmed. Her story is given below.

> I suffer with diverticulitis, which was diagnosed in 1992. Someone suggested that I try reflexology and recommended me to Jenny. After regular weekly, monthly and fortnightly treatments over a few years and changing to a less acid-base diet and reducing dairy produce, I have found the acid indigestion I suffered from has disappeared and the sinus problem is less acute. Reflexology has helped reduce the pain associated with my problems immensely and the relief gained justifies regular treatment.

I had also found congestion round the reproductive and bladder reflexes for some time and Lyn complained of a dragging feeling in the base of the pelvic area. Although Lyn's doctor could find nothing amiss during an examination, she sent her for a scan to check the pelvic area. Much to Lyn's surprise, she was found to have bladder warts, which she has since had removed.

Duodenal Ulcers

Eileen is an amazing lady at seventy-six who looks fifty and who came for reflexology complaining of gout, a history of digestive problems, culminating in a vagotomy for a duodenal ulcer, and other problems. She recognized that her diet could be improved and she was suffering high stress levels due to making a decision as to whether to move house on her own. She is a widow and does not feel she will be able to cope with living in a large house as she grows older. She had suffered from stress during her married life and her early childhood, which had left many emotional scars. Eileen felt it had been years of stress that led to her developing peptic ulcers and resultant surgery to ease the pain she suffered.

After several treatments, Eileen began to feel 'on top' of her stress levels and able to cope far more ably with life problems. She said she also felt more relaxed with a greater sense of well-being and reduced discomfort with her gout and digestive problems. Eileen continues to come for reflexology treatments and, with the time to talk through her problems during the treatment hour, she has made the decision to move house and make decisions, which before reflexology would, she said, have left her feeling uncertain that she had made the right choice.

Not only has she found the confidence to make one major life-changing decision with moving house, but she has begun her training in reflexology!

Gall-Bladder

Sheila has received regular treatments with reflexology over the last three years; this is her story about a troublesome gall-bladder.

221

I felt very ill over the Easter holiday and had a lot of knife-like pain near the waistline on the right side of my body. I knew I was seeing Jenny for a reflexology treatment on the following Tuesday, and had also made an appointment with my GP, so I wanted to hear what Jenny said about the pain from working on my feet. Jenny could hardly touch the right foot where the reflex point for the gall-bladder is found, it was so painful. She said she felt the pain was somehow linked to the gall-bladder and suggested I went to see my doctor as soon as possible. Jenny explained that reflexologists don't diagnose particular health problems, but energy blockages in the body that may reflect in the feet.

My GP referred me for a scan for a pulmonary embolism (a blood clot on the lung) and also thought that I may have bruised my ribs. The scan proved negative, although I was still in a lot of pain. My GP then made an appointment for ultra-sound, which was also negative. I continued with reflexology treatments that still gave the same message – the gall-bladder reflex was very painful when touched, reflecting how ill I felt!

Eventually, I saw a consultant who confirmed that it was the gall-bladder giving me so much pain and he referred me to a specialist for a scan. To my, the consultant's and Jenny's disbelief, the scan showed negative! I saw the consultant again after the scan and he confirmed, yet again, that it was my gall-bladder giving the pain, and as he was not satisfied with the results of the last scan, he would refer me to another specialist. I told him about the reflexology treatments, as I felt that my feet had shown all along where the problem was. From my experience, reflexology needs to be taken more seriously by the medical profession as a barometer for where problems may be in the body. I may not have been in acute pain for weeks before finding out what was wrong if reflexology had been taken more seriously!

I have great faith in reflexology and I have also felt a lot of benefit with my asthma since seeing Jenny for reflexology treatments.

CHAPTER 20
The Urinary System

Overview of the Urinary System

Regulation of electrolyte and water balance. Selective reabsorption
of nutrients; and filtration and elimination of toxins

Structures	*Functions*
Two kidneys	Regulate water and electrolyte balance; excrete waste products of cell metabolism; involved in regulation of blood pressure and production of red blood cells, and reabsorption of nutrients
Fatty sheath	Protects kidney structures
Hilum	Attaches the ureter tubes to the kidneys; lymph and nerves enter; blood enters and leaves kidney structures through the renal artery and vein respectively

FLOW OF SUBSTANCES THROUGH KIDNEY STRUCTURES

Cortex	
Bowman's capsule	Surrounds the glomerulus
Glomerulus	Reabsorbs blood cells and large protein molecules; contains an afferent arteriole that supplies the glomerulus with blood and an efferent arteriole that takes blood from the glomerulus to the capillary bed in the glomerulus
1st convoluted tubule	Reabsorbs hormones, glucose, amino acids, water and salts
Hormone: aldosterone	Regulates excretion of potassium and reabsorption of salt
2nd convoluted tubule	Regulates blood calcium levels and acid level present in blood
Hormone: parathormone	Regulates calcium levels in the blood
Juxtaglomerular apparatus	Produces the hormone renin to aid in controlling blood pressure; erythropoietin stimulates red bone marrow to produce red blood cells when kidneys do not get sufficient oxygen

Medulla	
Pyramids: contain over 1 million nephrons (tubules) in each kidney	Collect urine

Continued overleaf

Overview of the Urinary System *continued*

Structures	*Functions*
Medulla *continued*	
Loop of Henle	Regulation of water and salts
Collecting tubules	Regulate water balance
Hormone: antidiuretic hormone (ADH)	Regulates water reabsorption and excretion
Renal pelvis	
Calyces (muscular pouches)	Collect urine; push urine into ureter tubes
Two ureter tubes	Push urine toward the bladder
Bladder	Muscular reservoir for urine
Urethra	Tube from bladder to external environment

LINKS TO: digestive, endocrine, muscular, integumentary, respiratory and cardio-vascular systems.

EXCRETORY SYSTEM

Four interdependent systems are known as excretory systems because they excrete the waste products of metabolism.

- **The urinary system** regulates the volume of body fluids, the balance of pH and the electrolyte composition of fluids. It excretes water and waste products, which contain nitrogen and salts. These substances form urine.
- **The digestive system** excretes water, some salts, bile and a residue of digestion, all of which are contained in the faeces.
- **The respiratory system** excretes carbon dioxide and water, the latter appears as vapour and can be demonstrated by exhalation into cold air, or breathing onto a mirror.
- **The skin or integumentary system** excretes water, salts and very small quantities of nitrogenous waste. These appear in perspiration through evaporation of water from the skin.

URINARY SYSTEM

There are three main functions of the urinary system: selective reabsorption, secretion and filtration. The two kidneys lie against the muscles of the back in the upper abdomen and are about 10cm long, 5cm wide and 2.5cm (4 × 2 × 1in) thick. Each kidney is surrounded by fat, called the adipose capsule. This capsule is one of the chief supporting and protective structures of the kidneys. Each minute, 1 litre (1.8 pints) of blood passes through the kidneys with approximately 150–200 litres (270–360 pints) of fluid processed by the kidneys daily, with 1.5 litres (2.7 pints) leaving the body as urine. As they are situated under the dome of the diaphragm, they are protected by the lower ribs and the rib cartilages.

Blood supply to the kidney is supplied by a short branch of the abdominal aorta called the renal artery. Blood leaves the kidneys by the vessels that finally merge to form the renal vein. The renal vein carries blood into the inferior vena cava for return to the heart. Most of the substances filtered from the blood are still useful for the body, such as water. It is the function of the nephrons to reabsorb selectively the useful components in the filtrate, that is, to put glucose, hormones, amino acids, some salts and water back into the bloodstream. The tubule, therefore, separates the waste products from useful substances that can be used by the body. The amount of water and salts taken back into the bloodstream are constantly monitored and adjusted.

The structures of the kidneys are:

- the fatty sheath;
- the hilum;
- the glomerulus;
- the cortex;
- the medulla;
- the nephrons (encased in the pyramids);
- the pelvis.

The functions of the kidneys are to:

- excrete urine and maintain the balance of electrolyte and body fluids;
- excrete urea as a by-product of amino-acid metabolism;
- maintain water balance – as the amount of water consumed in a day can vary, the kidneys adapt so that the volume of body water remains stable;
- regulate acid-based balance in body fluids;
- reabsorb essential constituents, such as hormones, amino acids, glucose, water and salts;
- excrete urine, which consists of 96 per cent water, 2 per cent urea and 2 per cent sulphates and phosphates (salts);
- excrete urobilin, a bile pigment altered in the intestine, which is reabsorbed then excreted by the kidneys and which gives urine an amber colour.

Blood Supply

Blood enters the kidney via the renal artery. This artery divides into arterioles, then into a ball of capillaries called the glomerulus, which is surrounded by a renal capsule. Blood in the artery is already under pressure from the left ventricle of the heart, with pressure increasing as the vessel narrows. Blood entering the capillaries of the glomerulus is, therefore, under very high pressure.

Hilum

The hilum is the concave middle border of the kidney where the renal blood and lymph vessels and nerves enter the kidney structures.

Cortex

The cortex of the kidney is a reddish-brown layer of tissue lying immediately under the capsule and between the pyramids.

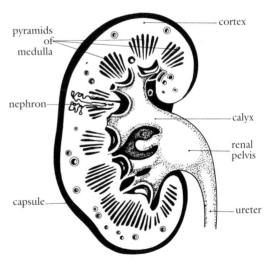

Fig 40. Longitudinal section through the kidney showing its internal structure.

225

Glomerulus

The closed end is indented to form a cup-shaped glomerular capsule (Bowman's capsule), which almost completely encloses a network of arterial capillaries. The process of urine formation begins in the glomerulus and Bowman's capsule. The membranes that form the walls of the glomerular capillaries are sieve-like structures, which allow water and soluble materials through them. Like other capillary walls, these are impermeable to blood cells and large protein molecules and leave the glomerulus through the renal vein. The capillary walls are one cell in thickness, so a solution containing the soluble

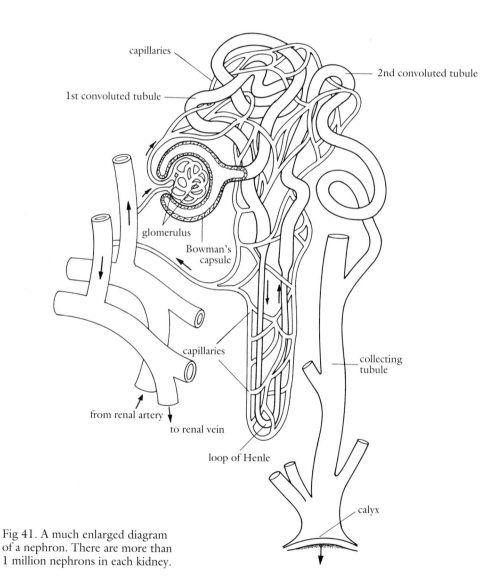

Fig 41. A much enlarged diagram of a nephron. There are more than 1 million nephrons in each kidney.

substances in the blood can squeeze out of the capillary. This process is called filtration. As the solution is squeezed out of the capillary and collected by the glomerulus, it enters the first convoluted tubule. In some cases, reabsorption of water and nutrients is regulated by hormones. In addition to water and nutrients, electrolytes (comprising sodium bicarbonate, potassium, calcium, magnesium and phosphate) are also passed into the nephron as part of the filtrate and may be returned to the body. Blood entering the glomerulus also consists of amino acids, glucose, hormones, urea, uric acid, toxins and drugs.

Medulla

The medulla is the innermost part of each kidney consisting of pale, conical-shaped striations called the renal pyramids. There are over one million tubules (nephrons) in each kidney, and a smaller number of collecting tubules. These tubules are closed at one end and supported by connective tissue containing blood, lymph vessels and nerves. The first convoluted tubule, the loop of Henle, and the second convoluted tubule lead into the collecting tubule. If all these tubes were separated, straightened out and laid end-to-end they would span approximately 120km (75 miles). Useful substances that can be used by the body either diffuse or are carried by active transport into tissue fluid surrounding the nephron. Selective reabsorption may be regulated by hormones.

First Convoluted Tubule

The first convoluted tubule selectively reabsorbs useful constituents that can be used by the body, such as hormones, glucose, amino acids, water and salts.

Hormone Function

The hormone aldosterone is secreted by the mineralocorticoid group of hormones in the cortex of the adrenal glands. Aldosterone influences the reabsorption of sodium and excretion of potassium. Waste products such as urea and uric acid are absorbed to a lesser extent.

Loop of Henle

As the filtrate continues into the loop of Henle and onwards, more waste materials and drugs are removed from the blood by the process of secretion. Water tends to flow across the partially permeable membrane into a salty solution by the process of osmosis in the loop of Henle. The solution entering the loop is permeable only to water, salts and urea. At this point in the tubule, the volume of fluid in the tubule has decreased and has a tendency to affect the speed at which the remaining fluid flows. The loop of Henle has a descending and an ascending tube. The cells of the ascending part of the loop are able to transport sodium salts from the tubule into the tissue fluid, and as a result there is a lot of salt in the tissue fluid around the base of the loop. Sodium is responsible for maintaining osmotic balance and body-fluid volume as water molecules and salt solutions bond. Nerve impulse conduction and maintenance of acid–base balance are also functions of salt.

Second Convoluted Tubule

The solution passes from the loop of Henle into the second convoluted tubule, where blood acidity and calcium reabsorption are adjusted by the cells of the tubule. From the second convoluted tubule the solution passes into the collecting tubule and at this point the concentration of urea is low. More water is reabsorbed as the filtrate flows down the collecting tubule.

227

Hormone Function

Parathormone secreted from the parathyroid glands and calcitonin secreted from the thyroid gland regulate the reabsorption of calcium and phosphates in the second convoluted tubule.

Collecting Tubule

Water travels from the collecting tubules into the tissue space of the medulla. Here, the amount of water reabsorbed from the collecting tubules depends upon the permeability of water to the cells of the tubule. If they are very permeable, a lot of water will be reabsorbed and the urine will be highly concentrated. If they are less permeable, less water is reabsorbed and the urine will be more dilute.

Hormone Function

The antidiuretic hormone (ADH), which is secreted from the posterior lobe of the pituitary gland, controls the permeability of the tubule walls. The regulation of water reabsorption is under the influence of ADH.

Pelvis

The renal pelvis is a funnel-shaped structure that receives urine formed by the kidney tubules. It has a number of branches called 'calyces', each of which surrounds the apex (point) of a renal pyramid. Urine formed in the kidneys passes through the apex of each pyramid into a calyx, then passes into a greater calyx before passing through the pelvis into the ureter. These pouches propel the urine into the ureter by peristalsis (muscular wave-like movements).

Ureters

The ureters are the tubes that convey urine from the kidneys to the urinary bladder and are about 25–30cm (10–12in) long. The ureter is continuous with the renal pelvis.

Bladder

The urinary bladder is a muscular pouch which acts as a reservoir for urine. When 200–300ml (⅜–½ pint) of urine has accumulated, autonomic nerve fibres in the bladder wall, which sensitize the bladder, expand and accommodate the increasing volume of urine. The bladder is pear-shaped when empty but becomes more oval in shape as it fills with urine.

Urethra

In the female, the urethra is short and is approximately 4cm (1½in) long. It runs downwards and forwards behind the symphysis pubis and opens just in front of the vagina. As a result females are more at risk from infections of the urinary tract. In the male, the urethra is much longer, some 19–20cm (7½–8in) long. It

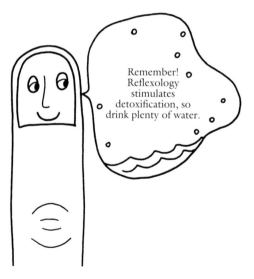

Remember! Reflexology stimulates detoxification, so drink plenty of water.

provides a pathway for the flow of urine and secretions from the male reproductive tract.

Additional Hormone Function

Other than the functions given above, the kidneys produce hormones, one of which is renin which is produced in the juxtaglomerular apparatus and is activated if blood pressure is low. This hormone activates a protein that causes blood vessels to constrict, causing blood pressure to rise.

When the kidneys do not get enough oxygen, the juxtaglomerular apparatus produces a hormone called erythropoietin. This stimulates the red bone marrow to produce red blood cells to prevent anaemia.

Dialysis

When the kidneys fail to do their job, the body gradually becomes poisoned by the increasing amount of urea in the blood. It must be removed or the body will die. Urea can be removed by dialysis. The alternative to this method of purifying the blood is by replacement of a diseased kidney with a transplanted kidney.

Hypertension

Hypertension (high) blood pressure can be caused by an abnormally high intake of sodium chloride, commonly known as salt. We need sodium chloride in blood plasma, but if we take in too much salt with our food the kidneys cannot maintain fluid balance and the following happens:

- water is added to the blood to dilute the salt from the collecting ducts in the kidneys;
- this increases the volume of blood;
- which means that more fluid goes to tissues;

- this causes the blood vessels to constrict in order to prevent the tissues being over-supplied with blood;
- which leads to increased pressure in the large vessels;
- which increases blood pressure.

Fluids in the Body

The human body is composed of 60–70 per cent water in adulthood and is higher in the young and in muscular people. As the amount of fat increases, with ageing, the percentage of water in the body decreases. Water is important to living cells as a solvent, as a transport medium and is involved in metabolic processes. Salts, nutrients, gases, waste products and special substances such as enzymes and hormones are dissolved or suspended in water. Body fluids are very important for internal environmental balance (homeostasis). Whenever the volume or chemical make-up of these fluids changes, disease can result.

- Intracellular fluid is contained within the cell – about two-thirds of body fluids are in this category.
- Extracellular fluid includes all body fluids outside of cells, including blood plasma, which constitutes about 4 per cent of body weight.
- Interstitial fluid, or tissue fluid, is located in the spaces between the cells of tissues all over the body. It is estimated that tissue fluid constitutes about 15 per cent of body weight.
- Fluid is found in special compartments, such as cerebrospinal fluid (CSF), the aqueous and vitreous humours of the eye, serous membrane fluid and synovial fluid in joints.

Functions of Water

Water can dissolve many different substances in large amounts. All the materials needed by the body, such as gases, minerals and nutrients, dissolve in water to be carried wherever they are needed. Water has many functions, for example:

- water provides a moist environment for all cells in the body, except nails, hair, the outer layer of teeth, and the superficial layers of skin;
- water is involved in chemical reactions both inside and outside of cells;
- water helps to regulate body temperature by sweat, which cools the body;
- water dilutes and moistens food in the digestive processes;
- water provides transport for substances around the body;
- water dilutes waste products and poisonous substances for excretion;
- water contributes to the formation of urine and faeces as part of the elimination process.

Water Balance and Thirst

Fluids are in a constant interchange and are transferred across semi-permeable cell membranes by diffusion and osmosis. In a healthy person, the quantity of water reabsorbed is about the same as the quantity eliminated. Water is lost through sweating, exhalation, urination, defecation, vomiting and crying.

The Sensation of Thirst

The control centre for the sense of thirst is located in the hypothalamus. A fluctuation in the concentration of body fluids stimulates the thirst centre and this causes an individual to drink more fluid, containing large amounts of water. Dryness of the mouth also causes the sensation of thirst as well as eating salty food, or in excessive sweating.

The salts that comprise the electrolytes are important substances dissolved in body water.

These are substances that separate into positively and negatively charged ions, which carry an electric current in solution.

Acid/Alkaline Balance

The pH-scale is a measure of how acid or alkaline a solution is. Normal body fluid is slightly alkaline at an approximate 7.4 on a scale from zero to 14. This scale must be kept within a narrow range of pH. The release of carbon dioxide from the lungs acts to make the blood more alkaline and increases the pH level. In contrast, a reduction in the release of carbon dioxide will act to make the blood more acidic.

SPECIAL INTEREST

High cholesterol levels can be caused by the production of abnormally high adrenalin release which is not used for physical activity. Refer to Chapters 14, 15 and 19, for chemical changes and effects on health. Refer to the liver reflex for sensitivity and the adrenal glands, as part of the endocrine system.

Skeletal misalignments may put pressure on the genito-urinary tract and prevent the bladder from emptying completely.

The bladder reflex and the surrounding area may be hard, red and swollen indicating possible fluid retention, urinary problems or the presence of diabetes. Extreme sensitivity can sometimes be felt as the thumb turns at right angles to work up the foot on the ureter reflexes. This can indicate the presence of strong smelling and dark amber coloured urine, cystitis and other genito-urinary tract infections. Remember that pressure from a swollen prostate gland or prolapsed uterus can put pressure onto the bladder, so that it cannot be fully emptied. Other disorders may be present in the bladder itself, which make micturition difficult.

Factors which play a part in developing the common disorder of cystitis are:

- synthetic underwear and/or tights;
- tight trousers;
- a full bladder after sexual intercourse;
- inadequate personal hygiene;
- inadequate cleansing of the genital area from front to back;
- emotional holding of deep-seated feelings in the unconscious related to sexuality or early childhood.

Recommend that your patients drink five pints of water a day to help the kidneys work efficiently in their task of eliminating toxins and the breakdown products of protein and hormones and other substances from the blood. Cranberry juice is also recommended for urinary infections and is doubly effective for bowel disorders if used to soak high-fibre cereals to assist the passage of faeces from the bowel.

The ureter tubes carry urine downwards, with gravity, to be expelled by the bladder. Consequently, we always finish working down the ureter tube as we do on the descending colon and sigmoid flexure.

The urethra is a deeply embedded reflex found at the base of the bladder on the sole of the foot. This reflex highlights inflammation and possible infection in this area, especially with cystitis, with men (as part of the structure of the penis) as well as women.

The adrenal glands are vital to life to such an extent that we cannot live without the hormones secreted by the cortex (outside) of the gland. These vital functions are easily upset by diet, stress and hormone imbalance elsewhere in the body. The medulla (middle) of the gland is responsible for muscle tone and sympathetic nerve response, as nerve fibres are the same as those found in the sympathetic nerve ganglia either side of the spine. Caffeine and nicotine act as stimulants, which induce this part of the gland to secrete adrenaline, which in turn speeds up the heart rate, leading possibly to hypertension. Excessive amounts of caffeine act as a diuretic and can lead to caffeine poisoning, and it is recommended that no more than five cups of tea or coffee be consumed a day. Recommend to your patients that they cut down their caffeine intake if the adrenal glands are sensitive without the presence of artificial steroids. Remember that the adrenal glands are indentations and need to be searched for.

The kidneys carry out the mammoth task of filtering the blood and in a 24-hour period it is estimated that 150–200 litres (270–360 pints) of blood pass through the kidney tubules, or nephrons, 99 per cent of which is reabsorbed by the tubules. The disease of arteriosclerosis (describing closed blood vessels) causes general blood pressure to rise, thus forcing the blood through the kidneys under extreme pressure. Eventually, the heart becomes affected by this type of renal disease, which is common with those suffering from diabetes mellitus. When the kidneys fail, waste substances accumulate in the blood resulting in a general poisoning known as uraemia.

By working the kidney reflexes in a general area from the top of the bladder to the adrenal gland reflex point, ensures that all possibilities of kidney problems are thoroughly worked by working round the cortex to stimulate the tubules and nephrons and the pelvis of the kidney to stimulate the calyces (muscular pouches) into squeezing the urine into the ureter tubes. Remember to plantar-flex the foot forward (towards you, the therapist) when working over the plantar tendon. When working the cortex of the kidney, a complete circle can be

231

worked from the top of the kidney reflexes, the adrenal gland, down the ureter tube and outwards over the bladder and the urethra tube as the final reflex. In severe cases of urinary infections, this has proved to be very effective. It cannot be stressed enough that your patient should be told to drink as much filtered water as possible, at least 3 litres (5.5 pints) daily and more if they suffer from urinary disorders.

WORKING THE REFLEXES

The Bladder, Urethra and Penis, Ureter Tube, Adrenal Gland and Kidney – Reflex Points 32, 33, 34, 35, 36, & 37 – Urinary and Endocrine Systems

Keeping the supporting hand over the ankle with the working fingers on the top of the foot, work in three pathways over the bladder area, beginning at the bottom of the raised area. From the topmost part of the bladder turn the thumb upwards on the medial side of the plantar tendon to work the ureter tube. Be careful not to work too closely to the spine or on the plantar tendon itself. Bring both supporting and working hands up the foot as you work towards the adrenal gland, which is situated underneath the diaphragm line. Turn your thumb sideways and massage the adrenal gland. Remember, it is an indentation, so look for a soft dip in the flesh of the foot. Now swap hands so that the working hand now becomes the supporting hand and support the foot from under the heel. Work down the ureter tube and out over the whole bladder area with the thumb, three times, to ensure that you have worked it thoroughly. Repeat these movements three times.

To work the cortex of the kidney, begin working from the top of the bladder, plantar-flex the foot towards you and work over the tendon, forming an arc as you work in

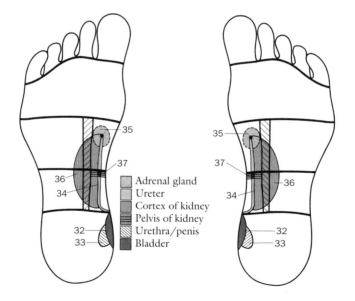

The urinary system, reflex points 32–37 (both feet). Refer to the Endocrine System and the adrenal glands.

The Urinary System

System(s)	Associated Reflexes	Disorders
REFLEX POINTS 32, 33 & 34: BLADDER, URETHRA AND PENIS, URETER TUBES		
Urinary	Ureter tube, bladder, urethra, kidneys	Ureteritis, cystitis, urethritis, physical and emotional tension
Muscular	Diaphragm	
Digestive	Pancreas, small intestine, large colon, sigmoid flexure, ileocaecal valve, liver, gall-bladder, duodenum	
Skeletal/joints	Innominate bones, spine	
Nervous	Brain, solar plexus	
Endocrine	Pituitary, hypothalamus, adrenal glands	

Nerve Innervations: 3rd and 4th Lumbar

System(s)	Associated Reflexes	Disorders
REFLEX POINT 35: ADRENAL GLANDS		
Endocrine	Hypothalamus, pituitary gland, ovaries and testes, thyroid and parathyroids	Addison's disease, Cushing's syndrome
Nervous	Brain, spine	
Urinary	Kidney	
Digestive	Pancreas, large colon, sigmoid flexure, ileocaecal valve	
Cardio-vascular	Heart, lymph nodes and ducts	

Nerve Innervations: 9th Thoracic

System(s)	Associated Reflexes	Disorders
REFLEX POINT 36 & 37: KIDNEY CORTEX AND KIDNEY PELVIS		
Urinary	Ureter, bladder, urethra	Oedema, nephritis, diabetic kidney, diabetes insipidus, renal failure, renal colic, polycystic kidney, hydronephrosis, ureteritis, cystitis, urethritis
Endocrine	Hypothalamus, pituitary, adrenal glands	
Muscular	Kidney, ureter tubes, urethra, bladder	
Digestive	Liver, gall-bladder, large colon, sigmoid flexure, ileocaecal valve	
Cardio-vascular	Lymph nodes and ducts, heart	
Skeletal	Spine	
Nervous	Brain, solar plexus	
Special senses	Eyes	

Nerve Innervations: 10th and 11th Thoracic

See Chapter 26 for a description of disorders related to the Urinary System

towards the adrenal gland. Massage the adrenal gland as before. Only work upwards for this reflex point.

Work the pelvis of the kidney medially to laterally on the waistline until you feel the plantar tendon. Then work two narrow pathways underneath the waistline and stop when you feel the plantar tendon.

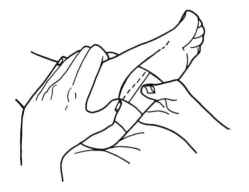 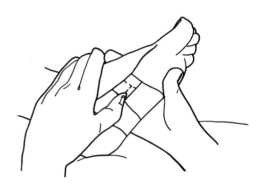

Hand position: the bladder, reflex point 32 (both feet). Working hand over supporting hand.

Hand position: the ureter tube, reflex point 34 (both feet). Working hand on top of supporting hand.

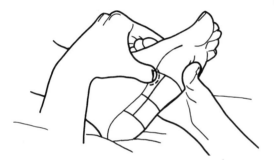

Hand position: massaging the adrenal gland, reflex point 35 (both feet). Working hand on top of supporting hand.

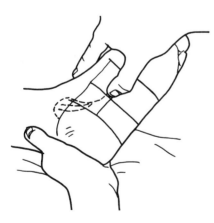 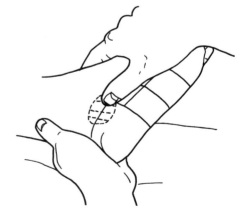

Hand position: the ureter tube, reflex point 34 (both feet). Supporting hand under the heel; working hand fingers on top of the foot.

Hand position: the bladder, reflex point 32 (both feet). Supporting hand under the heel; working hand fingers on top of the foot.

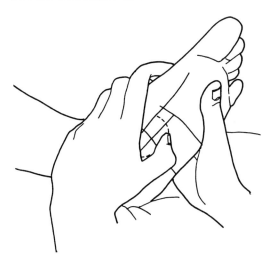

Hand position: the kidney cortex, reflex point 36 (both feet). Working hand on top of supporting hand.

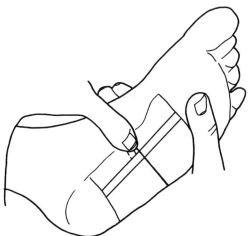

Hand position: the kidney pelvis reflex point 37 (both feet). Working hand on top of supporting hand.

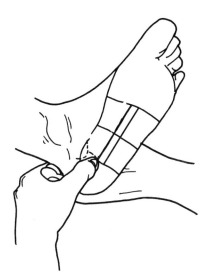

Hand position: the urethra and penis, reflex point 33 (both feet). Supporting hand under the heel; working hand underneath supporting hand.

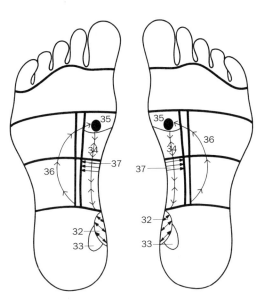

Directions for working: the urinary system, reflex points 32–37 (both feet).

235

CASE STUDY WITH CYSTITIS

Cilla came for reflexology treatment in a desperate attempt to wean herself off antibiotics, which she had taken for years for cystitis. Her following story is one of a remarkable recovery in a short space of time through reflexology and visualization practice.

I was aware even as a small child that I had a bladder which did not work properly. One of my earliest recollections was of nearly reaching home from school and having to walk with my legs crossed, suffering as I was from mild cystitis.

At the age of twenty-eight, married and with two small children, I suffered for weeks at a time with cystitis, with bleeding and great pain. I had to lie down with a towel between my legs as I felt the need to pass urine every two to three minutes. My doctor prescribed antibiotics every three to four weeks, which only succeeded in bringing me out in a rash.

After suffering this for over a year, I was sent to see a urologist who arranged for my admission to hospital, where a blockage was found and removed. This operation was performed twice and all went reasonably well until the age of forty-four when I had a full hysterectomy with the removal of both ovaries. The inevitable water infection flared up again during my stay in hospital and I had to be catheterized.

Six years later, at the age of fifty, I can only describe the pain and debilitation of cystitis as horrendous. Work was impossible, as I was unable to avoid going to the loo every ten minutes or so. The burning pain felt indescribable, keeping me almost housebound. I had two cystoscopies and bladder stretches in six months and was told each time that the bladder was inflamed. It was even more painful at night when lying down and would need to pass urine up to ten times in an hour. With the pain, dragging backache and depression the antibiotics put me out of my misery, so that I could get a few hours sleep. I was on antibiotics for over five years, during which time I would try to do without them but inevitably within two to three weeks the dragging, burning pain would return as though my insides were trying to push out.

Eventually, a friend recommended I try reflexology and I met Jenny. I was nurtured, counselled and advised with sometimes painful manipulation of my feet. After four weeks of reflexology treatments with Jenny and plenty of advice to drink at least five pints of filtered water a day, no tea, coffee or alcohol, I left off my antibiotics with a quaking heart and feeling fearful. However, I had great faith in Jenny and to my surprise and delight after four months I am still pain free and able to live a normal life again. I now see Jenny for one reflexology session a month.

Very often, visualization techniques practised by the patient whilst they are having treatment and at home can ease and accelerate healing. Learning to love the troublesome parts of our bodies is difficult, especially when they give a lot of pain. The mind is all-powerful and can be used by the client to speed the healing process.

CHAPTER 21

The Reproductive System

Overview of the Reproductive System

Reproduction of the human being.

Structures	Hormones	Functions
FEMALE REPRODUCTIVE SYSTEM		
Hypothalamus	Oxytocin	Uterine and mammary contractions
Pituitary gland	Follicle stimulating hormone (FSH)	Produces oestrogen in ovaries and is responsible for secondary sexual characteristics, such as development of breasts and sexual organs, and changes in the pelvis to an ovoid, broader shape
	Luteinizing hormone (LH)	Produces progesterone in ovaries
	Human chorionic gonadotrophin (HCG)	Assists in the maintenance of progesterone levels from the corpus luteum in the first trimester of pregnancy
	Prolactin	Produces milk in lactation (breast feeding)
Vulva/labia		External genitalia
Vagina		Muscular tube that transports spermatozoa to the cervix
Cervix		Receptacle for sperm and is connected to the vagina
Two Fallopian (uterine) tubes		Transport the ova (eggs) from the ovaries to the uterus
Two ovaries	Oestrogen and progesterone	Produce ova and hormones
Uterus		Provides a safe environment for the growing embryo and foetus
MALE REPRODUCTIVE SYSTEM		
Pituitary gland	FSH	Produces spermatozoa (testosterone is necessary in this process
	LH (known as interstitial cell-stimulating hormone (ICSH) in the male)	Produces testosterone
Penis		Ejaculates spermatozoa from the urethra into the vaginal tract
Scrotum		Sac containing the testes
Testes	Testosterone	Produce sperm cells
Epididymis		Coiled tube that store maturing spermatozoa

Continued overleaf

Overview of the Reproductive System *continued*

Structures	*Functions*
MALE REPRODUCTIVE SYSTEM	
Vas deferens	Transport spermatozoa to the ejaculatory ducts which lead into the seminal vesicles
Seminal vesicles	Produce semen and nutrients which prolong the life of spermatozoa
Cowper's glands	Produce mucus to aid in the lubrication and transportation of spermatozoa through the urethra
Ejaculatory ducts	Empty into the prostate gland and urethra
Prostate gland	Produces semen in which spermatozoa are aided through the vaginal tract; alkalinizes the acidity in the vaginal tract; aids in expulsions of semen from the body

LINKED TO: endocrine, muscular, circulatory, nervous, urinary and special senses systems.

INTRODUCTION

The reproductive organs of the male and the female differ, with both males and females producing specialized reproductive cells called gametes. These cells contain genetic material called genes, but half as many chromosomes as found in cells elsewhere in the body. During development of gametes a special process of cell division occurs which reduces the usual chromosome number from forty-six to twenty-three.

When an ovum (egg) is fertilized by a spermatozoan, the resultant zygote contains the full complement of forty-six chromosomes – twenty-three from the father and twenty-three from the mother. The zygote embeds in the wall of the uterus, where it grows and develops during the 40-week gestation period before birth.

The function of the female reproductive system is to form the ovum and, if this is fertilized, to nurture it through the various growth stages until the baby is born, then feed the baby with breast milk until it is able to take solid food. The function of the male reproductive system is to form the spermatozoa and transmit them to the female.

FEMALE REPRODUCTIVE SYSTEM

Female Reproductive Organs

Female reproductive organs are divided into external and internal organs. The external organ is known as the vulva in the female. The internal organs of the female reproductive system lie in the pelvic cavity and consist of the vagina, uterus, two Fallopian (or uterine) tubes and two ovaries.

Vagina

The vagina is a muscular tube that connects the external and internal organs of reproduction.

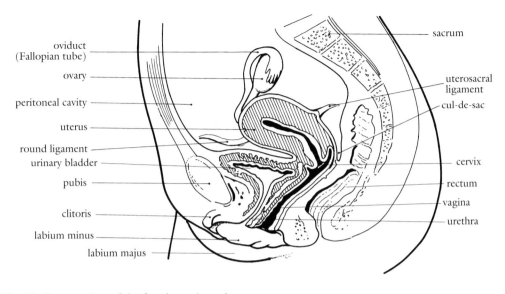

Fig 42. Cross section of the female genito-urinary system.

Uterus

The uterus is a flattened, hollow muscular pear-shaped organ. It lies in the pelvic cavity between the urinary bladder and the rectum, and leans forward almost at right-angles to the vagina, with its front surface resting on the bladder. When the body is in an upright position, it lies in an almost horizontal position. The walls of the uterus are composed of three layers of tissue: the perimetrium, the myometrium and the endometrium. The uterus and ovaries are suspended by the broad ligament, which incorporates the blood supply. Two sections of the peritoneum form a partition, which divides the female pelvic area into anterior and posterior sections.

Fallopian Tubes

The Fallopian tubes, or uterine tubes, are about 10cm (4in) long and extend from each side of the uterus. The end of each tube has finger-like projections called fimbriae. The longest of these is the ovarian fimbriae, which is closely associated with the ovaries. The function of the Fallopian tubes is to convey the ovum (egg) from the ovaries to the uterus by peristalsis of ciliary hair cells and the presence of mucus secreted by the lining membrane. Fertilization of the ovum usually takes place in the Fallopian tube, it then moves into the uterus where it embeds itself in the uterine wall.

Ovaries

The ovaries are the female gonads, or sex glands, which lie in a shallow dip on the lateral walls of the pelvis. Each ovary contains many ovarian follicles, containing ova. There are approximately 400,000 eggs present in the ovaries at birth. Before puberty, the ovaries are inactive, but already contain immature follicles. During childbearing years, one ovarian follicle matures, ruptures and releases its ovum during each menstrual cycle, unless fertilized.

The Cervix

The cervix lies at the neck of the uterus, and forms the lower, narrower part of the uterus. It separates the uterus from the vagina. The functions of the cervix are to:

- act as a reservoir for sperm and to secrete mucus, which protects sperm and provides them with energy;
- provide a receptacle for the foetus within the womb;
- secrete protective antibodies to prevent infection in the abdominal cavity;
- allow menstrual flow from the uterus;
- provide an opening into the uterus for spermatozoa.

A smear test allows the detection of abnormal changes in the cells of the cervix.

Hormones and the Menstrual Cycle

The ovarian follicle is matured by follicle stimulating hormone (FSH) from the anterior lobe of the pituitary gland. While maturing, cells lining the follicle produce the hormone oestrogen. After ovulation, the follicle-lining cells develop into the corpus luteum (yellow body), under the influence of luteinizing hormone (LH) from the anterior lobe of the pituitary. The corpus luteum produces the hormone progesterone.

If the ovum is fertilized, it becomes an embryo, travels along the Fallopian tubes and embeds in the wall of the uterus, where it grows and develops. The chorionic gonadotrophin hormone is similar to anterior pituitary luteinizing hormone and stimulates the corpus luteum in continuing to secrete progesterone for the first three months of the pregnancy.

If the ovum is not fertilized, the corpus luteum degenerates with the endometrium

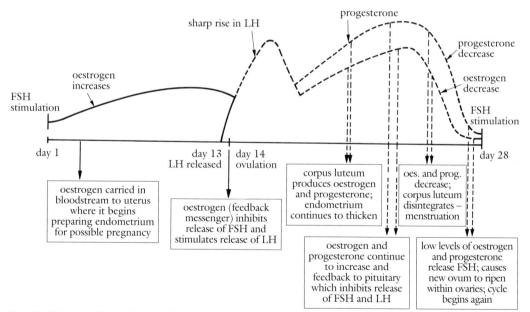

Fig 43. Hormone levels during the menstrual cycle.

and the menstrual cycle begins again. If the ovum is fertilized, there is no breakdown of the endometrium and therefore no menstrual flow.

Amniotic Fluid

Amniotic fluid is clear and contained within the amnion membrane that surrounds the foetus in the womb and protects it from external pressure. It is largely water and is produced by the amnion, being regularly circulated and swallowed by the foetus and excreted through its kidneys back into the amniotic sac. Towards the thirty-fifth week of pregnancy, there is about 1 litre (1¾ pints) of fluid, but this decreases to about 0.5 litre (⅞ pint) at the end of pregnancy. The amniotic sac normally ruptures early in labour, releasing the fluid or waters.

Development of the Placenta

Once the ovum has been fertilized by spermatozoa, the placenta develops and produces oestrogen, progesterone and the chorionic gonadotrophin hormone. The placenta provides an indirect link between the circulation of the mother and that of the foetus. The foetus obtains nutritional materials, oxygen and antibodies through the placenta, whilst getting rid of carbon dioxide and waste.

Mammary Glands

The function of the mammary glands is to provide the baby with milk after birth; they are only active during pregnancy. At puberty they mature in size under the influence of oestrogen and progesterone. During pregnancy these hormones stimulate further growth, and after the baby is born the hormone prolactin from the anterior lobe of the pituitary gland stimulates production of milk. Oxytocin is released from the posterior lobe of the pituitary, which stimulates the release of milk by muscle contraction in response to the stimulation of the nipples by the baby.

The mammary glands consist of glandular, fibrous and fatty tissue. Each breast consists of about twenty lobes of glandular tissue, with each lobe comprising of a number of lobules. The lobules consist of alveoli, which open into small ducts. These ducts unite to form large excretory ducts called lactiferous ducts. The lactiferous ducts converge towards the centre of the breasts, where they form reservoirs for the milk. Leading from these reservoirs are narrow ducts that open on to the surface of the nipple. On the surface of the nipples are many sebaceous glands, which lubricate the nipple in pregnancy and breast-feeding.

Menopause

The menopause usually occurs between the ages of forty-five and fifty-five and marks the end of childbearing years. It may develop suddenly or over a period of time. It is caused by the changes in the concentration of the sex hormones, as the ovaries gradually become less responsive to the hormones FSH and LH, and ovulation. The menstrual cycle becomes irregular, sometimes heavy, eventually ceasing. Depression and memory loss are also symptomatic of the menopause and may include unpredictable flushing, sweating and palpitations, which can cause discomfort and disturbance of the normal sleep pattern. The breasts begin to shrink, the axillary (armpit) and pubic hair become sparse, the sex organs shrink and episodes of uncharacteristic behaviour, such as irritability, sometimes occur.

MALE REPRODUCTIVE SYSTEM

Male Reproductive Organs

Scrotum

The scrotum is a pouch that is divided into two compartments, each of which contains one testis, one epididymis, and the testicular end of a spermatic cord.

Testes

The main part of the tissue in the testis is composed of tiny, coiled seminiferous tubules, where spermatozoa are developed by 'nurse' cells, known as sertoli cells. Between the tubules are groups of cells that secrete the hormone testosterone, which is also needed in the formation of spermatozoa. In the upper part of the testis, the tubules combine to form a single convoluted tubule called the epididymis, which leaves the scrotum as the deferent duct (vas deferens). The spermatozoa pass through the epididymis, deferent ducts (vas deferens), seminal vesicles, ejaculatory ducts and the urethra to be implanted in the female vagina during sexual intercourse. It is estimated that 200 million sperm cells are contained in each ejaculation.

Epididymis

In the epididymis and deferent ducts, the spermatozoa mature and become capable of independent movement through semen. If they are not ejaculated, spermatozoa are reabsorbed by the tubules.

The formation of spermatozoa takes place at a temperature of about 2–3°C lower than normal body temperature in the testes. A lower temperature is possible because the testes in the scrotum are covered by only a thin layer of tissue, which contains little fat.

Spermatic Cords

Blood and lymph vessels pass through the testes in the spermatic cord. There are two spermatic cords, one leading from each testis, consisting of one deferent duct (vas deferens) and nerves. The spermatic cord suspends the testis in the scrotum. Spermatozoa travel through the spermatic cords in the process of ejaculation.

Vas Deferens

The vas deferens pass upwards from the testes, through the inguinal canal and ascend towards the back wall of the bladder, where they are joined by the duct from the seminal vesicles. Together these parts form the ejaculatory duct.

Ejaculatory Ducts

The ejaculatory ducts are two tubes about 2cm (¾in) long, each formed by the union of a duct from a seminal vesicle and a deferent duct. They pass through the prostate gland and join the urethra.

Penis

The penis is formed by three elongated masses of erectile tissue and involuntary muscle. It contains the urethra (*see* Chapter 20, The Urinary System).

Seminal Vesicles

The seminal vesicles are two small muscular pouches lying to the back of the bladder. At its lower end, each seminal vesicle opens into a short duct, which joins with the corresponding deferent duct to form an ejaculatory duct. The function of the seminal vesicles is to produce a thick, yellow alkaline secretion that contain glucose and other substances to

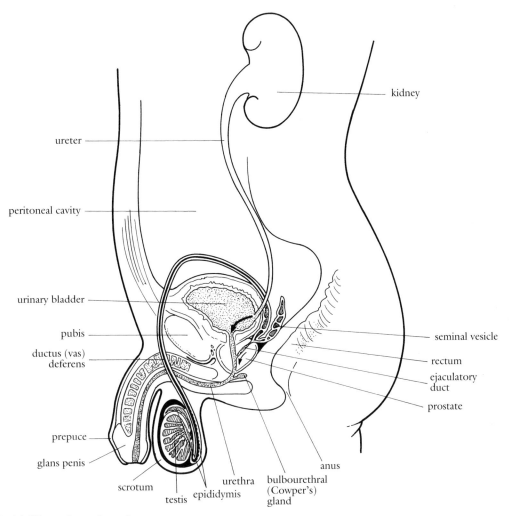

Fig 44. The male genito-urinary system.

provide nourishment for the long journey of the sperm through the female reproductive tract.

Semen is a fluid ejaculated from the urethra during sexual intercourse. It consists of: spermatozoa; a fluid that helps to nourish the spermatozoa secreted by the seminal vesicles; a thin, lubricating fluid produced by the prostate gland; and mucus secreted by glands in the lining membrane of the urethra.

Prostate Gland

The prostate gland is the size and shape of a walnut and is located at the base of the bladder. It surrounds the urethra and has two ducts which enter the urethra. The prostate can become inflamed due to infection, which causes irritation to the urethra and prompts a frequent desire to urinate. It may also become swollen and enlarged, thereby compressing

243

the urethra and obstructing the urine flow. This can result in the bladder becoming over-active to force the urine through the obstruc-tion, resulting in a desire to urinate frequently. The prostate gland produces an alkaline secre-tion, which neutralizes acidity in the vaginal tract and aids in the motility of sperm.

Cowper's Glands

Cowper's glands are mucus-producing glands, which are pea-sized organs, situated below the prostate gland. The secretions from these glands acts as a lubricant.

Urethra

The urethra provides a pathway for the flow of urine and semen, the secretions of the male reproductive organ. It is about 19–20cm (8in) long, and originates in the bladder; it is surrounded by the prostate gland.

Hormone Activity

In the male, as in the female, the reproductive organs are stimulated by the gonadotrophic hormones from the anterior lobe of the pitu-itary gland. The follicle stimulating hormone (FSH) stimulates the seminiferous tubules of the testes to produce sertoli cells (male sperm cells), and luteinizing hormone (LH), which stimulates the testes in the production of testosterone. In the male, luteinizing hor-mone is called the interstitial cell-stimulating hormone (ICSH).

SPECIAL INTEREST

The uterus and prostate gland are indenta-tions and, like all other indentations, work around the area until you are in the centre of the reflex point. These reflexes can feel lumpy

and swollen, due to possible adhesions and scar tissue left from surgery. Sometimes these reflexes need the thumb to be held in a static position, or massaging, with pressure devel-oping before you 'enter' the reflex – it can be described as 'breaking through' the resistance of any blocked energy held in this area. In the female, fibroids, hysterectomy or vaginal repair can show as a lumpy sensation; in the male, as prostate problems. I have found with some patients that locked-in feelings of grief surrounding child-bearing have an opportu-nity to be released by 'holding' the reflex when I have intuitively felt that resistance has been present. Offer an opportunity for your patient to talk about their experiences.

The Fallopian tubes give information about the lymph nodes in the groin (the inguinal nodes) to the medial edge of the foot and pos-sible problems with pregnancy from the fibia and talus joints to a little way over the ankle joint. In the male, the vas deferens appear to refer to the possibility of problems in the reproductive tract and scar tissue from a vasectomy operation.

The ovaries and testes refer to all hormonal, menstrual, libido and repro-ductive imbalances in both male and female and should

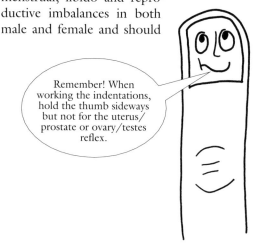

Remember! When working the indentations, hold the thumb sideways but not for the uterus/ prostate or ovary/testes reflex.

be worked in conjunction with all other endocrine glands, especially the pituitary, pineal and hypothalamus.

The mammary glands, or breasts, can relate to hormonal changes due to the menstrual cycle or menopause and associated lymphatic congestion. If a mastectomy (removal of one or both breasts) has been carried out, work all lymph nodes and ducts to assist the surrounding tissue in coping with lymph drainage. *See* Chapter 26 for more information before working with a patient who has or has had cancer.

WORKING THE REFLEXES

Ovaries/Testes – Reflex Point 39 – Reproductive System

On the lateral edge of the foot, you will need to remember to check with your patient if you can turn the leg into the middle of the body to look for the ovaries and testes reflexes at the mid-point between the fibula ankle joint and the lateral outside edge of the heel. Look for the reflexes with three fingers, as for the uterus/prostate reflexes.

At the mid-point you will find the ovaries and testes, which might show slight puffiness; massage gently with circular movements. Repeat working the pelvic cavity, as for the uterus/prostate, by working vertically from the back of the calcaneum (heel bone) to the fibula joint in a square shape ensuring that all reflexes are worked.

Remember to work only up to the ankle joint on both sides of the foot for the final movement in this area.

Uterus, Cervix, Vagina and Prostate – Reflex Points 38 & 38b – Reproductive System

Turn the foot outwards towards the lateral edge of the body, and on the medial side of the ankle look for the uterus/prostate reflexes between the tibia joint at the ankle and the edge of the calcaneum. There is a natural dip in the foot at

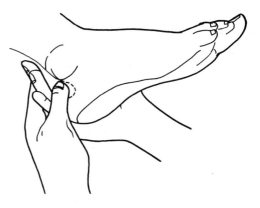

Hand position: the ovaries/testes, reflex point 39 (both feet). Working hand under supporting hand.

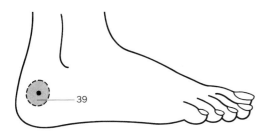

The ovaries and testes, reflex point 39 (both feet).

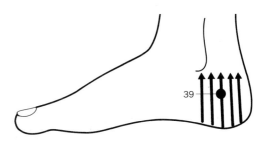

Directions for working: the ovary/testis supporter area, reflex point 39 (both feet).

The Reproductive System

System(s)	Associated Reflexes	Disorders

REFLEX POINT 38 AND 38B: UTERUS/PROSTATE GLAND, CERVIX AND VAGINA

System(s)	Associated Reflexes	Disorders
Reproductive	Ovaries and testes, fallopian tubes, vas deferens	Prolapse, impotency, obstetric cholestasis, inflammation and
Muscular	Uterus, mammary glands	infection of reproductive system,
Nervous	Brain, spine	venereal disease (VD),
Endocrine	Hypothalamus, pineal gland, pituitary, thyroid, parathyroids, adrenal glands	pre-eclampsia, atrophic dystrophy, cervicitis, endometriosis, adenomyosis, fibroids, salpingitis,
Urinary	Kidneys, bladder, ureter tubes, urethra	ectopic pregnancy
Digestive	Large colon, sigmoid flexure, ileocaecal valve	

Nerve Innervation: 3rd and 4th Lumbar

REFLEX POINT 39: OVARIES/TESTES

System(s)	Associated Reflexes	Disorders
Muscular and Nervous	All of the above reflexes and in addition, the uterus and prostate gland	Amenorrhoea, dysmenorrhoea, menorrhoea, oedema of the breast, reproductive vaginitis, ovarian
Endocrine		cysts, subfertility, mastitis,
Urinary		prostatitis, candidiasis
Digestive		

Nerve Innervation: 3rd and 4th Lumbar

REFLEX POINTS 40 & 41: FALLOPIAN TUBES, VAS DEFERENS, INGUINAL LYMPH NODES

System(s)	Associated Reflexes	Disorders
Reproductive	Ovaries, testes, uterus, prostate gland	Vasectomy, ectopic pregnancy,
Lymphatic	Lymph nodes and ducts	inflammation and infection of
Urinary	Kidneys, bladder, urethra, ureter	reproductive system, obstructed
Endocrine	Hypothalamus, pituitary gland, adrenal glands	Fallopian tubes, lymphatic oedema, inguinal hernia, femoral hernia,
Digestive	Large colon, sigmoid flexure, ileocaecal valve	constipation
Nervous	Brain, spine	

Nerve Innervation: 3rd, 4th and 5th Lumbar

REFLEX POINT 51: THE MAMMARY GLANDS (BREASTS)

System(s)	Associated Reflexes	Disorders
Reproductive	Uterus	Lymphoma, mastitis, lymphatic
Muscular	Diaphragm	oedema, emotional tension
Cardio-vascular	Lymph nodes and ducts, heart	
Skeletal	Spine, ribs	
Endocrine	Hypothalamus, pituitary, ovaries, adrenal glands	
Nervous	Brain, solar plexus	
Urinary	Kidneys	

Nerve Innervations: 3rd Thoracic

See Chapter 26 for a description of disorders related to the Reproductive System the mid-point between the two. You can check the area by placing your fourth finger on the heel edge and index finger on the ankle joint. The third finger should automatically fall into the dent between the joint and the heel edge. Once located, look for an indentation – it may feel like a dent, hard and lumpy or soft and hollow. Place the supporting hand palm (left hand, left foot) underneath the calcaneum. Massage gently with the thumb which should be at right angles to the ankle, facing up towards the patient's head. To work the cervix and vagina, massage the area at the base of the uterus reflex.

If surgery has taken place, check the area above the uterus towards the back of the heel for the deep muscles in the lower back and broad ligaments that support the uterus and ovaries, which are attached to the spine; massage gently if sensitive, to aid relaxation in this area.

To ensure that all reflexes have been worked, work vertically, gently with the thumb, over the whole of the back of the calcaneum to the bladder edge and up to the tibia joint, thus forming a square shape. This ensures that all reflexes have been thoroughly worked in the pelvic cavity.

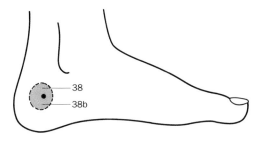

The uterus and prostate, reflex points 38 and 38b (both feet).

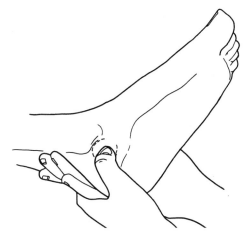

Hand position: the uterus/prostate gland, reflex points 38 and 38b (both feet). Working hand under supporting hand.

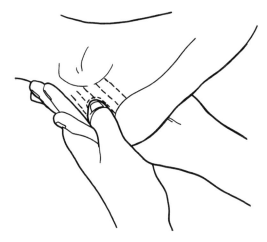

Hand position: the uterus/prostate, cervix and vagina supporter area, reflex points 38 and 38b (both feet). Working hand under supporting hand.

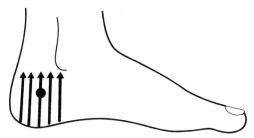

Directions for working: the uterus/prostate, cervix and vagina supporter area, reflex points 38 and 38b (both feet).

Reproductive Ankle Rotation – Working Reflex Points 38 & 39 Simultaneously

Place the third finger on the ovary/testes reflex point, the thumb on the uterus/prostate reflex and, gently holding the foot with the supporting hand underneath the heel, rotate the ankle in both directions, whilst applying appropriate pressure to the reflexes.

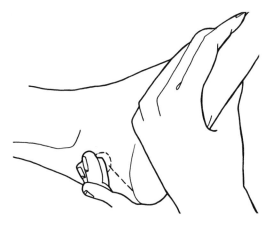

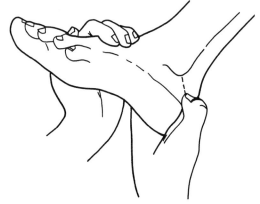

Hand position: the ankle rotation for the uterus/prostate (both feet). Working hand supports the heel; supporting hand supports the side of the foot.

Hand position: the ankle rotation, ovary/testis (both feet). Working hand supports the heel; supporting hand supports the side of the foot.

Fallopian Tubes/Vas Deferens/Lymph Nodes in the Groin – Reflex Points 40 & 41 —Reproductive System

Push the foot upright with the supporting hand (left hand/left foot and right hand/right foot), so that fingers are at the tips of the toes, making sure they do not hang over the toes – it looks very untidy from the patient's view of the foot. The reflexes are between the joints of the talus, tibia and fibula, and so it is important to dorsi-flex the foot as far as possible at right angles without causing discomfort. With two fingers, work in one direction only from the lateral side of the ankle joint (fibula) across to the medial side (tibia). Working medially to laterally pinches the skin. Work the helper area for these reflexes by working with two fingers in an upward movement only from inside the medial edge of the tibial ankle joint and work up the leg for about 7–9cm (3–3½ in).

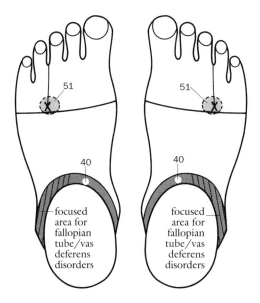

The reproductive system, reflex point 40 (both feet). Refer the to Lymphatic and Urinary Systems.

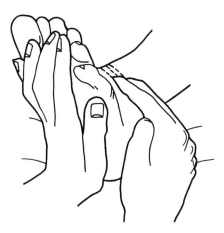

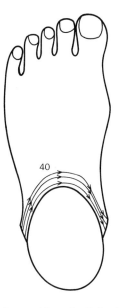

Hand position: the Fallopian tubes, vas deferens and inguinal lymph nodes, reflex point 40 (both feet). Supporting hand held against sole of the foot.

Directions for working: the Fallopian tubes, vas deferens and inguinal lymph nodes, reflex point 40 (both feet).

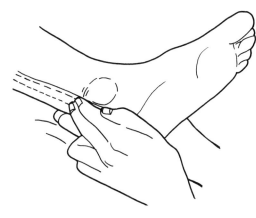

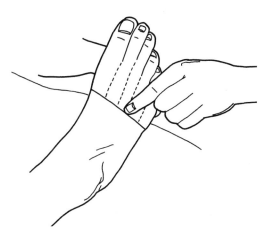

Hand position: the Fallopian tubes, vas deferens and inguinal lymph nodes supporter, reflex point 41 (both feet). Supporting hand cradles the heel and lateral edge of the foot.

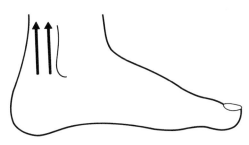

Hand position: the breast, reflex point 51 (both feet). Supporting hand makes a fist on the ball of the foot.

(Left) Directions for working: the Fallopian tubes, vas deferens and inguinal lymph nodes supporter, reflex point 41 (both feet).

249

CASE STUDIES WITH REPRODUCTIVE DISORDERS

Menopause

Carole came to see me for reflexology treatments complaining of the side-effects of HRT, which had made her put on a considerable amount of weight, gave her headaches and made her feel generally unwell. With regular treatments of reflexology and herbs (any prescription for herbs must be checked with the patient's doctor for any adverse effects with conventional medication or treatment before being taken) prepared by a medical herbalist for her, she managed to wean herself off HRT over a period of three months. Her weight decreased and the accompanying sugar-craving for sweet things to eat, and her general sense of well-being improved immensely.

Daphne complained of depression and dramatic mood swings, which left her feeling suicidal. She also suffered weight gain due to a craving for sweet things to eat. Again, with a high dose of prepared herbs for hormone imbalance problems and regular weekly reflexology treatments she found, for the first time in years, a greater sense of stability and relief from the dread of the depressive bouts and feelings of hopelessness and helplessness that accompanied her menstrual cycle in the menopausal years.

Amenorrhoea

Five years ago, Denise, a young woman, came for reflexology complaining of amenorrhoea (lack of menstruation), which she had suffered from for five years, probably due to stress and a general hormone imbalance. Her doctor had prescribed HRT and thyroxine to try and rebalance her endocrine system and encourage the return of her periods, but to no avail. In desperation she decided to contact me and in the first session her feet were so sensitive that only the lightest touch was bearable for her.

She recognized that her current work-related problems and relationship problems were the cause of her stress levels but that she had also suffered from stress for a considerable number of years beforehand, due to taking a degree and relationship problems.

After six months of treatment, she had a slight period lasting two days and a further one two months later. Slowly, over a period of two years, her periods have returned, usually arriving every six to eight weeks and now last three to four days.

Infertility or Subfertility

Many years ago, two couples came for reflexology because of infertility. Although in those days (the early 1980s) not much research had been carried out in regard to the effects of reflexology and infertility, they decided to give it a try as there was nothing amiss clinically with either couple. It may have been coincidence and both couples may have conceived regardless of the treatment, but when, after six and eight months, both couples gave me the welcome news that they were expecting a happy event, we were all convinced that reflexology was the cause of both couples conceiving and producing normal, healthy infants.

CHAPTER 22
The Nervous System

Overview of the Nervous System

Provides movement, leverage, and sensory perception within consciousness, and functioning of organs and glands beneath the level of consciousness.

Structures	*Functions*
CENTRAL NERVOUS SYSTEM (CNS)	
Brain (cerebrum, decision making)	Interprets nerve impulses received from sensory nerves from all parts of the body; decision making within conscious control
Spinal cord	Transmits sensory nerve impulses to the brain received from all parts of the body and transmits motor nerve impulses to voluntary (striated) and involuntary (smooth) muscles enabling movement and leverage under conscious control and enabling smooth muscle organ/gland functioning beneath the level of consciousness
SPECIAL SENSES	Provide information to the brain and spinal cord about the external environment
PERIPHERAL NERVOUS SYSTEM (PNS) 31 pairs of spinal nerves: sensory/motor nerves together are called mixed nerves, which form part of the autonomic nervous system (ANS) and the central nervous system (CNS)	Sensory nerve fibres from the periphery of the body (the skin) and organs/glands transmit nerve impulses via the spinal cord to the brain, which then relays motor impulses to the smooth muscle of the ANS of internal organs, glands and muscles at the edge of the body and skeletal muscle
12 pairs of cranial nerves originate in the brain and are sensory, motor and mixed nerves	Receive messages from the spinal cord and transmit impulses to muscles involved in the functions of smell, sight, hearing, chewing, sensory facial nerves, taste, balance, posture, secretion of saliva, and pharyngeal, laryngeal and neck/shoulder movements; the vagus nerve is the 10th cranial nerve and extends downwards through the neck, thorax and abdomen

continued overleaf

Overview of the Nervous System *continued*

Structures	*Functions*
AUTONOMIC NERVOUS SYSTEM (ANS)	Functions beneath the level of consciousness but can be influenced by decision making; finely balanced to provide optimum functioning; involuntary (smooth) muscle contains sensory and motor nerves; motor nerves stimulate glandular secretions and contractions of smooth muscle and sensory nerves transmit nerve impulses to the spinal cord and brain (*see* PNS above)

Sympathetic nerve impulses
hormones: adrenalin/noradrenalin

stimulate: a regular heart rate;
     secretions from glands in the alimentary canal;
     contraction of involuntary (smooth) muscle by motor nerves;
     dilation/contraction of pupils of the eyes

Parasympathetic nerve impulses
(work simultaneously with
sympathetic nerve impulses)

inhibit: facilitates adjustments to the external environment and maintains a normal temperature – called the 'peace-maker' as it calms activity to normal

CEREBELLUM (SMALL BRAIN)   Balance and coordination

MEDULLA OBLONGATA   Heart/respiratory rate; reflex actions and vasomotor centre

Endocrine (hormone) function responds to nerve impulses interpreted by the brain in response to the internal and external environment.

LINKS TO: endocrine, special senses, muscular, skeletal, digestive, respiratory, integumentary and reproductive systems.

INTRODUCTION

The nervous system conveys nerve impulses, which are tiny electrical charges. Neurons, or nerves, which contain a cell body, nucleus and nerve fibres composed of cytoplasm, are involved in conducting nerve impulses, with the strength of the impulse maintained throughout the length of the nerve. There are different sizes and types of each group of nerves.

There is always more than one nerve involved in the transmission of a nerve impulse from its origin to its destination. There is no continuity between nerves and the point at which the nerve impulse passes from one to another is called the synapse. The space between them is called the synaptic gap.

Remember! It is important to stay on the same spinal pathway when working down.

To keep a nerve impulse at a constant rate, stimulation can be described as electrical, mechanical and chemical:

- **Electrical** stimulation is found in sensory nerve endings, which move impulses quickly along nerves towards the brain.
- **Chemical** transmission of impulses crosses synapses with chemical neurotransmitters.
- **Mechanical** stimulation is found in motor nerve response where decision-making moves parts of the body.

Cells of some nerves initiate nerve impulses, while others act as relay stations where impulses are passed on or redirected. Nerve cells vary considerably in size and shape but are too small to be seen by the naked eye. They form the grey matter of the nervous system and are found at the periphery of the brain, in the centre of the spinal cord, grouped as ganglia outside the brain and spinal cord, and in the walls of organs. Nerve cells initiate irritability and conductivity.

- **Irritability** involves *stimuli* from outside the body (for example, touch) and inside the body, where changes in the level of carbon dioxide in the blood affect respiration. Decision-making may result in voluntary movement, under the control of the will.
- **Conductivity** involves *transmission* of impulses from one part of the brain to the other and from the brain to muscle, initiating voluntary muscle contraction; muscles and joints to the brain to aid in the maintenance of balance; from the brain to organs to provide the contraction of smooth muscles or glandular secretions; the regulation of body functions; from the outside world through sensory nerve endings in skin, stimulated by pain, temperature and touch; and, finally, from the external environment

to the brain through the special senses of ears, eyes, tongue and nose.

The nervous system is divided into three parts:

- the **central nervous system** (CNS), which includes the brain and spinal cord;
- the **peripheral nervous system** (PNS), consisting of nerves outside of the central nervous system, which extend to the periphery of the body;
- the **autonomic nervous system** (ANS), which controls functions beneath the level of consciousness.

THE CENTRAL NERVOUS SYSTEM (CNS)

Nerve cells in the central nervous system consist of up to a quarter to half the volume of brain tissue and, unlike other nerve cells, they continue to replicate throughout life. Movement is provided by nerve cells connecting with the part of the brain that influences control of the will and the spinal cord. The spinal cord is about 45cm (18in) long in an adult and is about the thickness of the little finger.

Mixed Nerves

In the spinal cord, *sensory* and *motor* nerves are arranged into separate groups or tracts. Sensory nerves belong to the PNS and motor nerves to the CNS. Outside of the spinal cord, sensory and motor nerves are enclosed in the same sheath of connective tissue, and are called mixed nerves. Most nerves in the body fall into this category.

Motor Nerves

Motor nerves begin in the brain, spinal cord and autonomic ganglia, and are involved in voluntary and reflex skeletal muscle contraction, involuntary (autonomic) smooth muscle contraction and the secretion of glands. Motor or efferent nerve impulses originate in the brain in response to sensory stimuli and nerve impulses transmit impulses towards muscle to provide movement. Motor nerves contain breaks in the myelin sheath, which are called the nodes of Ranvier. These nodes aid the rapid transmission of nerve impulses along the nerve fibres.

The motor end-plate is a sensitive area of muscle fibre. Nerve impulses are passed across the synaptic gap between the motor end-plates and the muscle fibres by chemicals called neurotransmitters. Movement is promoted by this process.

Axons and Dendrites

Each nerve consists of a nerve cell, which contains an axon and a dendrite. Axons and dendrites form the white matter of the nervous system. They are found deep in the brain and the periphery of the spinal cord.

Dendrites are processes or nerve fibres that carry impulses towards the cell and from the brain. They have the same structure as axons but are usually shorter and branch outwards, rather like branches on a tree. Each nerve has many dendrites.

Axons are longer than dendrites, sometimes as long as 100cm (39in). Axons carry nerve impulses from the cell to the brain. Axons have a membrane and a myelin sheath of fatty material surrounding them, which gives them a white appearance. The functions of the myelin sheath are to act as an insulator, speed the flow of nerve impulses through the axon and protect the axon from injury.

Spinal Cord and the Meninges

The spinal cord is the connecting structure between the brain and the rest of the body.

It is an elongated shape, is suspended in the spinal canal and is surrounded by the meninges and the cerebrospinal fluid (CSF). It continues upwards to become the medulla oblongata and extends downwards from the atlas vertebrae to the first lumbar vertebrae, and is approximately 45cm (18in) long in an adult.

Cerebrospinal fluid supports and protects the spinal cord and acts as a cushion or shock absorber between the brain, skull and vertebrae. It transports nutrients, white blood cells and waste products present in the CNS. The brain and spinal cord are surrounded by three membranes called the meninges. These membranes lie between the skull and the brain and between the vertebrae and the spinal cord. Named from the inside (nearest to the brain) to the outside of the brain, they are called the *pia mater*, the *arachnoid mater* and the *dura mater*.

The dura mater is the most durable as it provides a protective surface for the skull bones. It terminates at the coccyx at the tail of the spine.

The delicate web-like structure of the arachnoid mater lies between the dura and pia maters. It is separated from the dura mater and from the pia mater by a space containing cerebrospinal fluid (CSF). It envelops the spinal cord as it continues downwards and ends by merging with the dura mater at the level of the sacral vertebrae.

The pia mater is attached to the brain, which it completely covers. It contains blood vessels that transport nutrients to the brain; it continues downwards towards the base of the spine where it fuses with the coccyx.

Blood capillaries in the arachnoid mater return CSF to the circulating blood. The CSF consists of a clear, slightly alkaline fluid containing water, mineral salts, glucose, plasma proteins and waste products. The functions of CSF are to:

- support and protect the brain and spinal cord;
- maintain a constant pressure around the delicate structures of the meninges and brain;
- act as a cushion and shock absorber between the brain and the cranial bones;
- keep the brain and spinal cord moist.

The spinal cord ends between the third and fourth lumbar vertebrae at about the level of the hip bone. In a lumbar puncture, a sample of CSF is taken from between the third and fourth lumbar vertebrae, which can be analysed for the presence of disease or injury, for example in the case of meningitis.

PERIPHERAL NERVOUS SYSTEM (PNS)

The PNS is made up of all the nerves outside the CNS. Peripheral nerves constantly relay information to the brain by sensory nerves from the periphery of the body and from the brain by motor nerves to the muscles. The PNS consists of:

- Thirty-one pairs of spinal nerves that leave the spinal cord at the various parts of the vertebral column and supply all areas of the body below the neck. They consist of:
  - 8 cervical nerves;
  - 12 thoracic nerves;
  - 5 lumbar nerves;
  - 5 sacral nerves;
  - 1 coccygeal nerve.
- The autonomic nervous system;
- Twelve pairs of cranial nerves originate in the brain and are numbered in accordance with their connection to the brain. The cranial nerves supply the head, senses, organs, muscles, heart, respiratory and digestive tracts (through the vagus nerve) (*see* overview).

Sensory or Afferent Nerve Pathways

We have seen that nerves that transmit impulses from the periphery of the body to the spinal cord are called sensory or afferent nerves. These impulses may then pass to the brain or collect in the nerves of the reflex arc in the lumbar region of the spine.

The PNS is divided into two parts:

- *somatic* system: collects information about the external environment through the sensory organs of sight, hearing, smell and taste.
- *somatic* or '*common senses*': originate in the skin and comprise receptors that give external feedback on pain, touch, heat and cold.

The sensory nerves from the organs are grouped with those that come from the skin and voluntary muscles. Some sensory nerve endings are called proprioceptors. They originate in muscles, tendons and joints. The specialized nerve endings relay messages to the brain about the position, posture and balance of the body. The eyes and ears assist in coordination and maintenance of balance. These sensory or afferent nerves give us a sense of our external environment, for example, whether we are safe or in danger.

The sensory nerves terminate in skin and divide into fine branches called the sensory nerve endings. These are stimulated in the skin by touch, pain, heat and cold. Impulses are transmitted to the brain, where sensation is perceived and response activated.

Although the PNS is closely linked to the CNS, cranial and spinal nerves also carry impulses through the ANS to the organs in the thoracic, abdominal and pelvic cavities.

The internal organs such as the heart, lungs and stomach contain nerve endings and fibres for conducting sensory messages to the brain and spinal cord but most of these impulses do not reach consciousness.

AUTONOMIC NERVOUS SYSTEM

The function of the autonomic nervous system is reliant on sensory nerve input to the brain and motor response from the brain. Additionally, hormones play a key role in autonomic nerve reaction.

The autonomic nervous system regulates the action of glands, the smooth muscles of hollow organs and the heart. These actions occur automatically whenever changes are required in the maintenance of homeostasis, such adjustment being made without our conscious awareness.

The parts of the autonomic nerve system that stimulate and inhibit nerve response are called sympathetic ganglia, which stimulate organ and gland function, and parasympathetic ganglia, which inhibit organ or gland function. Sensory nerves originate in internal organs and tissues and are associated with reflex regulation of activity and visceral (organ or gland) pain.

Sympathetic Pathways and Ganglia

The sympathetic nervous system consists of a series of ganglia connected together by cords extending from the base of the skull to the coccyx, one on each side of the middle of the body, partly to the front and partly on each side of the vertebral column. The sympathetic nerve response has its base in the medulla oblongata and the hypothalamus.

Nerve fibre functions are to communicate with each other and with the spinal nerves, and to supply the internal organs and the blood vessels.

The sympathetic part of the autonomic nervous system tends to act as a stimulant for those organs when needed to meet a stressful situation. It promotes what is called the 'fight or flight' response.

There are more sympathetic ganglia than parasympathetic ganglia. The solar plexus ganglia are situated one on each side of the plexus and are the largest ganglia in the body. They are formed by irregular masses of smaller ganglia with spaces between them. These ganglia are situated in front of the diaphragm, close to the adrenal gland (*see* Chapter 13).

Parasympathetic Pathways and Ganglia

Parasympathetic nerve response is controlled by two nerves: one nerve is situated in the brain or spinal cord, and the other is situated in the organ or ganglion. Parasympathetic functions inhibit sympathetic nerve response.

Nerve Plexi

Nerves fibres are bundled into mixed neuron groups, called plexi. They leave the spinal cord to supply skin, bones, muscles and joints. There are five major nerve plexi called the cervical, brachial, lumbar, sacral and coccygeal. Each spinal nerve continues only a short distance away from the spinal cord.

- The **cervical plexus** supplies motor impulses to muscles and the neck, and receives sensory impulses from the neck and the back of the head.
- The **brachial plexus** sends numerous branches to the chest, shoulder, arm, forearm, wrist and hand. Nerve roots contain sensory, motor and autonomic nerve fibres.
- The **lumbosacral plexus** including the lumbar and sacral plexi supplies nerves to the lower extremities. The largest nerve in the body is the sciatic nerve, which is about 2cm thick; it leaves the pelvis, passes beneath the gluteus maximus muscle (muscle in the buttock) and branches down the back of the thigh to the knee, where it divides to supply each leg and foot, finishing on the dorsum

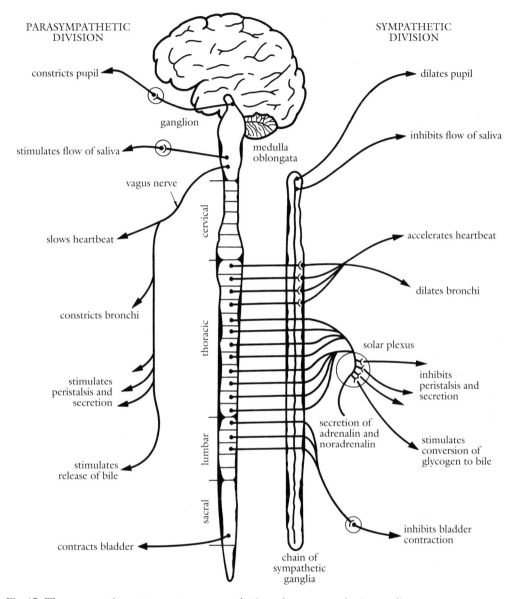

PARASYMPATHETIC
DIVISION

SYMPATHETIC
DIVISION

constricts pupil

dilates pupil

ganglion

stimulates flow of saliva

medulla
oblongata

inhibits flow of saliva

vagus nerve

cervical

slows heartbeat

accelerates heartbeat

dilates bronchi

constricts bronchi

thoracic

solar plexus

stimulates
peristalsis and
secretion

inhibits
peristalsis and
secretion

secretion of
adrenalin and
noradrenalin

stimulates
conversion of
glycogen to bile

lumbar

stimulates
release of bile

sacral

inhibits bladder
contraction

contracts bladder

chain of
sympathetic
ganglia

Fig 45. The autonomic nervous system: sympathetic and parasympathetic ganglia.

(top) of the foot and under the heel of the foot. The lumbosacral plexus also supplies the hip and pelvic cavity.

• The **coccygeal plexus** supplies the area surrounding the coccyx and muscles of the pelvic floor.

257

Vagus Nerve

The vagus nerve is one of the major nerves in the body. The parasympathetic vagus nerve branches to the thorax and abdomen.

The vagus nerve affects a large proportion of the organs and glands. The parts of the body controlled by the vagus nerve are the larynx, bile duct, ureters, intestines, heart, pharynx, trachea, kidneys, pancreas, stomach, oesophagus, gall bladder, spleen, lungs and liver. It contains motor, secretory, sensory and vasodilator fibres (meaning fibres that cause the blood vessels to dilate).

A vasovagal attack is a temporary loss of consciousness caused by an abrupt slowing of the heartbeat. This can happen following shock, acute pain, fear or stress. It is associated with fainting, as a vasovagal attack may be the consequence of over-stimulation of the vagus nerve, which is involved in the control of breathing and circulation.

Referred Pain

A referred pain is a pain felt at some distance from the site of the actual disorder, and can be found in the heart, referred to the left shoulder and arm, the liver, referred to the right shoulder, the uterus referred to the lower back, the lung, referred to the shoulder and upper arm, the spinal disc, referred to the leg or foot, the knee, referred to the spine, and the neck referred to the arm and hand.

Spinal Reflex Arc

Damage anywhere along the spinal reflex path causes loss of a tendon reflex. A reflex arc consists of a sensory and a motor nerve. The stretch reflex occurs when the muscle is stretched and contracts when tapped beneath the kneecap. Tapping large muscles produces the same effect, such as the gastrocnemius in the calf.

The 'Flight or Fight' Response

The medulla of the adrenal gland is made up of the same nervous tissue as the sympathetic nervous system and is, therefore, closely involved in stimulation from either the external or internal environment. The following is an example of how the special senses, the CNS, PNS, ANS and endocrine systems interrelate.

When an event is a potential danger to life, the brain interprets danger through peripheral nerves, which collect sensory information. Nerve impulses are relayed through the spinal cord to the brain where the message of danger is interpreted and a decision made, under the consciousness of the will, to run or fight the potential danger. The effect of the 'fight or flight' response is to stimulate the central portion of the adrenal gland to produce the hormone adrenalin, which prepares the body to meet emergency situations, and cortisol from the cortex of the adrenal gland. Sympathetic nerve response is stimulated by emotion and fear, hence sympathetic reflex action occurs with superhuman strength and/or speed. The sympathetic nerves and hormones from the adrenal gland reinforce each other.

The peripheral nerves react to the 'fight or flight' response in the following ways:

- the lens of the eye dilates, sharpening the focus of the eyeball onto the retina;
- the digestive and urinary functions shut down whilst in a state of emergency;
- the hormones adrenalin and cortisol are released to provide a quickened heartbeat, so that more oxygen supplies the body;
- the muscles in the bronchial tubes dilate to inhale more oxygen;
- increased glucose levels are released from the liver to be sent into the bloodstream to create energy for muscle;

- once the crisis is over, adrenalin is switched off and the heartbeat and other bodily functions resume normality.

Once acted upon and the crisis over, the parasympathetic part of the ANS slows the body to normal functions as noradrenalin is secreted through parasympathetic nerve action.

The sympatheticotonic type of person is less emotionally stable with a tendency to develop digestive disorders.

The vagotonic type of person is emotionally stable and balanced, and usually placid. These types possess a good digestion and are not easily disturbed.

BRAIN

The brain constitutes about one-fiftieth of the body weight and lies within the cranial cavity, where the skull bones protect it. It consumes 50 per cent of the glucose produced by the liver. Brain tissue reaches its maximum by age twenty years and then decreases throughout life. The parts of the brain are called:

- the cerebrum or forebrain;
- the cerebellum or hindbrain;
- the midbrain;
- the pons varolii;
- the medulla oblongata.

The midbrain, pons varolii and medulla oblongata form the brainstem.

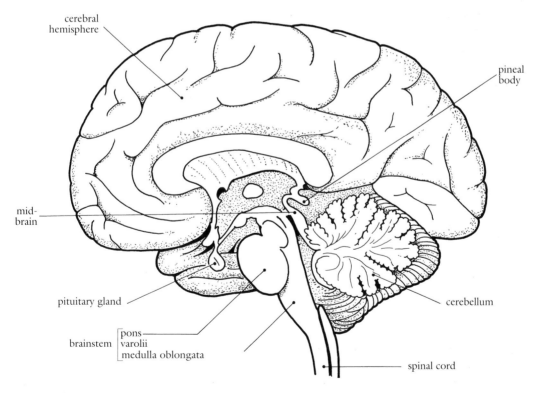

Fig 46. The brain.

The cerebrum is the largest part of the brain. The functions of the cerebrum are to do with decision-making and will. There are three main varieties of activity associated with the cerebral cortex, and these are:

- mental activities involved in memory, intelligence, sense of responsibility, thinking, reasoning, moral sense and learning;
- sensory perception, including the perception of pain, temperature, touch, sight, hearing, taste and smell;
- the promotion and control of voluntary muscle contractions.

The motor area of the brain lies in the frontal lobe, and nerve cells called 'betz cells' initiate the contraction of voluntary muscles. A nerve fibre from a betz cell passes downwards to the medulla oblongata, where it crosses to the opposite side and then descends into the spinal cord. This means that the motor area at the right hemisphere of the cerebrum controls voluntary muscle movement on the left side of the body and a motor area in the left hemisphere controls movement on the right side. Communication skills, such as talking and writing, are under the control of this area too.

In the frontal area of the brain there is a more highly developed area than in other animals. It is thought that communications between this and other regions of the cerebrum are responsible for behaviour, character and emotional balance.

The parietal lobe controls the sensory area in which impulses from the skin, such as touch, pain and temperature, are interpreted and judgement concerning distances, sizes and shapes takes place.

The temporal lobe is responsible for the auditory area, for receiving and interpreting impulses from the ear. The olfactory area is concerned with the sense of smell located in the medial (middle) part of the temporal lobe which is stimulated by receptors in the nose.

The occipital lobe lies behind the parietal lobe and extends over the cerebellum towards the back of the skull. This lobe contains the visual area for interpreting impulses arising from the retina of the eye.

The control of body movement and facial expressions is formed by the basal ganglia, which are masses of grey matter located deep within each cerebral hemisphere. A neurotransmitter, dopamine, is secreted from here. Dopamine has been linked to Parkinsonism.

Diencephalon

The diencephalon or inter-brain can be seen in the central section of the brain between the two cerebral hemispheres. It includes the thalamus and the hypothalamus. Almost all sensory impulses travel through the masses of grey matter that form the thalamus. The action of the thalamus is to process the impulses and direct them to particular areas of the cerebral cortex.

Hypothalamus

The hypothalamus is located in the mid-line below the thalamus and contains cells that help control body temperature and water balance. It controls hormonal secretions from the pituitary gland, body temperature, hunger and thirst, metabolism, genital functions and sleep. The hypothalamus influences the heartbeat and the contraction and relaxation of the walls of the blood vessels. Both the sympathetic and parasympathetic divisions of the autonomic nervous system are under the control of the hypothalamus and the pituitary gland (*see also* the Endocrine System).

Limbic System

The limbic system includes regions of the cerebrum and the diencephalon and is found running between the two. This system is involved in emotional states and behaviour. It includes the hippocampus (meaning shaped like a seahorse) and functions include the ability for learning and retaining information with long-term memory.

Midbrain

The midbrain is located just below the centre of the cerebrum. The midbrain is responsible for acting as a relay station between the pons varolii, medulla, cerebellum and spinal cord.

Pons Varolii

The pons varolii lies between the midbrain and the medulla and in front of the cerebellum. Its purpose is to connect the two halves of the cerebellum with the brainstem, as well as with the cerebrum above and the spinal cord below.

Medulla Oblongata

The medulla oblongata is located between the pons varolii and the spinal cord. The medulla oblongata forms the brainstem and is the control centre of the autonomic nervous system (ANS). The functions of the medulla oblongata are as follows:

- It is the centre of respiration, which controls the muscles of respiration in response to chemical reactions and other stimuli. It is here that the regulation of carbon dioxide and oxygen takes place within the brain. The brain requires carbon dioxide to be present for the successful regulation of the levels of oxygen in the blood.
- The cardiac centre regulates the rate and force of the heartbeat.
- The vasomotor centre regulates the contraction of smooth muscle in the blood vessel walls and thus controls blood flow and blood pressure. This also controls the reflex centres, for example vomiting, sneezing, yawning, coughing, blinking, shivering, the grasp reflex, and the response of the pupil to light.
- Controls the digestive process.

Pain Control

Control of pain is helped naturally from areas of the brain that produce endorphins and enkephalins. These substances are released by the hypothalamus, pituitary and other areas of the brain. Enkephalins are also believed to act as a sedative and mood changer. Endorphins have been shown to have an anti-psychotic effect and are of value in the treatment of major psychotic illnesses.

SPECIAL INTEREST

The brain reflex is interesting in how it can reflect the mental activity of the individual by the amount of 'crunchiness' of uric acid crystals present. Mental tiredness on one or other toes can relate to the type of activity, for example, a crunchy feeling on the left toe can relate to extreme creative activity, and sensitivity on the right toe to logical thinking. Remember that the nerves cross over from each side of the body as they enter the brain and thus the left side of the brain relates to the right side of the body, and vice versa.

With patients who have suffered a stroke, the toes round the brain area can appear to be red, a bluish colour, swollen or puffy. Again, a stroke suffered on the right side of the brain will affect the left side of the body and vice versa. (*See* Chapter 23 for special interest on the spine.)

Sciatica can be caused by psychological tension as well as physical misalignments of the pelvic girdle and spinal vertebrae. Make sure you work up and down these reflexes from under the fibia bone.

WORKING THE REFLEXES

Spinal Reflexes – Reflex Point 42 – Skeletal and Nervous Systems

Support the heel with the palm of the supporting hand (right hand on the left foot and the left hand on the right foot). Place the fingers of the working hand underneath the supporting hand. To work the coccygeal reflexes, begin at the back of the calcaneum (heel bone) and work vertically with the thumbs pointing up the leg for about 2.5cm (1in) and along the foot towards the bladder for about 2.5–4cm (1–1½in). Work back towards the heel edge of the calcaneum and repeat movements twice more. At the edge of the calcaneum, turn the thumb so that the tip is facing up the foot towards the big toe and decide which pathway you wish to begin working, for example the pathway on the curve of the foot or on the bony ridge of the foot. Begin working up the pathway from the heel edge of the calcaneum and when the thumb can no longer reach, bring both the supporting hand and the working hand fingers over the ankle on top of the foot – making sure that the fingers of the working hand are on top of the supporting hand. Continue to work the spine by bringing both hands up

---

The Nervous System

System(s)	Associated Reflexes	Disorders
REFLEX POINTS 8, 42: THE BRAIN AND SPINAL CORD		
All systems, especially nervous, skeletal, muscular	Whole foot for all systems and nerve innervations	Multiple sclerosis, epilepsy, meningitis, motor neurone disease, Parkinson's disease, polio, stroke

Nerve innervations: brain, 1st Cervical; spinal cord, all innervations

System(s)	Associated Reflexes	Disorders
REFLEX POINT 18: FACE AND NOSE		
Nervous	Brain, spine, solar plexus	Neuralgia, Bell's palsy, neuritis
Muscular	Diaphragm	rhinitis, olfactory desensitization,
Special senses	Ears, eyes	skin disorders, head cold, sinusitis,
Endocrine	Pituitary, hypothalamus and pineal glands	skeletal misalignments
Respiratory	Lungs, sinuses	
Skeletal/joints	Skull bones, spine	

Nerve innervations: 1st, 2nd, 3rd, 4th Cervical

System(s)	Associated Reflexes	Disorders
REFLEX POINTS 29, 45: THE SCIATIC NERVE		
Nervous	Brain, solar plexus	Sciatica, skeletal misalignments,
Muscular	Diaphragm	psychogenic factors, lower motor
Skeletal/joints	Spine, innominate bones, arms, legs, all joint reflexes	neurone lesions

Nerve innervations: 4th, 5th Lumbar and Sacrum

See Chapter 26 for a description of disorders related to the Nervous System

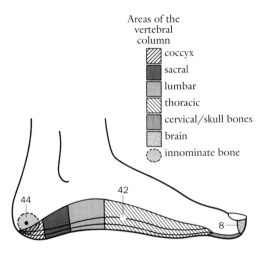

The spinal vertebrae and spinal cord, reflex points 42 and 44 (both feet).

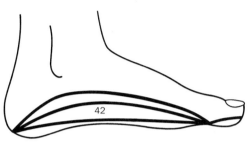

The nervous system, reflex point 42 (both feet).

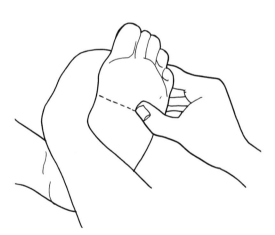

Hand position: the solar plexus and diaphragm, reflex point 1 (both feet). Working hand over supporting hand. Refer to the Nervous, Respiratory and Digestive Systems.

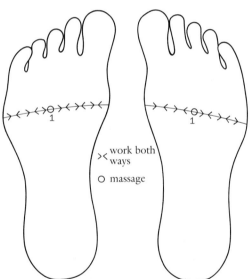

Directional working: the solar plexus and diaphragm, reflex point 1 (both feet).

the foot together so that the foot is correctly supported as you move towards the big toe.

At the neck reflex at the 7th cervical vertebra (base of the big toe), swap the working finger to the index finger to work the cervical vertebrae. Flip the supporting hand over the big toe to cradle it firmly between the thumb and index finger. This stops the toe from

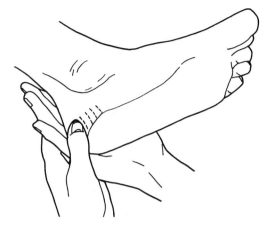

Hand position: working the coccyx and the spinal cord, reflex point 42 (both feet). Working hand under supporting hand.

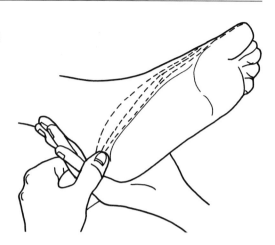

Hand position: Working the spinal pathways, reflex point 42. Working hand under supporting hand.

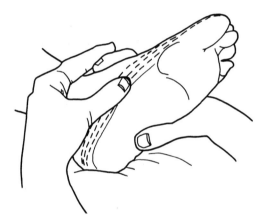

Hand position: working the spinal pathways, reflex point 42. Working hand over supporting hand.

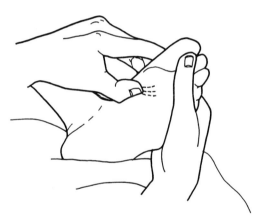

Hand position: the neck supporter when working the spinal pathways, reflex point 54a (both feet). Working hand over supporting hand.

moving. Make small ripple movements with the index finger up to the top of the big toe and rock the brain as before.

To work down the same spinal pathway, use the top of the left hand on the left foot to support the sole of the foot with the tips of the fingers supporting the big toe firmly and place the palm of the working right hand over the big toe, supporting the toe firmly from above. This way the big toe resembles 'meat in a sandwich' with the working hand thumb free to work down from the tip of the toe. Work down the same pathway as you worked up, sliding the supporting hand down the sole of the foot as you work down the spine to the edge of the calcaneum.

Repeat these movements on the second pathway between the curve of the foot and the

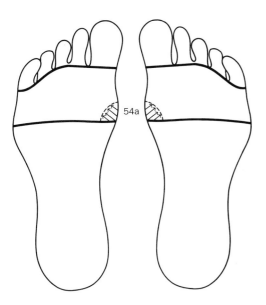

54a

Directions for working: neck supporter area from spinal pathways, reflex point 54a (both feet).

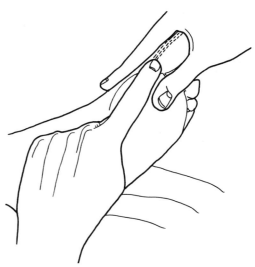

Hand position: the spinal pathways, reflex point 42. Supporting hand cradles the big toe.

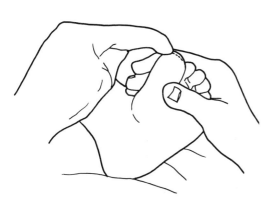

Hand position: the brain reflex and the spinal pathways, reflex point 8 (both feet). Supporting hand is held across the tips of the toes.

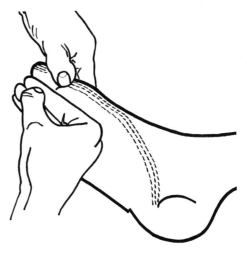

Hand position: the spinal pathways towards the heel, reflex points 42 and 43 (both feet). Supporting hand and working hand fingers 'sandwich' the big toe between them.

bony ridge of the metatarsal and tarsal bones, then repeat the movements on the bony ridge itself. It may be helpful to run a finger over the bony structure to be sure where you need to work. Refer to skeletal system for further information relating to the spine.

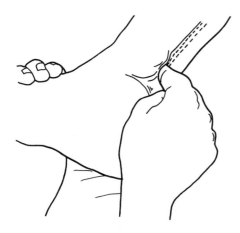

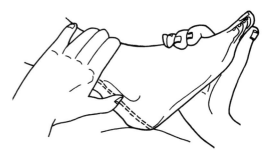

Hand position: the sciatic nerve, reflex point 45 (both feet). Supporting hand supports the medial edge of the foot.

Hand position: the sciatic nerve, reflex point 45 (both feet). Supporting hand supports the medial edge of the foot.

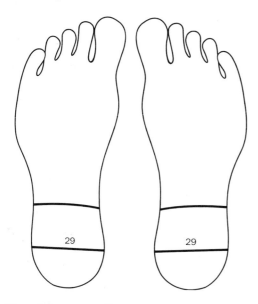

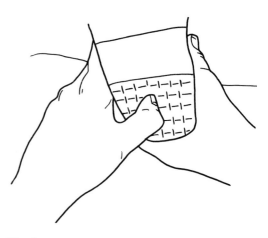

The sciatic nerve, reflex point 29 (both feet).

Hand position: the sciatic nerve, reflex point 29 (both feet). Supporting hand is held under the heel; working hand fingers are placed on top of the foot.

Reflex Point 54a – Chronic Neck and Shoulder Supporter

This reflex can be worked when working the spinal pathways as it affects the muscles, nerves and vertebrae between the shoulder blades, which are associated with neck pain. From the base of the ball of the big toe, work diagonally into the middle of foot, for approximately halfway up the side of the fleshy part of the 1st metatarsal joint.

CASE STUDY WITH A STROKE PATIENT

This gentleman came for treatment many years ago, on recommendation by his wife. He had suffered a stroke to the left side of his brain, which meant that the right side of his body was affected. His right arm was bent at the elbow and twisted in towards the body, with wrist and hand bent into the underarm. Amazingly, the big toe on the right foot was completely blue, whilst the left big toe appeared to be quite normal.

In the first few treatments he felt little or no pain in the foot reflexes, then after a few more treatments he began to find movement at the wrist and pain on the foot reflexes. Unfortunately, just after this point he ceased coming for treatment because of personal reasons and I never did know the outcome of his condition. I would like to think that his condition improved but I shall never be sure. Very often, this situation happens with patients – they begin to get good results from reflexology treatments, they stop coming and you are left wondering about the outcome of their health problem.

All we can do as complementary practitioners is be there for our patients and do the best we can and hope that they receive benefit from treatment – no matter how long or short the course of treatment.

CASE STUDY ON EPILEPSY

A multidisciplinary case where three other complementary therapies were introduced to speed-up the healing process had spectacular results for a young epileptic woman some years go. She was one of a pair of twins and was slightly brain-damaged at birth and suffered her first epileptic fit when she was two years old.

Her fits gradually worsened, and by the age of seven and a half her medication had increased to almost 500mg daily. This had the side-effects of weight gain, early pubescent development, she felt mentally slow, found school difficult and had no friends. Her parents divorced when she was still a young child and she went to live with her father, whilst her other twin and a brother lived with her mother.

By the age of nineteen she was put on 1200mg daily of medication. This caused her bowel to stop functioning, depression, suicidal feelings and desperation, headaches, an inability to cope with daily life and pains all over her body.

She came for reflexology initially, but after the consultation I decided that other therapies, such as colonic irrigation to swiftly clear the bowel, cranial osteopathy, to gently correct skull bone misalignments, polarity therapy, to help rebalance and calm energy pathways, would aid the healing process. It was with grateful thanks that she received these therapies freely by therapists as, most importantly, what she had never felt given was love and genuine care from others.

As reflexology and the other therapies progressed, her periods, which had stopped for five years, appeared spasmodically, her bowels became normalized, the depression lifted, she felt more interest in life and as a result more confident and able to take her place in society. Because she had spent all of her twenty-two years on medication, her life had become a haze of living from one fit to the next.

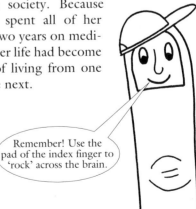

Remember! Use the pad of the index finger to 'rock' across the brain.

Much to her gratification, her *grand mal* fits were reduced from eight fits a day to one a day, and eventually none. She was, however, suffering from *petit mals* but was not always conscious of having suffered a minor fit. Her partner monitored her improvement and supported her throughout her involvement with myself and the other therapists.

Within three months, as a result of a combination of therapies, she felt able to reduce her medication under her doctor's supervision. At this stage of recovery she felt more present in the world, which created another problem – her emotional immaturity to cope as an adult. As she had never had the opportunity for healthy mental and emotional development from babyhood, her next therapeutic encounter would necessarily involve psychotherapy or counselling.

Unfortunately, I have lost touch with her over the last few years but I hope she continues to stabilize and find herself and her place in the world.

CHAPTER 23

The Skeletal System and Joints

Overview of the Skeletal System and Joints

Provides movement and leverage, protection of internal structures, attachments for muscles, forms boundaries between the cranial, thoracic and pelvic cavities and is weight bearing.

Two hundred and six bones form the human skeleton, with twenty-six bones in each foot and twenty-seven bones in each hand.

Structures

COMPACT BONE
Appendicular skeleton:
   Limbs, pelvic and shoulder girdles
   Shape: long bones

CANCELLOUS BONE
Axial skeleton:
   Skull, sternum, ribs and vertebrae
   Shape: short, flat and irregular

SESAMOID BONE
Develop in tendons and joint capsule
   Found in the patella
     (knee cap) and feet

Functions

Provide movement, leverage and is weight bearing; store calcium, manufacture erythrocytes (red blood cells) in red bone marrow at the ends of long bones; give attachment to (voluntary) muscles

Manufacture erythrocytes in red bone marrow; give protection to internal structures; movement; attachment to muscles

Act as shock absorbers

THE JOINTS

SYNOVIAL JOINTS
Freely moveable
   Types: gliding, hinge, saddle,
     condyloid, pivot, ball and socket

Provide movements of flexion, extension, circumduction, rotation, adduction, abduction, inversion and eversion; allow angular and free movement

FIXED (OR IMMOVABLE) JOINTS
Found in the skull bones

No movement; protect internal structures

CARTILAGINOUS JOINTS
   Found in the symphysis pubis
   and vertebrae

Act as shock absorbers and allow slight movement

LINKS TO: muscular, urinary, circulatory, lymphatic, nervous, respiratory and endocrine systems.

INTRODUCTION

There are 206 bones in the human body, including twenty-six bones in each foot and twenty-seven bones in each hand. Bone is the hardest connective tissue in the body and when fully developed it is composed of 20 per cent water, 30–40 per cent organic material and 40–50 per cent inorganic material. There are two types of bone tissue called compact and cancellous.

BONE TISSUE

Compact Bone

Compact bone appears to be solid but on microscopic examination an extensive number of Haversian canals can be seen. These consist of minute tunnels in which blood vessels, lymphatics and nerves maintain and repair bone. Surrounding the Haversian canals are plates of bones called 'lamellae', which are separated from one another and contain lymph and bone cells (osteocytes). This tubular arrangement gives bone greater strength than a solid structure of the same size. Tendons, ligaments and muscles are attached to bone.

Compact bone is found in the limbs. The shaft of the bone is composed of dense bone, which forms a hard tube and which is surrounded by a membrane of periosteum that houses fatty yellow bone marrow. The end of a long bone is called the 'epiphysis' and is formed of cancellous bone and red bone marrow.

Cancellous Bone

Cancellous bone has a spongy appearance and the Haversian canals are much larger than in compact bone. There are fewer plates of bone so that the bone structure has a honeycomb appearance. Red bone marrow is always present in cancellous bone.

Periosteum

Bones are almost completely covered by periosteum. In the deeper layers of the periosteum, there are osteogenic (bone) cells that increase the thickness of compact tissue and maintain the shape of the bones. Periosteum gives attachment to muscles and tendons and protects the bone from injury. Periosteum is replaced by hyaline cartilage on the articulating surfaces of the synovial joints, and by the *dura mater* meninge on the inner surface of the cranial bones.

Bone Growth

The development of bone tissue begins before birth and is not complete until between the twenty-first and twenty-fifth year of life. Bones develop in thickness from fibrous tissue and lime salts deposited in bone cells.

Shapes of Bone

There are five shapes of bone:

- **sesamoid**: patella and feet;
- **irregular**: cranium, vertebrae;
- **flat**: sternum, scapula;
- **long**: fibula, tibia;
- **short**: phalanges.

Irregular, flat and sesamoid bones are composed of a relatively thin outer layer of compact bone with cancellous bone inside. Long, short and irregular bones develop from cartilage, flat bones from membrane and sesamoid bones from tendons.

There are two divisions of the skeleton.

- The **axial skeleton** forms the bony core of the body and includes the ribs, sternum, vertebrae and skull.
- The **appendicular skeleton** forms the shoulder and pelvic girdles and the limbs.

The functions of bones are to:

- provide a framework for the body;
- give attachment to muscles and tendons;
- allow movement of the body by forming joints to give attachment to muscle;
- protect the organs and form boundaries in the cranial, thoracic and pelvic cavities;
- provide a reservoir for red bone marrow in which blood cells develop;
- provide a reservoir for calcium;
- provide a reservoir for fluorine, phosphorous and magnesium salts.

Sesamoid Bones

Sesamoid bones are cartilaginous in early life and calcified (harden) in the adult. They develop in tendons such as the knee, and in the feet which are weight-bearing joints.

THE SPINE

The vertebral column consists of thirty-three vertebrae in total, with twenty-four separate movable irregular bones. The twenty-four separate bones are divided into three groups, known as:

- seven cervical;
- twelve thoracic;
- five lumbar;

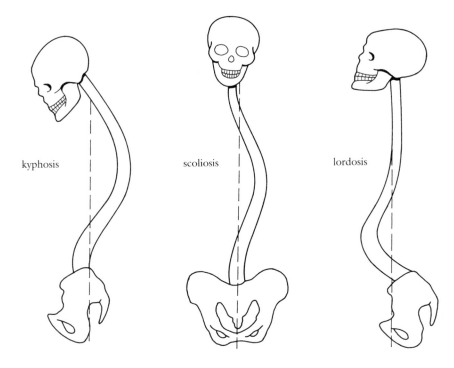

Fig 47. Curvatures of the spine.

- the sacrum consists of five fused bones, thereby forming one bone;
- the coccyx is composed of four bones fused together to form one. The coccyx is named after the shape of a cuckoo's beak.

Some groups of vertebrae have distinguishing features and their size varies with where they are found. They are smallest in the cervical region and become larger toward the lumbar region. The atlas is the first cervical vertebra and consists of a ring of bone. We obtain the nodding movement of 'Yes' from the atlas. The axis is the second cervical vertebra and gives the movement of the head turning from side to side in the movement of 'No'.

The longitudinal ligament in the vertebral canal helps to keep the vertebrae in place. Cartilaginous joints have a shock-absorbing function by acting as a form of cushioning between the vertebrae. They contribute to the flexibility of the vertebral column as a whole. When viewed from the side, the vertebral column presents four curves. These are found in the curve of the cervical, thoracic, sacral and coccyx areas of the spine. Individual bones of the vertebrae give little movement with the cervical and lumbar regions providing the most.

The functions of the vertebral column are as follows:

- the vertebral canal provides a strong bony protection for the delicate spinal cord lying within it;
- the spinal nerves, blood vessels and lymph vessels pass either side through the vertebrae;
- movement is obtained because of the large number of individual bones;
- it supports the skull;
- the intervertebral discs act as shock absorbers so protecting the brain;
- it forms the axis of the trunk, giving attach-ment to the ribs, shoulder girdle and upper limbs and pelvic girdle and lower limbs.

The spinal canal follows the curves of the spine and is largest where the spine has most movement – in the neck and in the pelvis, where it is wide and triangular for weight bearing. The narrower the curve of the spine, the narrower and more rounded the spinal canal becomes, for example, in the neck where motion is limited.

THE SKULL

The weight of the skull is approximately 5.5kg (12lb), and without the sinuses present we would find it extremely difficult to lift the head in an upright position. The sinuses communicate with the nose and are lined with ciliated mucus membrane. Their functions are to:

- give resonance to the voice;
- lighten the bones of the face and cranium, thereby making it easier for the head to balance on top of the vertebral column;
- provide release of mucosal congestion from the mucous membrane.

THE JOINTS

A joint is a site where two or more bones come together. There are three main types of joints called synovial, fixed and cartilaginous. Some joints have no movement and are called 'fixed', some have only slight movement and are called 'cartilaginous', and some are freely movable, known as 'synovial joints'. Fibrous or fixed joints are also called 'immovable joints' and have fibrous tissue between the bones, for example the bones between the skull and those between the teeth and the jaw bones.

Immovable or Fixed Joints

Examples of fixed joints are those between the tibia and fibula, hip bones and cranial bones; they are bound together by ligaments and fibrous tissue. Fixed joints do not have a cavity and, therefore, do not contain fluid.

Cartilaginous Joints

In cartilaginous joints, discs of cartilage containing a jelly-like substance separate the bones, as in the vertebral column and symphysis pubis. These joints have a pad of white fibrocartilage between the ends of the bones. This allows very slight movement, caused by compression of the pad of cartilage.

Synovial Joints

Synovial joints are freely moveable joints and are covered in hyaline cartilage. They are strong enough to bear the weight of the body. Synovial joints have a cavity that is filled with synovial fluid. This fluid helps to nourish the cartilage, which covers the surfaces of the bones and removes damaging substances from within the joint cavity.

Small, fluid-filled sacs called bursae are present in the shoulder, elbow, knee, back of the heel and the metatarso-phalangeal joint (big toe). They act as cushions to prevent friction between a bone and a ligament, tendon or skin, where a bone in a joint is near the surface.

Examples of synovial joints are as follows:

- **Gliding joints** allow the movement of carpal bones in the hand and between the tarsal bones of the feet. The articulating surfaces glide over each other.
- **Hinge joints** allow the movements of flexion and extension only. These can be found in the elbow, knee, ankle, the joints between the atlas and the occipital bone, and the joints of the fingers and toes.
- **Ball and socket joints** are found at the hip and shoulder and allow for a wide range of movement.
- **Pivot joints** are found at the radius and ulna at the elbow joint, and between the atlas and the axis.
- **Saddle joints** articulate the carpal and metacarpal bones of the wrist, hands and the phalanges (finger joints).

Ligaments

Ligaments are strong bands of fibrous tissue, which are flexible and only slightly elastic. They join bone to bone, bind ends of bones together, prevent over-exertion of joint movement and support various organs.

SPECIAL INTEREST

Spinal Pathways

The spine is the most important reflex for affecting every part of the body. The bony structure of the vertebrae connects muscles, nerves, blood and lymph vessels to every part of the physical body and, thus, should be worked thoroughly to find as much information as possible about other conditions that may exist.

From my experience of working the spinal pathways, I have discovered that there are three pathways that can relate to muscles attached to the vertebrae, innervations to viscera from the spine and the bony ridge of the vertebra itself. In all spinal problems, all three pathways should be worked as bone, nerves, muscles and viscera are all connected via the spinal nerves and autonomic nervous system ganglia along each side of the spine. However, by concentrating on specific problems and spinal pathways, greater detail can be obtained that can aid in giving professional advice on reflexology treatments and, possibly, other therapies which may be beneficial for the patient. It is amazing to see just for how many years individuals will walk about with their skeletal frame twisted and lopsided, and then wonder why they develop serious knee and hip problems in later life!

It is important to remember to check the spine when visceral problems are present; for example, with kidney problems check the 9th, 10th and 11th thoracic innervations for tenderness.

Find the spinal pathways as follows:

- The first pathway is found on the curve of the medial arch of the foot. Care should be taken not to work on the sole of the foot as this represents the reflex area for the ureter tube.
- The second pathway is found a little above the curve of the medial arch and the first pathway.
- The third pathway is found on the bony arch of the foot that forms the ridge of the instep.

All three pathways begin at the heel, at the coccyx reflex point, and converge at the base of the great toe for the 7th cervical vertebra. Once at the 7th cervical vertebra, the thumb should swap to the index finger (for sensitivity) to work these tiny vertebrae.

The cervical vertebrae in the neck and shoulders are a common position for stress, emotionally, by hunching the shoulders, physical tension through holding the head in one position for long periods of time, and injury, such as whiplash. Everybody suffers from some form of neck and shoulder tension and so work all related reflexes thoroughly. The effort alone of keeping upright and

balancing the head on the pivot joints of the atlas and axis create stiffness in the large muscles in the neck. The reflexes here are concerned with the skull, neck and innervations from the spinal cord for the upper part of the chest.

The thoracic vertebrae tend to show muscular problems as the six major abdominal muscles keep us upright and, therefore, take most of the strain of standing and bending. The reflex pathway for muscles is on the curve of the medial edge of the foot and a pathway a little above it. Be careful not to work onto the sole of the foot where you would be on the reflex for the ureter tube. The reflexes here are connected to the thoracic and abdominal cavity and include the digestive and urinary systems, the transverse colon and the ribs. The diaphragm muscle separates the two cavities and plays an important role with breathing and relaxation.

The lumbar vertebrae are the largest and strongest bones in the spine and take the body weight, along with the pelvis and legs. Thus, bad posture and lack of exercise can create nerve pain, such as sciatica and pelvic misalignments. At the 5th lumbar vertebra, the pelvic girdle and sacroiliac joint are joined by strong ligaments and it is at this point that most of the body weight is distributed. It is therefore no surprise that this is a common area for extremely painful problems.

The sacrum is the name given to the bone that joins the pelvic girdle and the 5th lumbar vertebra, and is directly linked to the lumbar area of the spine. I have found that mothers who have not had their pelvic girdle realigned after giving birth, walk around for years with one leg longer than the other! I cannot emphasize enough the importance of attending regular sessions with a good and gentle chiropractor to correct any misalignments in this area. There may be no pain in youth but by middle-age tell-tale signs of knee and hip problems indicating misalignments can develop into major surgery in later life with knee and hip replacements. Everyone should visit a chiropractor, like having a dental check-up, regularly! We look after our teeth, which are bone, why not our whole bony structure? Work all three pathways and check the sacral area of the spinal column for tenderness and the innominate bones to find possible problems with the pelvic girdle.

The amazing accuracy of finding skeletal misalignments from the feet is a skill that a proficient practitioner can master at a relatively early stage in training. As I have said before, the art of good reflexology is precision. With a retentive memory and an accurate idea of the patient's life-style, habits and medical records, the practitioner can discover which bones in the vertebrae may be out of alignment, with, for example, the ribs, skull bones, sacral iliac joint, pelvis and joints. If all joint reflexes are painful, this could be an indication that acid is present in joint cavities.

The most common problems connected to the spine are sciatica, low back pain, involving the sacroiliac joint, and neck-related problems. The way we sit, move, stand, drink our tea (by bringing the head to the cup, rather than the cup to the head), put pressure onto the nerves surrounding the spine which then give us pain. The movement of bone is only fractional, in most cases, but sufficient to put pressure onto the nerves and to bruise them.

The skull weighs approximately 5.5kg (12lb), with most of the weight centred from the mandible (jawbone) forwards. This lightness of the front of the skull is created by the sinuses, which extend from the ears and surround the eyes. This lightening effect means that we can keep our head erect. We know how this is pronounced when we have a cold and our head feels 'heavy' with blocked sinuses.

The old regimental posture of shoulders back, head up, stomach and bottom in is the worst stance for damaging and compressing the vertebrae and nerves of the spine. The spine should be slightly extended, so that the cartilaginous joints and nerves can move freely. To keep the correct posture for the spine the chin should drop forward slightly, so that the vertebral column can extend. Exercises that loosen the pelvic and shoulder girdles and stretch the spine, such as swimming, yoga and walking, are excellent for developing strong back muscles and a healthy spine. It is by no chance that the bony structure of the spine itself is represented on the bony ridge of the medial arch of the feet. I have found that tenderness on these reflexes relate directly to vertebral problems and the two underlying pathways to muscles, the spinal cord innervations and viscera.

Check the spinal vertebrae. Remember the innervations from the spinal cord that connect to organs and glands – it is possible that a visceral problem can affect the vertebrae. To work the innervations, keep your thumb at a pressure comfortable to the patient and hold until any pain or discomfort has disappeared. If the sacral vertebrae reflexes are painful on the spinal pathways, especially the bony ridge, with the innominate bones (laterally and medially) painful on both feet, then a sacro-iliac problem is likely to exist. The patient will probably have already had such a problem diagnosed by their doctor, because of extreme vertebral pain and connected sciatica.

The ribs are found on the tops of the feet and should be worked laterally to medially under the toes to the base of the metatarsal joints. The ribs in the neck (which sit under the clavicle bone) are, therefore, found under the toes and the lower ribs at the base of the metatarsal joints on the waistline.

The skull bones are found from the base of the big toe up to the brain reflexes on the top of the toe. This area is also the cervical vertebrae reflex area and the skull bones and vertebrae are usually linked, as I have found, especially with migraine and epilepsy.

The joint reflexes in the triangular shaped area on the lateral edge of the foot include the lower back (towards the apex in the ankle), the knee, hip and elbow. The reflex for all joints is found on the lateral edge of the foot, on, just below and just above the cuboid notch. The reflex just above the cuboid bone represents the arm and the reflex underneath, the leg. Pain on the cuboid bone itself represents acid sitting in joint cavities anywhere in the body.

To find out if acid is present in the digestive tract, as well as the joints, check the reflexes in the anatomical oesophagus, the duodenal reflex and the oesophageal supporter reflex.

Drink plenty of pure water (preferably 3 litres (5¼ pints) per day) and cider vinegar made from apples, which is an alkaline once in the body and which neutralizes acid held in the joints. Relief from joint pain is a major benefit of this simple age-old remedy and it cleanses the digestive system, including elimination of waste products via the large colon and kidneys. To drink cider vinegar, dilute it in pure water and add honey if desired to make it more palatable.

Through researching extensively with skeletal problems and referring the patient to a chiropractor, findings of misalignments with reflexology have proved to be accurate in every case. Most people have shoulder and neck tension through sitting with their head in one position for long periods of time, so work these reflexes often throughout treatment.

The shoulder girdle at the diaphragm boundary includes the axillary lymphatic nodes.

The teeth reflexes extend from the lateral edge of the root of the toes and represent the wisdom teeth. The molars and premolars are the teeth most affected by mastication in adult life and sensitivity between the first/second and second /third toes can indicate problems in this area of the teeth. Tooth abscesses affect

the facial nerve (trigeminal nerve) and so check the face reflex when sensitive tooth reflexes are found.

The placement of callouses on the feet can indicate pelvic misalignments. For example, callouses found on the lateral edge of the foot can indicate a pelvis which is tipping to the lateral edge of the body and callouses found on the medial edge of the foot can indicate the possibility of the pelvis tipping forwards into the middle of the body. A young student came to me for treatment and I found callouses on the lateral edges of both feet, and found his spinal reflexes in the sacral and coccygeal areas of the spine and all four innominate bone reflexes to be very sensitive, especially the innominate bone reflexes on the lateral edges of the feet. I puzzled over this as, although born in Australia, he had lived in England for some years and had not led a particularly active life. I imagined he had learnt to ride a horse in the Outback as a child and when I asked him if this was the case, he replied 'No', but he had been taught to ride a motorbike from the age of five! Sitting astride from a tender age had developed his pelvis in a 'fixed' position and created bandy legs. He was a student in chiropractic and amazed that I could discover his secret childhood passion from his feet!

Callouses on the spinal pathways can also indicate imbalances with the chakras (energy centres) along the spine. For example, callouses found at the base of the big toe can indicate that the throat chakra is out of balance. The positions of the chakras on the spinal reflexes are as follows:

- **Crown Chakra**: the brain reflex point. May represent intense thought patterns, mental overactivity or blocked creativity.
- **Third Eye Chakra**: the spinal pathways in line with the pineal gland reflex point. May represent 'blocked' spiritual development and ability.

- **Throat Chakras**: the spinal pathways in line with the reflex point for the trachea and the thymus gland The throat chakra represents unexpressed words and the thymus chakra represents confusion about feelings about what one does want to express.
- **Heart Chakra**: spinal pathways in line with the heart reflex point. (*See* reasons for chakra imbalance below.)
- **Solar Plexus Chakra**: spinal pathways in line with the diaphragm line. May represent emotional tension and holding on to situations and feelings.
- **Sacral Chakra**: the spinal pathways over the sacral area reflex points of the spine. May mean insecurity and fear about life situations. Anxiety can affect the sacral chakra.
- **Root Chakra**: the spinal pathways over the coccygeal reflexes of the spine. May represent ungroundedness and an inability to 'keep feet on the ground' in the practicalities of life.

An example of Chakra imbalance is with a client who came for treatment with a callous over the solar plexus chakra. Her life at the time was full of emotional tension; when the tension disappeared, the callous disappeared with it.

Callouses over the heart reflex point on the left foot can indicate a defence mechanism where the client has developed an armour with which to protect themselves from emotional pain. Those who have suffered heart disease may develop a callous as the heart is an emotional organ in which feelings are stored. When feelings are unexpressed, the effect is similar to a pressure cooker where pressure builds up until it explodes, if not allowed to release slowly.

Feelings, which have remained unexpressed over a period of time, can explode in a physical heart attack. It is important to encourage clients to talk about their feelings, or go into counselling as a route in exploring their feelings. Encouraging them to talk by asking questions relevant to each chakra, with, for example 'do you find it hard to express your feelings?' in the case of throat chakra imbalance or 'do you feel you wish to spend more time on your spiritual development?' in the case of the third eye chakra imbalance.

The possibilities outlined above are to be used as examples and it is recommended that for those who wish to learn more about the chakras, meditation, Tai Chi', yoga classes and other Eastern practices and disciplines are a good way of experiencing the energy centres and the theory behind them.

WORKING THE REFLEXES

Refer to reflex point 42 (*see* Chapter 22) for working the spinal pathways.

Reflex Point 44 – Skeletal System, Innominate Bone

Search for a dent in the bone on the calcaneum, with the thumb on the lateral and medial sides of the feet. This reflex is difficult to find; it is located beneath the reproductive reflexes towards the back edge of the heel. The reason for the difficulty is that there is muscle and skin covering this area and the dent in bone can be obscured. Massage and make a mental note which sides of the feet are the most painful, for example, if the lateral reflexes are the most tender the pelvis could be tilted outwards, resulting in a 'bow-legged' effect. If the medial reflexes are tender, then the pelvis may be tipped forward resulting in a 'knock-kneed' posture. In cases where reflexes on the one foot are generally more tender than the other, a difference in leg length may

The Skeletal System and Joints

System(s)	Associated Reflexes	Disorders

REFLEX POINTS 6, 46, 52, 54A: THE SHOULDER GIRDLE

System(s)	Associated Reflexes	Disorders
Skeletal/Joints	Neck (all reflexes), joints, arms, spine, innominate bones, ribs, whiplash	Bursitis, neuritis, capsulitis, tension
Muscular	Diaphragm	
Nervous	Solar plexus	

Nerve Innervation: 6th, 7th Cervical

REFLEX POINT 42: THE SPINAL VERTEBRAE

All systems, especially nervous, skeletal, muscular	Whole foot for all systems and nerve innervations	Skeletal misalignments, slipped disc, psychogenic factors

Nerve Innervation: all innervations

REFLEX POINT 43: THE TRACHEA

Muscular	Diaphragm	Laryngitis, pharyngitis
Respiratory	Lungs, sinuses	
Lymphatic	Lymph nodes and ducts	
Skeletal/joints	Neck, spine	
Endocrine	Thyroid, parathyroids	
Special senses	Ears, eyes, nose	
Nervous	Brain, solar plexus	

Nerve Innervation: 5th, 6th, 7th Cervical; 1st, 3rd Thoracic

REFLEX POINT 44: THE INNOMINATE BONES

Skeletal/joints	Spine, sciatic nerve, skull bones, legs, arms, ribs, all joint reflexes	Skeletal misalignments, polymyalgia, rheumatica, arthritis, lumbago, sciatica, pressure from viscera onto spinal nerves, paralysis
Genito-urinary tract	All reflexes of the urinary and reproductive systems	

Nerve Innervation: 4th Lumbar; Sacrum

REFLEX POINT 46: SHOULDER SUPPORTER; REFLEX POINT 47: THE JOINTS – HIP, ELBOW, KNEE; LOWER BACK

Skeletal/joints	Spine, arms, legs, 'all joints'	Cartilage disorders, spinal misalignments, housemaid's knee, tennis elbow, gout, arthritis (rheumatoid and osteoarthritis), lupus, polymyalgia rheumatica, acidosis, alkalosis
Muscular	Shoulder, diaphragm, innominate bones	
Digestive	Oesophagus, stomach, duodenum, liver, gall-bladder, large colon, sigmoid flexure, ileocaecal valve, pancreas	

Nerve Innervations: 4th Lumbar; 1st Thoracic; 3rd Lumbar; 4th, 5th Lumbar; Sacrum; Coccyx

The Skeletal System and Joints *continued*

System(s)	Associated Reflexes	Disorders
System(s)	*Associated Reflexes*	*Disorders*

REFLEX POINT 48: REINFORCEMENT OF REFLEXES FROM THE SOLE OF THE FOOT

Digestive, nervous, skeletal, joints, muscular	All reflexes in the thoracic, abdominal and pelvic cavities and pelvic extension to the lateral edge of the foot	Disorders associated with reflexes on the sole of the foot, relative to each cavity

Nerve Innervations: refer to the Pelvic, Abdominal, Skeletal and Thoracic Cavities

REFLEX POINTS 49, 49A AND 49B: ALL JOINTS, ARMS AND LEGS
Systems, reflex points and disorders as for Reflex Point 48

Nerve Innervations: all of the above joints, plus Arms 1st Thoracic; Legs 3rd and 5th Lumbar; Skull Bones 1st Cervical

REFLEX POINTS 17, NECK AND TEETH; 53, WHIPLASH; 54, CHRONIC NECK; 54A, CHRONIC NECK AND SHOULDER SUPPORTER; AND 55, NECK AND TEETH

Nervous	Brain, solar plexus	Caries, torticollis, bursitis,
Lymphatic	Lymph nodes and ducts	neuritis, capsulitis, muscle strain,
Special senses	Face, nose, ears, eyes	injury, ankylosing spondylitis,
Muscular	Diaphragm, trachea	spondylosis, fibrositis,
Skeletal/joints	Neck, all joint reflexes, ribs, shoulders, arms, legs, spine	fibromyalgia, arthritis, tooth abscess, periodontal gingivitis, emotional and physical tension

Nerve Innervations: Whiplash 1st to 7th Cervical; 1st, 2nd, 3rd Thoracic; Neck and Neck/Teeth – 3rd, 4th, 5th, 6th, 7th Cervical

REFLEX POINT 56: THE RIBS

Skeletal/joints	Shoulder girdle, spine, all joint reflexes, neck	Bruised and fractured ribs, asthma, bronchitis, pleurisy
Muscular	Diaphragm	cough, skeletal misalignments,
Respiratory	Lungs	emphysema
Nervous	Solar plexus, brain	
Reproductive	Breast	
Cardio-vascular	Heart, lymph nodes and ducts	

Nerve Innervations: 1st, 2nd, 3rd Thoracic

See Chapter 26 for a description of disorders related to the Skeletal System

be putting pressure onto the side of the body where the leg is slightly longer. In this case the body can be described as 'listing' to one side. Where continual pain is present, the patient may compensate body weight onto the other side of the body; hence, discomfort and pain begin on the opposite side of the body. There are many permutations for the reasons of back/hip sciatic pain and consultation with a proficient practitioner who can realign the skeletal frame is essential. In some instances it is not possible to correct the skeletal frame entirely but regular reflexology and skeletal checks can provide maintenance, act as preventative medicine and give immense relief from pain and discomfort.

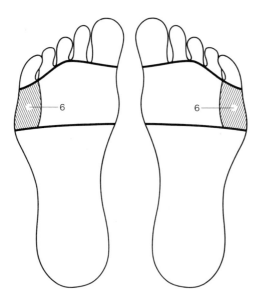

The skeletal frame. The shoulder, reflex
point 6 (both feet).

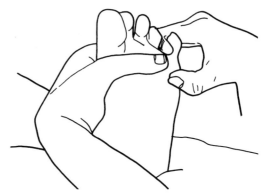

Hand position: working the shoulder, reflex
point 6. Working hand over supporting hand.

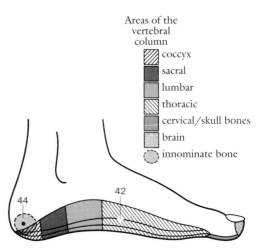

Areas of the
vertebral
column

- ▨ coccyx
- ■ sacral
- ▦ lumbar
- ▨ thoracic
- ▥ cervical/skull bones
- ⣿ brain
- ◯ innominate bone

The spinal vertebrae, spinal cord and innominate
bone, reflex points 42 and 44 (both feet).

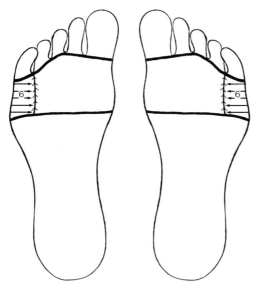

Directions for working: the shoulder, reflex
point 6 (both feet).

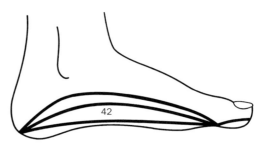

The nervous system, reflex point 42 (both
feet).

280

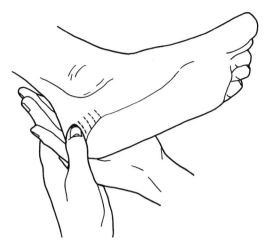

Hand position: the vertebral pathways, reflex point 42 (both feet). Supporting hand under the heel; working hand under supporting hand.

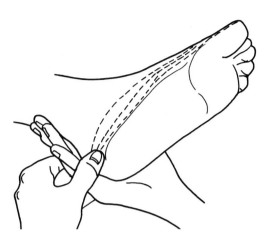

Hand position: the vertebral pathways, reflex point 42 (both feet). Supporting hand under the heel; working hand under supporting hand.

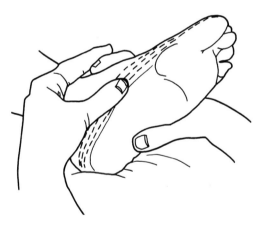

Hand position: the vertebral pathways, reflex point 42 (both feet). Working hand over supporting hand.

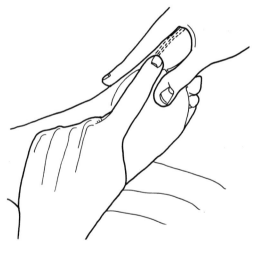

Hand position: working the vertebral pathways, reflex point 42 (both feet). Supporting hand cradles the big toe.

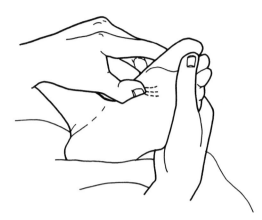

Hand position: the neck and shoulder supporter when working the spinal pathways, reflex point 54a (both feet). Working hand over supporting hand.

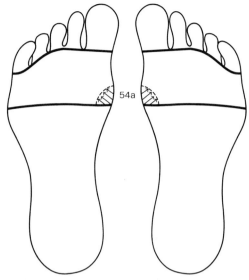

Directions for working: neck and shoulder supporter area from spinal pathways, reflex point 54a (both feet).

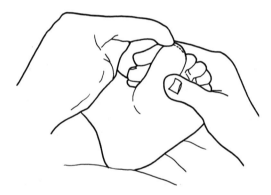

Hand position: the brain, reflex point 8 (both feet). Supporting hand supports across the tips of the toes.

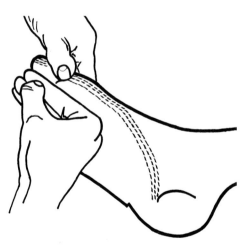

Hand position: the vertebral pathways towards the heel, reflex point 42 (both feet). Supporting and working hands' fingers 'sandwich' the big toe.

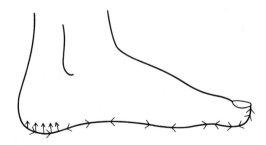

Directions for working: the vertebral pathways, reflex point 42 (both feet).

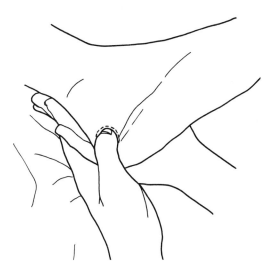

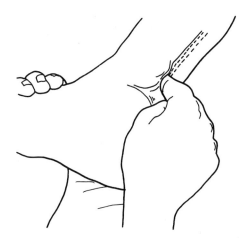

Hand position: massaging the innominate bone, reflex point 44 (both sides of both feet). Working hand under supporting hand.

Hand position: the sciatic nerve, reflex point 45 (both feet). Supporting hand supports the medial edge of the foot.

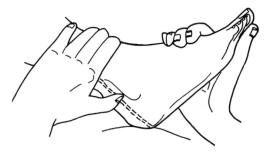

Hand position: the sciatic nerve, reflex point 45 (both feet). Supporting hand supports the medial edge of the foot.

Sciatic Nerve and Shoulder Supporter – Reflex Point 45, 46 – Nervous and Skeletal Systems

Whilst working the lateral edge of the foot, you will need to check with your patient if it is comfortable for them to turn the leg in towards the centre of the body. With two fingers, work up the leg from the lateral edge of the foot, underneath the fibula bone, for

about 9cm (3½in). If there is no pain, turn the hand and work down in the same way with the thumb. Make sure you begin working down the leg where you stopped and that the fingers of the working hand rest on the leg.

As well as continuing to work the sciatic nerve under the heel of the foot, the thumb can work round the lateral fibula joint at the ankle, finishing round the curve of the bone for the supporter shoulder reflex.

Reflex Point 47 – Joints (Lower Back, Hip, Elbow, Knee)

Find the triangle from the cuboid notch on the lateral edge of the foot and imagine a 45-degree angle, upwards into the ankle joint. Imagine a second 45-degree angle taken from the ankle joint down to the outside edge of the heel (avoiding the ovaries/testes). Work with two fingers within the triangular shape, ensuring that you finish working into the ankle joint where a pressure point for the sacroiliac joint can be worked at the apex of the triangle.

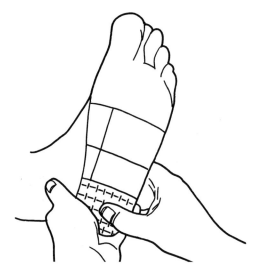

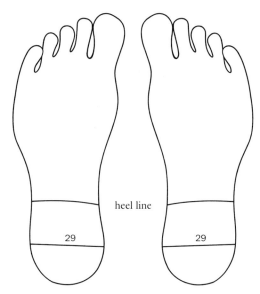

Hand position: the sciatic nerve, reflex point 29 (both feet). Supporting hand is held under the heel; working hand fingers are placed on top of the foot.

The sciatic nerve, reflex point 29 (both feet).

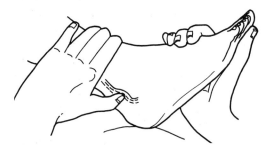

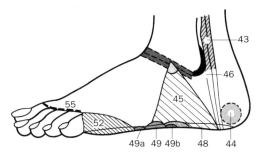

Hand position: the shoulder supporter, reflex point 46 (both feet). Supporting hand supports the medial edge of the foot.

The sciatic nerve, innominate bone, all joints, shoulder supporter areas, legs, arms and neck, reflex points 44, 46, 49, 49a, 49b and 55 (both feet).

Skeletal and Digestive Systems Reflex Points 6, 48 & 49 – Shoulder/All Joints/Reinforcements of Reflexes from the Sole of the Foot

Reflexes overlap from the sole of the foot on to the lateral edge of the instep. To ensure that all reflexes related to the anatomical cavities on the sole of the foot are worked thor-

oughly, we can work as follows. Turning the foot and leg into the middle of the body, with the thumb work upwards from the bottom of the lateral edge of the heel. Massage the cuboid notch for all joints on the way up to the base of the little toe. Continue to work up the outside edge of the foot into the base of the little toe to cover all reflexes.

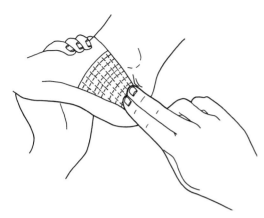

Hand position: the joints, reflex point 47 (both feet). Supporting hand supports medial edge of the foot.

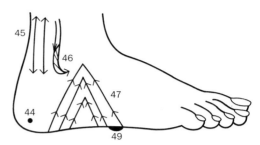

Directions for working: the sciatic nerve, shoulder supporter, innominate bones, and all joints, reflex points 44, 45, 46, 47 and 49 (both feet).

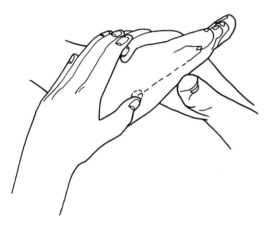

Hand position: all joints, reflex point 49 (both feet). Working hand over supporting hand.

Respiratory, Reproductive, Skeletal/Joints – Reflex Points 50–54 – Working the Top of the Foot for Lungs, Breast, Shoulder, Whiplash, Chronic Neck

Using the left hand on the left foot and the right hand on the right foot, hook the thumb of the working hand into the back of the supporting fist to give control and pressure for the working index finger. With the working hand over the foot and the finger pointing towards the ankle, begin working from the medial edge of the foot. Point the index finger in a downward direction from the base of the big toe and first toe, and work down towards the base of the metatarsal joints, ensuring that the finger is between the joints as you work down. Do not allow the finger to work in a sideways position as you will not contact the reflexes but sit on top of them.

Continue to work across the width of the foot, working down from the base of the toes to the base of the metatarsal joints. Remember that the breast reflex is found between the third and the fourth toes towards the base of the metatarsal joints. Once on the lateral edge of the foot, swap hands to work back to the medial edge of the foot with identical movements as before.

In the fifth zone, between the third and fourth toes, extending to the lateral edge of the foot, are the shoulder reflexes. To give reinforcement to these reflexes, work down as described but with the index and third fingers together. Working with two fingers in this way saves time and the reflexes are thoroughly worked. Change hands, then revert to

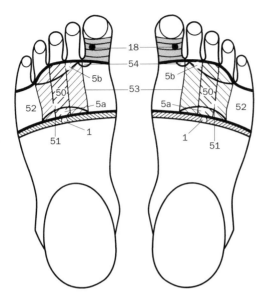

The respiratory tract (top of foot), reflex points 1, 5a, 5b, 18, 50 51, 52, 53 and 54.

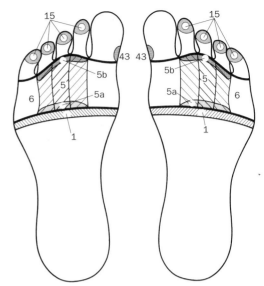

Respiratory tract (sole of foot) and diaphragm, reflex points 1, 5, 5a, 5b, 6, 15 and 43.

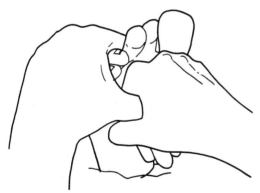

Hand position: working the reflexes on top of the foot (rear view/both feet). Supporting hand makes a fist on the ball of the foot.

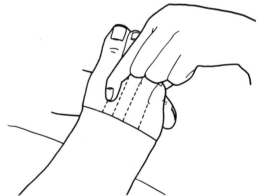

Hand position: working down the whiplash reflex, lung and heart, breast and shoulder, reflex points 5, 5a, 5b, 50*, 51, 52 and 53 (both feet except for the heart reflex which is found on the left foot). (* Heart referral pain on left foot and lungs.) Supporting hand makes a fist on the ball of the foot. Refer to the Circulatory System.

working with the index finger only as before back towards the medial edge of the foot.

Once the joint between the great toe and

first toe have been worked, turn the working hand thumb upwards (right hand on the left foot), so that it points towards the toes whilst

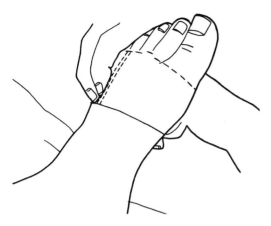

Hand position: the shoulder, reflex point 52, on top of the foot (both feet). Supporting hand makes a fist on the ball of the foot.

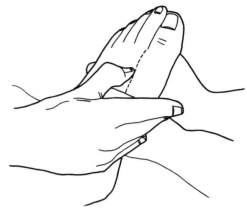

Hand position: working up the whiplash, reflex point 53 (both feet). Supporting hand makes a fist on the ball of the foot.

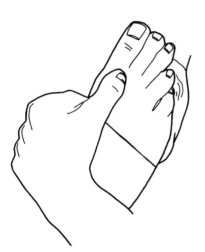

Hand position: the chronic neck, reflex point 54 (both feet). Supporting hand makes a fist on the ball of the foot.

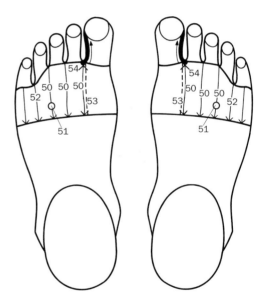

Directions for working: the shoulder, breast, lungs, whiplash and chronic neck, reflex points 50 to 54 (both feet).

keeping your working fingers over the medial edge of the foot. Massage between the base of the great toe and the first toe for chronic neck problems and continue working up the inside of the great toe whilst moving the supporting fist up behind the toe. This way the toe is kept steady by being held firmly between the fist and working thumb and fingers.

Neck/Ribs – Reflex Points 55 & 56 – Skeletal System

Push the ball of the foot in with the supporting hand fist (*see* metatarsal massage, relaxation technique) and see the metatarsal joints

open out on top of the foot. With two fingers, work across the foot at the base of the toes, laterally to medially.

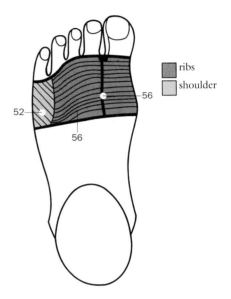

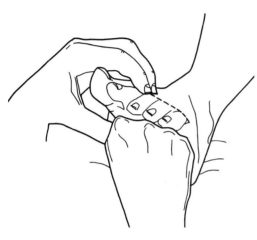

Hand position: the neck and teeth, reflex point 55 (both feet). Supporting hand makes a fist on the ball of the foot.

The ribs and shoulder, reflex points 52 and 56 (both feet).

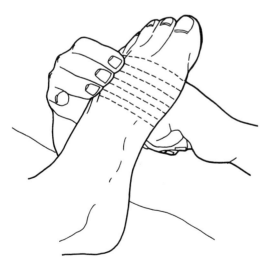

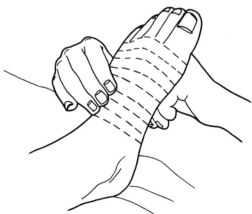

Hand position: the shoulder and ribs, reflex points 52 and 56 (both feet). Supporting hand makes a fist on the ball of the foot.

Hand position: continuation of working reflex points 52 and 56, completing working the feet into the ankle (both feet). Supporting hand makes a fist on the ball of the foot.

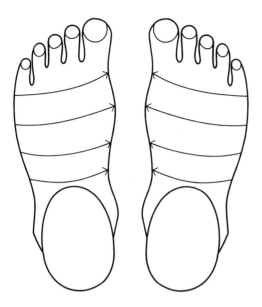

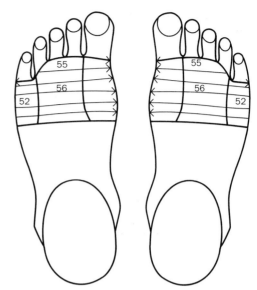

Directions for working: completing working into the ankle (both feet).

Directions for working: the neck, shoulders and ribs, reflex points 52, 55 and 56 (top of feet/both feet).

Swap hands and work medially to laterally in the same way. Work across the foot from the lateral edge with three fingers, bearing in mind that the ribs are between the big toe and extend to the third toe, down to the base of the metatarsal joints (waistline). Continue working down in this way into the ankle joint, thereby ensuring that all reflexes are thoroughly worked.

Finishing Treatment of Both Feet

Place the thumbs into the solar plexus and make a 'V' with the fingers on top of the foot, ensuring that the index fingers stay together. Work down the foot with the ripple motion into the ankle joint. Massage around the ankle joint.

The Electromagnetic Field

To take away negativity and tiredness, use both hands and stroke downwards from the knee with the hands held about 5cm (2in) above the leg and foot, and work around the foot and ankle. To re-energize, stroke upwards towards the knee in the same way as you worked down.

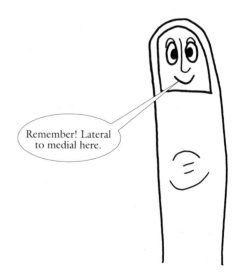

Remember! Lateral to medial here.

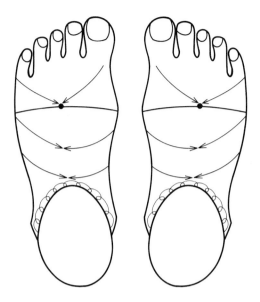

Directions for working: finishing the treatment (both feet).

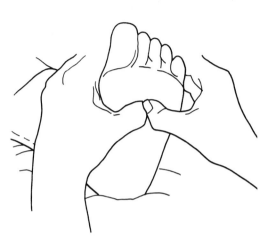

Hand position: finishing the treatment (both feet). Hands form an inverted 'V' on top of the foot, with thumbs on the solar plexus.

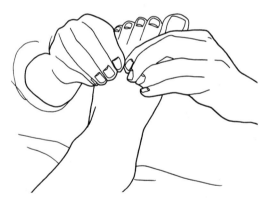

Hand position: finishing the treatment (both feet). Thumbs are placed on the solar plexus reflex on the sole of the foot.

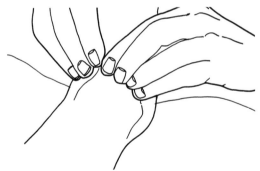

Hand position: finishing the treatment (both feet). Massaging round the ankle, with thumbs over the sole of the foot.

Relaxing with Deep Breathing

Place your thumbs on the solar plexus on both feet and ask your patient to breathe in slowly through the nose, expanding their stomach as far as possible as they do so. As they breathe in, press in on the reflex point.

Then, ask your patient to breathe out slowly through the mouth, emptying the lungs as much as possible until their head rests forward. As they do this, release the pressure on the solar plexus. Repeat about six times, or longer as necessary. Suggest to them that they

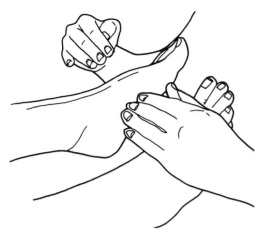

Hand position: finishing the treatment; working the electromagnetic field.

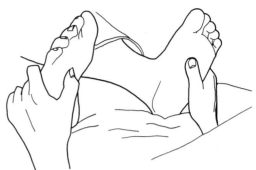

Hand position: finishing the treatment; relaxing with deep breathing – thumbs on the solar plexus.

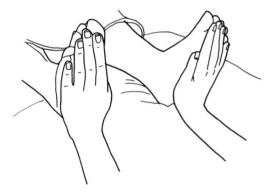

Hand position: finishing the treatment, giving healing.

visualize tensions and anxieties leaving the body as they release the breath slowly through the mouth.

Healing

Finish the treatment by placing the palms of your hands on the soles of the feet. Visualize healing white light flowing through the top of your head, through your body, down through your arms and hands and into your patient's

body until you are both filled with white light. Practice 'seeing' the auric/ vital bodies and check with your patient that they can relate to your sense of perception.

Neck and Shoulder Massage

If necessary, and time permitting, offer to massage your patient's neck and shoulder muscles to ease tension in these areas. Use essential oils for maximum benefit, such as lavender mixed into a base oil. (Obtain professional advice before use of essential oils as some are highly toxic.) Pay particular attention to the *sternocleidomastoid* muscles in the neck, which bring the head forward onto the chest and tilt and rotate the head; these muscles extend from the sternum across both sides of the neck to the mastoid process. When the neck is fixed in one position to the left or right, torticollis is present.

The *trapezius* muscle extends into the neck where it aids in keeping the head upright and turns it from side to side; it also raises the shoulders. This large muscle extends across the back of the shoulder and inserts into the

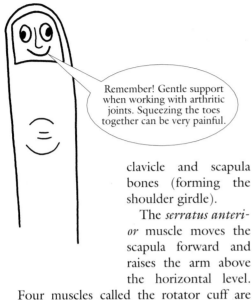

Remember! Gentle support when working with arthritic joints. Squeezing the toes together can be very painful.

clavicle and scapula bones (forming the shoulder girdle).

The *serratus anterior* muscle moves the scapula forward and raises the arm above the horizontal level.

Four muscles called the rotator cuff are deep muscles located in the shoulder joint. They aid in extensive movement, such as when playing sport. As a result, they may become torn through injury.

It is recommended that you acquire at least a basic training in massage so that massage techniques can give your patient a wonderfully calming and relaxing end to the reflexology treatment.

CASE STUDY ON SCIATICA

Ann came with sciatica and received weekly reflexology treatments for several months then, over a period of time, treatments were reduced to once a month. The following is her story, written in her own words:

I had been suffering from sciatica, due to a trapped nerve that had become damaged. I had been taking pain killers in large doses for the whole of 1993, plus two epidurals that didn't work. By January 1994 the pain was so bad I couldn't get downstairs and at that point it was suggested that I try bed-rest, which I did for three-and-a-half weeks. My doctor sent me for a scan and an operation was suggested, to which I said 'No'.

I had already tried a chiropractor, which seemed to make it even worse. However, I continued investigating alternatives and had read of reflexology. I rang a couple of practitioners and felt confidence in just speaking to Jenny, so booked my first appointment. Jenny worked on my feet, treating all areas, especially the spine and sacroiliac joints. I soon began to feel the benefit from my weekly treatments, which gave me a feeling of all-over well-being and helped me cope with the pain.

I continued with treatments weekly at first and then reduced them to monthly appointments as I began to feel improvement. I also went to a hydrotherapy pool and a McTimoney chiropractor on Jenny's recommendation.

I am now completely off pain killers but still feel the need for my four- and six-weekly treatments of reflexology. These treatments have covered problems that begin to develop, and as Jenny works on these everything seems to even out and there is little or no pain, unlike four years ago when treatments were painful.

From this Case Study, we can see how reflexology can aid skeletal and nerve problems, especially when combined with the gentle McTimoney technique of chiropractic.

CHAPTER 24

Hand Reflexology

YOU NEED HANDS ...

Hand reflexology is a parallel method of working with reflexology, when, for various reasons the feet cannot be worked at all or where there is restricted access due to injury which could mean that working the reflexes would be less effective. A brief overview of *when* and *how* to work the hands is given below and the practitioner or student who wishes to know more about hand reflexology will find many good books on the subject in their local book store (*see also* the Hindu hand charts in the colour section).

HEART AND HANDS

We greet, hug, caress, talk, hit out and protect ourselves with the arms and hands. These expressive parts of the body are closely related to the heart centre and feeling nature, and can be described as spiritually expressive, for example the hands together in prayer, or the spiritual message of ballet. It is therefore logical for us to consider that the hands give the dimension of feeling expressiveness and give us a gentle tool to work with in reflexology.

Hand reflexology can be described as working on the mental, emotional and subtle bodies, with the ancillary benefit of working on the physical. Foot reflexology worked with as described in this book will give benefits on the physical body first with the emotional, mental and subtle bodies receiving ancillary benefits.

When to Work the Hands

It may be preferable or necessary to work the hands in the following situations:

- if a limb has been amputated;
- when the feet are contraindicative through infection, disease or injury;
- if the feet are inaccessible;
- when hand reflexology is more suitable to work with the presenting condition of the patient;
- when the patient can work on their own hands as an ancillary aid to an overall treatment plan between foot reflexology treatments.

How to Work the Hands

To work the hands, the sitting position of the reflexologist is important because the hands are a more intimate part of the body. The practitioner is closer to the patient's face and has entered personal space, which can extend from 0.5–1m (2–3ft) or more away from the body. It is a good idea to experiment in finding your own personal space by allowing someone who you do not know too well to move in towards you so that you can sense when you begin to feel that they are uncomfortably close. An additional consideration is

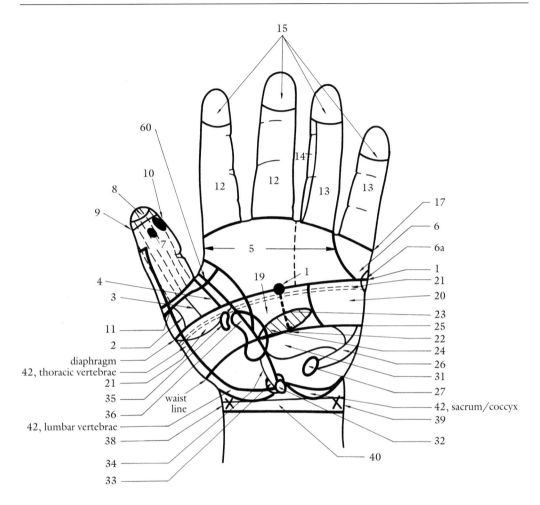

Fig 48. Left hand, palm up.

that of *touching* the hands, which are an intimate part of the body. A sensitive and confident approach to working with a feeling and expressive part of the body must be present so that trust can be engendered with the patient.

Once foot reflexology has been mastered, hand reflexology becomes easy to understand when transposing the reflexes found in the anatomical cavities on the feet to the hands. Study the hand reflex points on the diagrams in this chapter and work with the ripple move-

ment horizontally, vertically and diagonally, making a mental note of sensitive reflexes as you work. As the reflexes are closer together than on the feet, more concentration will be required. It may feel a little strange to begin with as the intimate zone of the patient and practitioner becomes involved in the healing process. However, practice will develop ease and confidence for both parties!

If it is appropriate to treat the hands rather than the feet, request permission from your

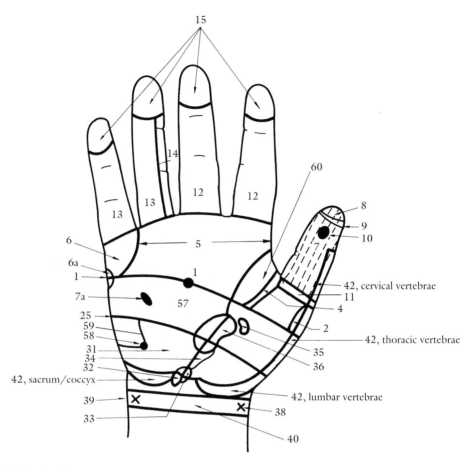

Fig 49. Right hand, palm up.

patient before beginning treatment and explain the reasons why you think it advisable to work on the hands.

The following guidelines will ensure an enjoyable and soothing hand reflexology treatment:

• Sit opposite or by the side of your client on a swivel chair so that you can change the position of working. Remember that sitting opposite is more confrontational than sitting at an angle or sideways, so experiment with the sitting position before beginning the treatment. Sitting opposite the patient can feel threatening for them, so have a table or tray between you, on which is placed a pillow, towel and paper roll on which to rest the hand. An elbow support will be necessary to steady the arm and to prevent strain and tension occurring to the arm muscles.

• Use cornflour or talc lightly rubbed over the hands before beginning the treatment, and

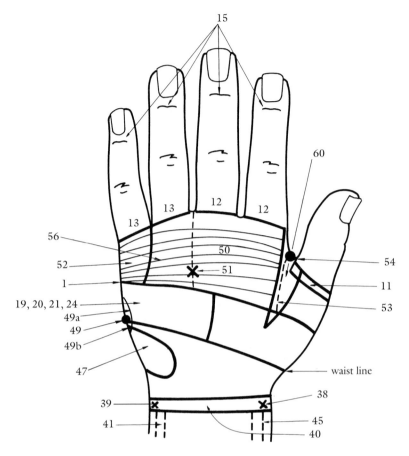

Fig 50. Left hand, palm down.

at the end massage with hand cream and gently pull each finger and thumb between your index and third finger, giving a gentle shake to loosen ligaments and joints.

• Remember – you are entering the patient's intimate zone. Anyone in our intimate zone increases the heart rate, adrenalin levels increase and more blood is pumped to the brain and muscles. Ensure that your own intimate zone is fragrant and remember to protect yourself from 'vampire' clients by practising visualization before beginning treatment!

• Apply the hand positions used on the feet, where possible.

• Be careful with eye contact – keep it gentle, direct and occasional – staring straight into your client's eyes will unnerve them and will not engender trust!

• Ensure your client does not lean forward but reclines with a well-supported neck, shoulders and spine.

• Ensure that the patient's ankles are not crossed as energy flow and circulation round the body will be impeded.

• Ideally, allow them to have their back to the

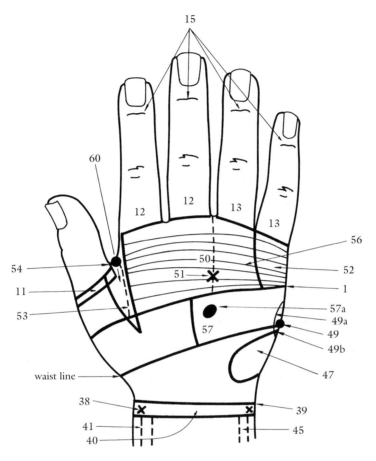

Fig 51. Right hand, palm down.

wall – this will make them feel more secure – try it and see!

- Hold the reflexes for longer as the hands are more resistant to work than the feet. Reflexes, therefore, take longer to stimulate.

CONDITIONS OF THE HANDS

There are several conditions that can be found on the hands:

- eczema
- Raynaud's disease
- osteoporosis
- osteoarthritis
- rheumatoid arthritis
- physical injury
- warts
- fungal infections
- callouses
- carpal tunnel syndrome
- ganglion
- cyst and various nail disorders
- dermatitis.

297

RELAXATION TECHNIQUES

At the beginning, during the treatment and at the end, the following movements will aid the patient in relaxation:

• stroking the hands, cleansing the auric field and the electromagnetic field (*see* page 289);
• thumb and finger pulls and rotations;
• wrist rotations;
• opening out the metacarpals by pressing with the thumbs on the solar plexus;

• hand massage.

Apply professional practice and observations of the hands as you would when working with the feet. Hand reflexology is pleasurable and soothing to give to others and beneficial as a self-treatment tool for the practitioner as well as the patient! You can identify and demonstrate reflex points to patients to work in between regular foot reflexology, which will give them a sense of involvement in their treatment.

Section 4

Diseases, Dying and Drug Misuse

*Beyond the senses is the mind, and beyond mind is reason, its
essence. Beyond reason is the Spirit in man, and beyond this
is the Spirit of the universe, the evolver of all.*

The Upanishads, Katha Upanishad

This section of the book is mainly concerned with treating the terminally ill, and drug and alcohol misuse. A comprehensive list of systemic diseases, with a glossary that explains the more unusual words, is included to assist the student in training. Finally, a list of training and accredited bodies in complementary medicine and a bibliography are included to provide ongoing education for the student in training, or those thinking of training in a complementary therapy.

CHAPTER 25
Treating the Terminally Ill

What do we mean by the word 'terminal'? Is there such a thing – not if we believe in life after death. In the Western culture, there is a great terror surrounding death and a drive to maintain youth and health, whereas in the Eastern philosophies death is an accepted and inevitable part of living.

We often think of terminal illness in relation to cancer, but it can include any number of conditions where the patient is not expected to survive. There are cases of spontaneous remission, where the patient recovers completely, and I am left wondering, as are many involved in health-care, how this comes about. It may be determination, visualization practice, prayer and other methods that are responsible for such a dramatic and miraculous recovery, However, on the whole, the function of the reflexologist asked to give treatment to someone who is dying will be palliative, as pain relief and comfort giving.

If the patient's feet are so painful that working them gives them even more discomfort, work the hands or massage both the feet and hands. Visualize giving healing in your own way as you work and, if involved in healing, send absent healing to them when at home.

For those interested in pursuing the Eastern Buddhist philosophy, *The Tibetan Book of Living and Dying* by Sogyal Rinpoche can be of great comfort to those who know their life expectancy is short-lived, to their family and friends, and to the carers who have the responsibility for looking after them whilst sick and making their last days as comfortable as possible. There are also many other self-affirmation and support books available, such as *On Death and Dying* by Elisabeth Kubler-Ross, *Getting Well Again* by O. Carl Simonton, Mathews-Simonton and Creighton, *The Holistic Approach to Cancer* by Ian C. B. Pearce and *You Can Fight For Your Life* by Lawrence LeShan. Look in your local bookstore to find a book you feel able to relate to.

MEDICATION, IMMUNIZATION AND ILLICIT DRUGS

Medication

In our culture, drugs are a necessary part of health-care, for pain relief, regulation of body functions, emotional and mental disturbances and other conditions of the human being. For thousands of years, herbs have provided the panacea for disease, and modern-day drugs have become a derivative of the essential goodness of herbs, or have replaced them altogether with chemical compounds, which are merely synthetic replacements.

It is important for the practitioner, student or layperson to be aware that reflexology is not an alternative to medication but an additional method, which encourages the body's natural healing mechanisms impact imbalances held within the psyche, thereby restoring internal balance and a sense of well-being.

Drugs are suppressive to the body's immune system and, as such, tend to deal with symptoms and not the cause of a problem. The reflexologist or other holistic practitioner, on the other hand, aims to deal with the cause. Sometimes, the balance of medication and reflexology can alter when a condition begins to improve and the body no longer requires a certain level of medication and, with liaison with the patient's GP, medication levels can be lowered.

The side-effects of drugs are difficult to determine and are, unfortunately, all too common. However, there are common side-effects, such as nausea, bloatedness, dizziness, feeling the condition is worsening, disturbance in the menstrual cycle, weight gain and, most importantly, additional medication, which seeks to decrease side-effects but creates secondary symptoms and health conditions.

The area of when medical drugs are useful in the treatment of disease and when avoidance is the best course of action is a wide and controversial topic. Generally, avoid antibiotics as far as possible, as they debilitate the body's natural immune defences and can create side-effects such as thrush, nausea and allergy response, which kill off healthy bacteria in the intestine. If the condition is not that serious, after consultation with your GP, consult a medical herbalist in the first instance who will prepare a remedy of pure herbs suited to you as an individual and the presenting condition. Remember that any medication, whether prescribed by your GP or bought over the counter at the local pharmacist, can have long-term effects in the body, which can take considerable time to eliminate through the body's excretory systems. If reflexology and any other complementary therapies have been tried but not helped, then consult your GP further for advice.

Reflexology boosts the immune system naturally, and having regular treatments with a good practitioner will ensure that your body can fight any possible germs to the best of its ability.

Drug Misuse and Abuse

Any abuse is not only harmful to the body but to the psyche as a whole. The nuclear family structure has generated more isolation in our society than ever before and one of the negative results is the increase in the use of narcotic drugs by the young. This is a reflection of their feelings of isolation, inadequacy, stress, frustration, depression and other psychological symptoms. The pressure and stresses of our age, especially for the young, are immense and life is highly competitive. Peer-group pressure with children and adolescents leads to the need to affirm their 'Okayness' with the use of soft and, increasingly, hard drugs, such as heroin.

The drug trade is an international multi-billion pound industry with turnover estimated at 8 per cent of total international trade. This equates to approximately the same as textiles, oil, gas or world tourism. Well over £1 billion a year is spent by central and local government in coping with the drug problem in the UK. Yet, despite expenditure, the number of addicts and availability of drugs and drug-related crime are on the increase. Drugs misuse is most common amongst young people in their teens and early twenties and the average age is becoming younger with almost half likely to take drugs at some point in their lives. Boredom, curiosity or peer-group pressure, and a combination of factors, are the major factors for young people beginning to misuse drugs. There is increasing evidence to suggest that the younger a person starts taking drugs the greater the chance that he or she will develop a serious drugs problem. Cannabis is the most commonly used drug amongst young people, followed by amphetamines,

---

Classification under the Misuse of Drugs Act

Class A	*Class B*	*Class C*
Cocaine, crack, ecstasy, heroin, LSD (acid), magic mushrooms (if prepared for use), speed (amphetamines – if prepared for injection)	Cannabis, speed (amphetamines), barbiturates (sedatives, codeine and sleeping pills)	Anabolic steroids, benzodiazepines group (tranquillizers, e.g. possession of Temazepam/Diazepam/Nitrazepam)

Class A drugs carry the heaviest penalty under the law, class B, the second heaviest and class C, the mildest.

POSSESSION AND SUPPLY
Guidelines for the penalties for possessing or supplying drugs are as follows:

Class A	Maximum penalty:	possession – 7 years' prison and/or a fine Supply – life imprisonment and/or a fine
Class B	Maximum penalty:	possession – 5 years' prison and/or a fine supply – 14 years' prison and/or a fine
Class C	Maximum penalty:	possession 2 years' prison and/or a fine Supply – 5 years' prison and/or a fine

---

poppers, LSD and ecstasy. It appears that the trend is towards indiscriminate use, based on availability and price.

Drugs enter the body through drinking, eating, snorting, inhaling, injecting and contact. They travel through the bloodstream to the brain and central nervous system, where the control of all body functions and emotions takes place. In this way, they affect every system in the body. The liver is the principal organ involved in neutralizing drugs, and the kidneys for filtering drugs from the body. Just how much these organs will be affected depends on the amount absorbed into the bloodstream and, although the body will try and adapt, eventually an increasing tolerance

level means that more drugs are necessary to obtain the same 'high'. When drugs are withdrawn from the body, the user experiences withdrawal symptoms, the body readjusting to how it would have functioned before the drug intake caused these symptoms. Some withdrawal symptoms from drugs and alcohol include sweating, palpitations, depression, anxiety, craving, diarrhoea, loss of concentration, sleep disturbance, panic attacks and joint and muscle pains.

Drugs are divided into the following categories:

- 'Uppers' which include speed, cocaine and crack and ecstasy;

- 'downers' include heroin (a pain killer) and methadone, barbiturates and benzodiazepines which are tranquillizers such as Temeazepam and Diazepam;
- psychoactive drugs (those that alter perception), such as LSD (acid), magic mushrooms (prepared for use) and cannabis;
- solvents, such as glue, paint, varnish removers, propellant gases in aerosols, or fuels such as cigarette lighter fuel, all of which are sniffed with the head inside a plastic bag.

It is important to realize that a 'cocktail' of alcohol and valium can be as lethal as any classified drug. Likewise, sniffing solvents found in aerosol cans, such as glue and other products bought off the counter at the local supermarket, are as dangerous, if not more so, because they can be bought so easily.

Social changes and the divorce rate, which can result in children being left alone until the parent or parents arrive home from work, have created a younger generation that feel no connectedness within the family unit. The infiltration of computers and television into the home, school and office have isolated those who are 'addicted' to them and who, as a result, have lost the art of communication, self-expression and a deadened imagination. Whenever possible, encourage children to read, listen to music, talk about feelings and needs, so that they develop a sense of self-discipline and inner resources. Children are sponges and soak up their environment like water!

Alcohol Abuse

Drinking alcohol is not illegal, and because of this it is a growing problem with young people with up to 28,000 dying at a young age in England each year through alcohol abuse. On average, it takes one hour for one unit to be cleared from the body through the functions of the liver and kidneys. Although drinking an excess of alcohol is detrimental to the body there are positive benefits for men over the age of forty from drinking a moderate amount and for women who have been through the menopause.

Alcohol is measured in units and the following classification acts as a guide to a low, increased and harmful risk level, based on units per week:

Men: low risk 0–21;
increased risk: 22–50;
harmful: 50+.
Women: low risk: 0–14;
increased risk: 15–35;
harmful: 35+.

One unit is equal to ½pt of ordinary strength lager, cider or beer; 1 small glass of sherry or port; 1 small glass of wine or one measure of spirits.

Over the last twenty years, loneliness, lack of purpose in life, stress and the change of women's role in society has created more drink-related problems with women than ever before. The rise in unemployment, caused through redundancy, the economic climate or ill-health, has also contributed to the rise in alcohol consumption, which has many side-effects, such as depression, suicidal tendencies, a sense of hopelessness and helplessness that lead to feelings of being out of control of life events. This leads eventually to feelings of despair.

The reasons why addictions of this kind exist needs caring investigation.

There is insufficient research into benefits of reflexology with an addictive type of personality, but as awareness and understanding increases for both addict and personal and professional carers we will be able to assess the role of reflexology and other complementary therapies as an integrated route for treatment of the individual.

For further information about national organizations that can help with enquiries about drug and alcohol related problems, *see* Organizations.

Those who wish to stop their addictions should consult their GP, their local Alcoholics Anonymous Group, Al-Anon, and Drug and Alcohol Abuse Agency or similar, who will be able to support, help and provide counselling to find out the root cause of the addiction.

Immunization

The topic of immunization has become increasingly controversial over the last few years. We have managed to destroy life-threatening childhood diseases since the advent of penicillin and injection of vaccines containing live bacteria. However, although immunization saves lives, it has also been found to create serious side-effects and although consultation with your GP is recommended before making a decision whether or not to vaccinate your child, it remains ultimately the parents' personal decision whether or not to immunize their child. A primary concern with non-vaccination is that the disease may reappear in its original form or as a mutation of the original disease in the future.

CHAPTER 26

Systemic Disorders

SKIN DISORDERS

Acne is due to an inflammation of the sebaceous glands in which blackheads and pustules appear.

Alopecia is another term for hair loss or baldness.

Arterial ulcers occur in skin away from the ankle region and are commonly associated with arterial disease. There is an arterial insufficiency in the affected areas.

Cellulitis is caused by inflammation and infection in subcutaneous tissue. It has become incorrectly associated with excessive fat deposits in the arms, thigh of the leg and buttocks.

Dermatitis is an inflammation of the skin and can be due to many causes. Some features of the condition are: red and hot skin, affecting the epidermis and superficial dermis; oedema in acute stages and weeping of fluid onto the skin surface; excoriation, produced by intense itching. Dermatitis can be caused by irritants, to which there may be an allergy.

Ecthyma is a condition where pustular eruptions are accompanied by surrounding inflammation. The pustules burst and discharge, leaving pigmented scars.

Eczema means 'flowing over', which describes similar inflammatory changes in the skin as in dermatitis. Unlike dermatitis, eczema is not caused by irritants but may be due to diet, genetic factors, heat, humidity, contact with woollen clothing, drying of the skin, house-dust mites and airborne allergens, such as pollen.

Impetigo is an acute and contagious crusted eruption of pustules on the skin, commonly seen on the face and limbs of children. It is caused by staphylococci, streptococci or a combination of the two. It is unclear why it is limited in some children and with others it is widespread.

Leucoderma is a condition of the skin where white patches appear, due to the presence of various skin diseases.

Melanoma is a tumour of the skin arising from the cells that produce melanin; a highly malignant form may develop from moles on the body.

Molluscum contagiosum is a condition where papules (small, solid elevations of the skin or pimples), not larger than the size of a pea, develop on the surface of the skin. It is due to a virus and is highly contagious, being most commonly conveyed from one person to another by wet and warm conditions, such as swimming baths and steam rooms. The papules may disappear spontaneously.

Neurodermatoses or neurodermatitis are grouped as disorders of the skin in which stress is the important factor, such as is found in pruritis (itching) and rosacea. In atopic eczema and lichen, stress is a secondary factor but nonetheless important with mental and emotional stress and strain exacerbating the condition.

Podopompholyx is a form of eczema characterized by deeply set vesicles (small blisters containing serum) on the soles of the feet. It is called cheiropompholyx when it occurs on the fingers and palms of the hand.

Psoriasis is a chronic, recurrent skin disease, characterized by reddish marginated patches with profuse silvery scaling on joint surfaces, such as elbows and knees, but which can become more widespread. The cause is unknown and is thought to be related to hereditary factors.

Seborrhoea describes a group of diseases of the skin in which the oil-forming or sebaceous glands are at fault. It can manifest by an accumulation of dry scurf or an excessive oily deposit on healthy skin. On the scalp, it is called seborrhoeic dermatitis or eczema.

Systemic lupus erythematosus is an inflammatory disease that affects the internal organs and the skin. It is thought to be an autoimmune reaction to sunlight, infection, or other unknown causes.

Urticaria or nettle-rash is a disorder of the skin characterized by eruptions resembling red and white patches, as result from the sting of nettles, which can occur in parts of the body or the whole body and which is extremely irritating, causing itching. It can manifest in an acute or chronic form and is sometimes linked to digestive malfunctioning or with a possible allergy to protein, the bite of an insect, exposure to cold temperatures, the use of penicillin, or through stress. Because of the link to allergy forming conditions, it is includes in the categories of asthma and hay-fever.

CIRCULATORY SYSTEM

Angina pectoris is due to an inadequate supply of blood to the myocardium of the heart and is generally linked to thrombosis or coronary spasm. Symptoms: a feeling of suffocation and severe pain in the thorax (chest cavity), which encompasses the heart, shoulder and left arm.

Angiomas are benign tumours of either blood or lymph vessels.

Aneurysm is a dilatation of the artery due to the vessel wall stretching by pressure of the blood flow. The causes are strain and weakening (the most important cause) of the arterial wall.

Arrhythmia is a contraction of the heart muscle fibres in a disorderly sequence. The chambers do not contract simultaneously and the pumping action of the heart is disrupted.

Arteriosclerosis is the common term for 'hardening' of the arteries. Artery walls lose elasticity and thicken, thereby restricting blood flow. Most commonly found in the elderly.

Atherosclerosis is due to fatty deposits accumulating in the arteries (atheroma), and although this complaint is similar to arteriosclerosis, it can be found in younger people. Bad (fatty) diet, smoking, alcohol and stress are major factors involved.

Bruise: this is a discoloured area under the skin, often painful and swollen, caused by leakage of blood from damaged capillaries.

Coronary heart disease *See* page 133.

Coronary occlusion is due to attacks usually caused by muscular exertion and emotional stimulation, followed by interference or obstruction of the flow of blood through an artery because of a thrombosis or embolus, causing the blood vessels to narrow (see arteriosclerosis). Lack of oxygen and a build-up of metabolic substances stimulate afferent nerves (nerve impulses that are sent back to the brain from the periphery of the body). The agonizing chest pains result in angina pectoris, which is a disease of the coronary arteries.

Embolism is caused by an embolus, which forms as an abnormal mass of substances in the blood and which are large enough to block blood vessels, e.g. fragments of tumour, blood clot, fat or an air bubble.

Endocarditis occurs when infecting organisms damage the endocardium (innermost layer of the heart muscle), nearest the valves.

Erythromelalgia is characterized by fingers, toes or parts of the limbs becoming bloated in appearance, purple and painful. Attacks are common in the summer and worse when the affected parts become warm; it is linked to vascular disease, such as hypertension, diseases of the central nervous system and metallic poisoning. Avoidance of hot climates and aspirin can give relief.

Fainting is a temporary loss of consciousness caused by an inadequate supply of blood to the brain resulting in nausea, sweating, loss of vision and ringing in the ears. It is caused by the pooling of blood in the extremities, which reduces the venous supply to the heart, thereby reducing cardiac output. It is induced by hot weather or prolonged standing.

Heart murmur is due to a faulty action of heart valves when blood leaks back from the ventricle into the atrium. A narrowing of a valve opening is called stenosis.

Heart failure is due to a deterioration of heart tissue, which results from disorders of long duration, such as high blood pressure.

High cholesterol is a condition where atheromas (fatty deposits) are a contributory factor in heart and circulatory diseases. *See* The Circulatory System and notes on cholesterol formation in The Digestive System.

Hypertension is due to high blood pressure, which is above the norm (120 over 80). Causes are emotional stress, alcohol and trauma (physical and emotional).

Hypotension means blood pressure that is below the norm. The elderly are at risk if BP is too low as hypothermia is the result of chronically low BP.

Myocarditis is an inflammation of the muscular wall of the heart.

Pancarditis is simultaneous inflammation of the pericardium, myocardium and endocardium muscles of the heart.

Phlebitis is usually found in the lower extremities and involves inflammation of a vein, which can be accompanied with pus formation and can lead to a thrombosis (thrombophlebitis). If the infected embolus breaks loose it can travel to other parts of the body. Usually found in patients who have given birth or received abdominal surgery and are therefore confined to bed.

Polyarteritis is a disease linked to any system of the body causing fever and inflammation and other symptoms.

Polycythaemia is due to an increase in the number of red corpuscles in the blood.

Raynaud's disease is due to obstruction of the circulation in the periphery of the body, due to the spasm of small arteries in the affected area. Symptoms are numbness and whitening (or blanching) of the skin, especially the fingers, toes, ears or nose.

Rheumatic fever is an auto-immune disease, which can occur two to four weeks after a throat infection. The antibodies that develop fight infection and cause damage to the heart.

Septicaemia is a serious form of blood poisoning due to the multiplication in the blood of bacteria, resulting in an infection of the blood. Symptoms are very high temperature, with shivering, profuse sweating, and joint and muscle pains.

Stroke is when a blood vessel ruptures and/or a blockage occurs in a blood vessel in the brain. Paralysis, loss of speech, motor activity and consciousness may result.

Tachycardia is a condition where the heart beats at an excessively high rate. Paroxysmal tachycardia is where the heart beats at around 150 beats per minute.

Thrombosis can affect veins and arteries. In the former, sluggish blood flow and a tendency for blood to coagulate are the cause. In this type of thrombosis, the deep veins of the leg are affected, which are found round the venous valves and which form 'red thrombi' consisting of red cells and fibrin. The growing thrombus is formed of platelets and fibrin and is likely to form an embolus (*see* Embolism). Chronic venous obstruction in the deep veins in the leg cause swelling in the limb and lead to ulceration. Arterial thrombosis occurs in association with atheroma, which tends to form at areas of rapid blood flow. Platelets become attached to the damaged walls of the vessels and form a 'white thrombus'. Blood coagulation may result in a complete closing of the vessel or embolization that produces obstruction at another point in the artery. This condition is linked to atherosclerosis and the heart.

Varicose veins occur when the walls of the veins become weakened, either through obesity, pregnancy, constipation (the most common reason) and hereditary factors. Knotted, swollen and torturous veins cannot return the flow of blood to the heart, which stagnates in the vessels, resulting in inefficient working of the one-way valves. It can affect people of any adult age.

LYMPHATIC SYSTEM

AIDS–HIV is caused by a retrovirus (meaning to turn back on itself), human immunodeficiency virus or HIV, affecting ribonucleic acid (RNA). The target of the HIV virus is the T4 lymphocyte (produced in the thymus gland), where it sends an enzyme to convert viral RNA into deoxyribonucleic acid (DNA), or provirus. HIV has an affinity for cells with a protein membrane, other than T4, macrophages, monocytes, some B-lymphocytes and neurogial cells in the brain. This effectively converts the T4 lymphocytes into a virus factory. HIV infection results in a decline of the white cell count, causing suppression of the immune system and most

clinical consequences result from this deficiency. The principle modes of transmission are: sexual (homosexual or heterosexual), blood transfusion, organ transplant, sharing of needles by drug users and infection from mother to child before birth, during birth or during lactation. Presence of antibodies to HIV indicates exposure but not necessarily the presence of AIDS. A few weeks after infection, flu symptoms develop followed by remission for two to three years without further symptoms.

Breast lumps occur when lymph nodes in the breast become infected and cause benign growths, cysts and mastitis and malignant carcinoma.

Head colds are caused by a virus (antigen), which tricks the immune system into believing it is harmless and colonizes cells, which in turn burst and colonize other cells. Lymphocytes produce antibodies to destroy the virus. Because a virus can change its outer coat and outwit the lymphocytes for a time, we continually contract new virus strains. A breakdown of the virus leads to congestion of mucus in the sinuses, nose, ears and eyes and possibly pharynx and larynx. Temperature and muscle weakness can accompany a head cold, with flu-like symptoms. There are over 100 viral strains of the common head cold.

Hodgkinson's disease is a form of cancer in which the lymph nodes become increasingly enlarged over the entire body. Fever and anaemia is symptomatic with this condition and the body becomes gradually weaker.

Hydrocephalus is an enlargement of the skull due to an abnormal collection of cerebrospinal fluid around the brain.

Infections are caused by bacteria, microbes and viruses invading the body (antigens), causing the immune system to produce antibodies which destroy the invaders.

Leukaemia is a condition caused by an increase in leucocytes and their precursors in the blood, which cause disease. Increased production of leucocytes enlarges the lymphoid tissue in the spleen, lymph glands and bone marrow. It can affect any age.

Lymphadenitis is an inflammation of the lymph glands.

Lymphagenitis is an inflammation of the lymphatic vessels.

Lymphocytosis is an increase in the number of lymphocytes in the blood due to a response to infection or lymphatic leukaemia.

Lymphoedema is a swelling due to an accumulation of fluid in an organ or part of the body caused by an obstruction in the lymph vessels draining the part.

Lymphoma is a tumour of lymphoid tissue.

Lymphosarcoma is a malignant growth of the parts of the lymph system characterized by enlargement of the lymphatic glands, spleen and liver.

Mumps is an infectious disease characterized by swelling of the parotid and other salivary glands. Its name comes from the old verb 'mump', meaning to mope or assume disconsolate appearance. It is caused by a viral infection and is highly contagious.

Swollen ankles are due to oedema and fluid retention in the tissue spaces, usually around the ankles, but can develop anywhere in the body. Spaces become swollen with large amounts of fluid and attributing conditions are bad circulation, diabetes mellitus, kidney dysfunction, removal of lymph glands and pregnancy. It can affect any age group and used to be known as 'dropsy'.

Tonsillitis is the inflammation of the tonsils, commonly caused by a bacterial infection.

RESPIRATORY SYSTEM

Asbestosis is a form of pneumoconiosis, caused by the inhalation of asbestos dust.

Asthma is a narrowing of airways within the lung, with the main symptom of breathlessness and inflammation of the bronchial tubes present resulting in coughing. A major feature is the variability of airways passages and reversibility may occur spontaneously. Swelling in the walls of the airways narrows the space for air to flow into, resulting in contraction of smooth muscle in the airway. Narrowing of airways in the lung is responsible for difficulty in breathing. Irritants, such as pollen, skin scales, animal fur, house mites and industrial irritants with dietary foodstuffs may be important, especially food additives or colourings. The illness can be worse in the early hours of the morning or may be related as an allergen to feather pillows, eiderdowns, etc. Non-specific factors, such as cold air, emotional disturbance and stress, may exacerbate asthma. Hay fever and eczema may also be present as allergic factors. The amount of airway narrowing can be monitored by a peak expiratory-flow meter. Exercise or life-threatening situations can also cause an attack. Peak expiratory-flow readings usually show a gradual decline for some days before an acute attack. In a severe attack, the patient is often more able to breathe by sitting up. There are two main forms of drug treatment: bronchial-dilator drugs to dilate the airways and relieve breathlessness; and anti-inflammatory drugs, which suppress the conditions that trigger an attack. Corticosteroids are given to adults and need to be taken regularly to be effective. Hereditary and genetic factors are being researched as predisposing factors with the disease.

Atopy, meaning out of place, is a form of hypersensitivity to certain antigens, which can have hereditary tendencies and which are responsible for asthma, hay fever and eczema. It affects a large proportion of the population.

Bronchitis can manifest in either an acute or chronic form. Acute bronchitis often develops by exposure to cold, particularly if accompanied by damp or a sudden change of temperature, or inhaling irritating dust particles or vapour. Symptoms show as the onset of a common cold or catarrh with the onset of feverishness and general debility. A short, painful, dry cough, wheeziness and pain in the throat with a feeling of tightness across of the chest mark the early stages of the disease. Acute bronchitis is dangerous at extremes of life and collapse of the lung(s) may occur. Chronic bronchitis occurs in the elderly and reasons for it being present are: exposure to irritants; dust; smoke or fumes; excessive cigarette smoking; bad housing; a cold, damp, foggy climate; obesity; recurring respiratory infections. A cough can disappear completely in summer but changes in the weather can cause reoccurrence.

Croup is a condition caused by acute obstruction of the larynx caused by allergy, foreign body, infection or new growth. It affects infants and children.

Emphysema means an abnormal presence of air in certain parts of the body, usually the lungs. There are two forms that affect the lungs: over-distension of air-cells of those of the lungs with destruction of the walls; this is the most common form of the disease. The second form is where air is infiltrated into the connective tissue beneath the pleura and between the pulmonary air-cells. This produces an acute form of the disease called 'acute interstitial (fluid) emphysema'. In the case of bronchial asthma and bronchitis, numbers of the smaller bronchial tubes become obstructed, the air in the pulmonary vesicles remains imprisoned, with the result that the force of expiration is insufficient to expel it. A stronger force of inspiration creates distention of the air-cells and permanent alterations in their structure, including emphysema, is the result. This disease is linked to whooping cough. Smoking is an important cause of emphysema.

Hay fever or seasonal rhinitis is the most common of all allergic diseases. Nasal irrita-tion, sneezing and watery discharge are the most troublesome symptoms. There can also be itching of the eyes and soft palate and, occasionally, itching of the ears.

Head cold – *see* Lymphatic system

Influenza starts abruptly with shivering, fever and generalized aching in the limbs. There is also headache, soreness of the throat and a persistent dry cough. Influenza viruses can cause a prolonged period of debility and depression that may take several weeks or months to clear.

Laryngitis is an inflammation of the mucous membrane of the larynx. Its cause can be viral or bacterial, or may be due to voice abuse.

Nasal polyps are round, smooth, semi-translucent glistening structures, which are attached to the sinus by a narrow stalk. They cause nasal obstruction, loss of smell and taste, and mouth breathing, but rarely sneezing.

Pharyngitis is an inflammatory condition affecting the wall of the pharynx or throat proper. It is commonly due to a viral upper respiratory tract infection.

Pleurisy (pleuritis) is an inflammation of the pleura surrounding the lungs. It may be caused by infection, injury or tumour. There are several types of this condition.

Pneumoconiosis is an industrial disease of the lungs, due to inhalation of dust particles over a period of time.

Pulmonary embolism is a condition where a blood clot (embolism) is lodged in the lungs caused by a clot in the abdomen or lower limbs as a result of thrombophlebitis.

Pulmonary oedema occurs when the lungs become waterlogged caused by narrowing of the opening between the chambers of the left side of the heart, where the mitral valve develops rigidity and adhesions.

Rhinitis is the presence of sneezing attacks, nasal discharge or blockage, occurring for more than one hour a day.

Silicosis is due to an industrial hazard where

silica is present, for example, potteries, sand-stone and sand-blasting, metal grinding, tin-mining, coal mines. Inhaled into the alveoli of the lungs, silica produces fibrosis. Diminished efficiency of the lungs produces shortness of breath. The main complication is that of the development of tuberculosis.

Sinusitis is inflammation of the linings of the sinuses in the head.

Tuberculosis is a disease recognized since the time of Hippocrates. It consists of a group of diseases, of which pulmonary tuberculosis is the most common. It may invade any organ, being seldom found in muscles or tissues with few blood-vessels, like cartilage. The disease spreads by way of the lymphatic system and its severity can vary considerably. The most dangerous type is where the meninges of the brain are affected and is found in infants and young children. Chronic inflammation of the joints with white swelling is a symptom of the disease. Enlargement of the glands, usually in the neck, gives a pig-like expression. Many chronic abscesses can be tuberculous in origin and lupus vulgaris is another manifestation of a disfiguring skin disease. Other sites are the bowels and genito-urinary tract, the kidneys, bladder and epididymis.

SPECIAL SENSES

Blepharitis is a microbial or allergic inflammation of the eyelid margins. Common causes are staphylococcal infection or allergy to dandruff.

Caries of the teeth or dental decay. The precise cause of caries is still uncertain but it is generally believed to be caused by acid produced by oral bacteria from dietary carbohydrates, particularly refined sugar, which dissolves the enamel.

Cataracts occur when the lens, or its capsule, becomes cloudy, restricting vision.

Choroiditis is due to a spread of infection from the front of the eye or a variety of systemic conditions, such as rheumatoid arthritis, Reiter's disease or ulcerative colitis.

Conjunctivitis is due to microbial or allergic inflammation. Infection may spread to the cornea and cause ulceration. Allergic conjunctivitis may be a complication of other autoimmune diseases or antigens in the environment, such as dust, pollen, spores, fungus, cosmetics, soaps, hair spray and animal fur.

Diabetic retinopathy is where the retina is damaged as blood vessels haemorrhage.

Eyestrain is fatigue of the eye, which may result from over-use or improper conditions for reading, such as poor lighting or small print.

Gingivitis is an inflammation of the gums and may occur as an acute or chronic condition.

Glaucoma describes a group of conditions in which there is increased pressure due to defective drainage of aqueous fluid through the canal of Schlemm in the angle between the iris and cornea.

Glue ear is the commonest inflammatory condition of the middle ear and is caused by persisting sticky discharge in the middle ear.

Iritis is due to an inflammation of the iris and ciliary body. Infection may spread from the outer eye but in most cases the cause in unknown. Symptoms are moderate to severe redness, pain and an excessive secretion of tears from the lacrimal glands.

Labyrinthitis is due to a spread of infection from the middle ear. In some generalized viral diseases, the organ of Corti is destroyed, causing sudden total nerve deafness. Causes of infection include mumps, measles, chicken-pox and influenza.

Meniere's disease or syndrome is caused by attacks of vertigo and tinnitus, which causes progressive deafness.

Otalgia is the medical term for earache.

Otitis is an inflammation of the ear.

Otomycosis is due to a fungal infection of the auditory canal.

Otosclerosis is the formation of spongy bone in the labyrinth of the ear, causing the ossicles to become fixed and less able to pass on sound waves to the inner ear. It is thought to be hereditary, related to vitamin deficiency or otitis media. It is accompanied by ringing in the ears and a progressive loss of hearing.

Periodontal disease is the spread of gingivitis to involve the periodontal membrane of the tooth and its florid form used to be called pyorrhoea.

Retinal detachment is where the retina becomes detached from the underlying layer as a result of trauma or an accumulation of fluid or tissue between the layers.

Strabismus is where the muscles of the eyeball do not co-ordinate, so that the two eyes do not work together.

Stye is due to an inflammation of the sebaceous glands of the eyelashes.

Tinnitus is a ringing, buzzing or roaring sound in the ears, caused by damage to the auditory pathway. The most common part of the canal to be damaged is the cochlea.

Tooth abscess is an infection that arises in or around a tooth and spreads to involve the bone.

Trachoma is due to an inflammatory condition caused by microbial infection in which fibrous tissue forms in the conjunctiva of the eye and cornea, leading to eyelid deformity and possibly blindness.

Vertigo is loss of balance and spatial sense giving a false sensation of body movements. Due to interference with the fluid in the semicircular canals in the inner ear.

ENDOCRINE SYSTEM

Acne – *see under* Skin Disorders.

Acromegaly is a tumour of the pituitary gland causing widening of the bones in the hands, face and feet.

Addison's disease is a deficiency of cortisol, aldosterone and androgens due to the destruction of the adrenal cortex. A common cause is autoimmune damage.

Cushing's syndrome is due to hypersecretion of cortisol, where there may be an adrenal tumour secreting cortisol or from a pituitary tumour secreting the ACTH hormone, which stimulates the adrenal cortex to produce an excess of cortisol.

Diabetes insipidus is characterized by the passing of a large volume of urine and is due to the lack of the antidiuretic hormone (vasopressin).

Diabetes mellitus – there are two types of this disease: insulin-dependent (juvenile, or early onset) and non-insulin-dependent (late onset). In the former, children and young adults are affected and the onset is usually sudden. The deficiency or absence of insulin is due to the destruction of islet cells. The causes are unknown but may be genetic. The latter form usually affects obese women over the age of 65 and the cause is unknown. Insulin secretion may be below or above normal. A reduced healing ability causes loss of sensation, flexibility and elasticity of the skin so that it becomes cracked, brittle and thin; caused by damage to peripheral nerves and an excess of sugar in the blood, which produces an increase in bacteria; symptoms are excessive sweating, poor circulation, oedema and greater risk of infection through skin lesions, which increases the possibility of gangrene developing.

Grave's disease is characterized by goitres, overactive thyroid, protruding eyes and loss of weight. Intolerance of heat and a rapid heart rate (palpitations), irritability, tremors, muscle weakness and hyperactivity can result.

Hyperthyroidism is caused by excessive activity of the thyroid gland and is connected with Grave's disease and goitres.

Hypothyroidism is caused by an insufficiency of thyroid gland secretion and is connected with myxoedema.

Myxoedema is a disease caused by underactivity of the thyroid gland.

Pituitary tumours are the commonest form of pituitary disease. Problems may be caused by excessive or inadequate hormone release.

DIGESTIVE SYSTEM

Acidosis is caused by a faulty metabolism of fat, which results in the production of abnormal acids. It can occur in diabetes mellitus, nephritis or as a milder form in children who have a fever.

Alkalosis means an increase in the alkalinity of the blood due to large doses of alkalis for the treatment of gastric ulcers.

Anaemia is condition of the blood characterized by inadequate red blood cells and/or haemoglobin in the blood. There are four types of anaemia and causes can be due to: loss of blood, menstruation, childbirth, bleeding from the gastrointestinal tract, blood diseases; defective blood formation, toxins (such as uraemia), drugs; inadequate intake of iron, inadequate absorption of iron. Symptomology includes pallor of skin, weakness and giddiness, rapid breathing and pulse with low blood pressure. In chronic cases, the tongue may be sore and fingernails become brittle, and difficulty in swallowing may be present with an accompanying huskiness.

Anorexia nervosa is caused by a complete lack of appetite for food, resulting in extreme emaciation. It occurs more frequently in young women and is generally due to psychological reasons.

Appendicitis is an inflammatory disease starting in the vermiform appendix. In its acute form, the condition is usually due to a combination of infection and obstruction, e.g. faeces.

A grumbling appendix is a much less common form and the person is troubled by repeated slight attacks of pain or discomfort in the right iliac region.

Bulimia is due to an abnormal increase in the sensation of hunger, resulting in 'binge eating' or episodes of uncontrolled and compulsive overeating occurring in response to stress. Induced vomiting or abuse of laxatives to avoid increase in weight reveal a fear of obesity. Bulimic binges often occur in anorexia nervosa.

Cirrhosis is the result of long-term inflammation of the liver. It may be due to viruses, micro-organisms or toxic substances. The commonest cause is alcohol abuse. Fibrosis, or scar tissue, forms and interferes with the working of the organ.

Coeliac disease is due to abnormal amounts of mucosa in the small intestine, which improves with a gluten-free diet and which can relapse when gluten is reintroduced. Gluten is contained in cereals, wheat, rye, barley and, possibly, oats.

Constipation is a condition where the bowels are not opened on most days. The difficult passage of hard stools is also considered to be constipation, irrespective of stool frequency.

Crohn's disease is an inflammation of an area in the small intestine. It is accompanied by colicky abdominal pains, irregularity of the bowels, loss of weight and a slight fever.

Cystic fibrosis is one of the most common genetic diseases. It is associated with the accumulation of excessively thick and tenacious mucus and abnormal secretion of sweat and saliva. It may cause intestinal obstruction in the newborn and the extremely thick mucus causes a predisposition to repeated infection leading to chronic lung disease.

Diarrhoea is the passing of increased amounts of loose stools and is different from the frequent passage of small amounts of stool, which may be seen in bowel disease.

Watery stools of large volume are always due to an organic cause. Bloody diarrhoea usually implies colonic disease and can be classified as acute or chronic: the former indicates infective causes.

Diverticulitis is an inflammation of the diverticulum and is commonly found in the colon. Symptoms are lower abdominal pain with colic and constipation.

Dyspepsia or indigestion is a term used to describe symptoms of nausea, heartburn, acidity, pain or distension that occur through eating and drinking or the ability to digest food.

E. Coli is the abbreviated name for *Escherichia coli* and is a form of bacteria found in the intestine. Under normal circumstances, *E. coli* and other forms of bacteria are necessary in the human gut to remain healthy by providing necessary vitamins for absorption, such as the vitamin K and B complex. A rare strain of *E. coli* (0157:117) is a toxin which causes damage to the cells in the intestinal walls, resulting in loss of water and salts and damaged blood vessels causing haemorrhaging. The condition can be lethal in small children who are too small to tolerate excessive blood and fluid loss. It is also dangerous for the elderly and infirm if they come into contact with the bacteria. A secondary condition is haemolytic uraemic syndrome characterized by kidney failure and loss of red blood cells. *E. coli* can be contracted from the surface of meat; it takes only ten bacterial cells in raw meat for transmission of infection. Once meat is ground, such as in hamburgers, bacterial cells become distributed throughout the meat. Thorough cooking of all meat until the juices of the meat run clear, not pink, is essential to reduce the risk of infection. Contaminated water, or persons, can pass the bacteria into other foodstuffs, so thorough washing of fruit and vegetables is essential. In view of the seriousness of the condition, medical attention should be sought as soon as possible.

Enteric fevers include typhoid fever, paratyphoid fever, food poisoning and salmonella infections due to ingestion of microbes from either water or food.

Flatulence is a term used to describe excessive wind through belching via the mouth or passing of wind through the rectum.

Food poisoning is characterized by abdominal pain, diarrhoea, vomiting; it results from eating food contaminated by metallic or chemical poisons, micro-organisms or undercooked food. Bacteria are the main cause of food poisoning, such as *Salmonella* and *E. coli*.

Gastritis is an inflammation of the lining of the stomach.

Gallstones consist of deposits of the constituents of bile, most commonly cholesterol. There are three types of stone: cholesterol, pigment, and mixed, depending upon their composition. Stones are usually mixed and may contain calcium deposits. The cause in most cases is not clear but sometimes gallstones will form around a foreign body within the bile ducts or gall-bladder.

Gastritis occurs when the amount of mucus in the stomach is insufficient to protect the surface from the destructive effects of the hydrochloric acid contained in gastric juice.

Heartburn is a form of indigestion marked by a burning sensation in the oesophagus, often accompanied with regurgitation of acid fluid.

Hepatitis (A, B, C, D, E) is an inflammation of the liver. Hepatitis A is the commonest type and arises from the ingestion of contaminated food. Hepatitis B is caused by the intravenous route, for example, transfusion of infective blood or blood products by contaminated needles used by drug addicts, tattooists, or acupuncturists, or by close personal contact, such as sexual intercourse, particularly in male homosexuals. Hepatitis C is transmitted by blood or blood products and there is a high incidence in intravenous drug abusers and male homosexuals. Hepatitis D is seen in intravenous drug abusers but can affect all risk routes for HIV infection. Hepatitis E causes waterborne hepatitis and epidemics have been seen in many developing countries.

Hiatus hernia is where a part of the stomach protrudes through the oesophageal opening in the diaphragm.

Hiccups are caused by the involuntary spasmodic contraction of the diaphragm, causing an abrupt inspiratory sound.

High density lipoproteins (HDLs) are produced in the liver and intestine. HDL particles are capable of carrying cholesterol away from the periphery of the body to the liver, unlike LDLs which are carried round the body. HDL particles have been shown to protect against atheroma formation and it is thought that this is because particles have the ability to transport cholesterol from the peripheral tissues to the liver. HDLs have important effects on platelets, thereby arresting haemorrhage and the causes of thrombosis.

Hyperglycaemia is an excess of sugar in the blood and is a condition accompanying diabetes mellitus.

Hypoglycaemia is a condition where there is a deficiency of blood sugar. It may occur in states of starvation or after the administration of insulin in too large doses, causing symptoms of weakness, tremors, nervousness, breathlessness and excitement followed sometimes be unconsciousness. Symptoms are removed by an intake of sugar or adrenaline, which antagonizes the action of insulin.

Irritable bowel syndrome is due to constipation or diarrhoea with the passage of small-volume stools and a feeling of incomplete emptying of the rectum. Pain is found on the left side of the large colon and is usually relieved by defecation or the passage of wind. The pain may be variable and occur in any part of the abdomen and the bowel habit may be normal.

Jaundice is a yellow discoloration of the skin, due to the presence of bile pigment in the blood. There are four types of this condition.

Low density lipoproteins (LDLs) are the main carriers of cholesterol, which is delivered to the liver and peripheral cells. Not all cholesterol synthesized by the liver is packaged immediately into lipoprotein particles, some are converted into bile salts, and both bile salts and cholesterol are excreted in bile and reabsorbed through the last section of the small intestine. There is a strong association between LDL cholesterol concentration and coronary heart disease.

Oesophageal varices is due to the veins at the bottom end of the oesophagus becoming distended and there is a likelihood that the veins may be ruptured by increased venous pressure or by bulky food passing through the oesophagus.

Pancreatitis is thought to be caused by alcoholism and gallstones. When a gallstone obstructs the ampullae there is a reflex of bile into the pancreas and the spread of infection.

Peptic and duodenal ulcers can be caused by ulceration of the mucosal lining of the stomach and duodenum by acid in the gastric juice. Ulcers are more rarely found in the oesophagus.

Peptic reflux oesophagitis is caused by the regurgitation of acid gastric juice into the oesophagus, causing irritation and ulceration.

Pernicious anaemia is caused by a lack of vitamin B12 due to a failure of absorption of B12. It is common in the elderly and is also common in fair-haired and blue-eyed people, more common in females than males. This form of anaemia has an association with other autoimmune diseases, particularly thyroid disease, Addison's disease and vitiligo. Symptoms of patients with pernicious anaemia are a yellowy colour due to a combination of pallor and jaundice caused by excess breakdown of haemoglobin due to the ineffective production of red blood cells in the bone marrow, and a sore red tongue.

Rectal polyps are due to nodules, tags of skin or cauliflower-like excrescences, which give rise to watery discharge, pain and itching.

Splenomegaly may be caused by blood diseases. The spleen enlarges to deal with the extra workload associated with removing damaged, worn-out and abnormal blood cells.

Thrush is caused by yeast (*Candida albicans*) and is usually spread to the oesophagus from the mouth and pharynx. It is most common in bottle-fed babies. The vagina is another common site.

Ulcerative colitis is an inflammation and ulceration of the colon and rectum.

Vagotomy is an operation where nerves to the stomach are cut.

URINARY SYSTEM

Cystitis may be due to the spread of microbes to the bladder via a short urethra, its proximity to the anus and moist conditions. Infection may also be caused by blood. The effects are small haemorrhages, inflammation and oedema of the mucosa in the bladder, with sensitivity of sensory nerves in the bladder wall which are stimulated by the inflammation, before the bladder completely fills, which leads to artificial desire and frequency to pass urine, accompanied by pain.

Diabetic kidney is so-called because renal failure is linked to early-onset, insulin-dependent diabetes. The cause is unknown but there may be an immune reaction to insulin.

Hydronephrosis is a chronic disease in which the kidney becomes distended with fluid which is caused by obstruction to the flow of urine into the pelvic area of the kidney and ureter tube. If the obstruction is in the ureter tube, the surrounding area will dilate and pressure will be transmitted back to the kidney.

Obstruction may also occur at the neck of the bladder or in the urethra. In the male, enlargement of the prostate gland is a common cause for obstruction round the neck of the bladder. If the condition is not relieved, the stagnation of urine infection can lead to cystitis and polynephritis.

Nephritis (Bright's disease) is an inflammation of the kidney, which is commonly sited in the glomerulus.

Nephrocalcinosis is caused by calcium deposits in the renal tubules, resulting in kidney-stone formation and renal insufficiency.

Polycystic kidney is due to cysts forming at the distal convoluted and collecting tubules. The cysts slowly enlarge and cause ischaemia and death of a portion of tissue (necrosis) of the nephrons. Associated abnormalities include polycystic liver disease, cysts in the spleen, pancreas, lungs and berry aneurysms in cerebral arteries.

Pyelitis is an inflammation in the part of the kidney called the pelvis, which is connected to the ureter tube. Infection involves kidney tissue promoting pyelonephritis.

Renal calculi are stones formed in the kidney and bladder. Once in the pelvis of the kidney, they may increase in size and become too large to pass through the ureter, thereby obstructing the flow of urine. Sometimes, stones originate in the bladder.

Renal colic – increased activity of the parathyroid glands is considered a possibility in causing renal calculi (kidney stones).

Uraemia is caused by renal (kidney) failure and is symptomatic of excess amounts of urea in the blood.

Ureteritis is due to the upward spread of infection in cystitis.

Urethritis is due to microbe infection spread by sexual intercourse directly to the urethra in the male and the perineum (tissue between the anus and external genitalia) in the female. In many cases, there is no known cause.

REPRODUCTIVE SYSTEM

Amenorrhoea is the absence of menstruation. Secondary causes can be due to pregnancy or disease.

Balanitis is an inflammation of the penis.

Candidiasis or thrush, is caused by small fungi (*Candida albicans*), which can infect moist, warm areas such as the vagina, mouth and skin folds.

Dysmenorrhoea means painful periods without apparent cause. Onset is usually shortly after puberty.

Eclampsia is a condition applied to convulsions arising in pregnancy, which can occur in the later months of pregnancy, during the delivery or after. Although the cause is not known, the kidneys are affected and cerebral oedema is thought to occur.

Ectopic pregnancy is the implantation of a fertilized ovum outside the uterus, most commonly in the Fallopian tube. As the foetus grows, the tube ruptures and its contents enter the peritoneal cavity, causing acute inflammation with the possibility of severe haemorrhage.

Endometriosis is the growth of endometrial tissues outside the uterus, found in the ovaries, Fallopian tubes and other pelvic structures. Tissue reacts to sex hormones, as does uterine endometrium, causing menstrual-type bleeding and the formation of cysts. Pain is present due to swelling.

Fibroids (myoma) are multiple, benign tumours of masses of smooth muscle encapsulated in compressed muscle fibres, which vary greatly in size. They develop during the reproductive period, regressing at the menopause.

Genital Warts are caused by a virus and the condition has been linked to cancer of the reproductive tract, especially cervical cancer.

Hypogonadism (female) is due to impaired ovarian function, which leads to oestrogen deficiency and abnormalities of the menstrual cycle, resulting in the absence of menstruation altogether. The absence of periods or irregular and infrequent periods (oligomenorrhoea) are a common symptom of amenorrhoea.

Hypogonadism (male) may be due to a complaint or occur through investigation for subfertility. Except with subfertility the complaints are usually of an androgen deficiency rather than semen production. Sperm only makes up a small proportion of seminal fluid volume.

Hysterectomy is where the uterus (partial hysterectomy) and possibly the ovaries (full hysterectomy) have been removed.

Mastalgia is a pain in the breast.

Mastitis is due to microbes entering through a nipple abrasion caused by the baby sucking. Infection spreads along mammary ducts and may become chronic or abscess forming.

Menopause is due to the ovaries ceasing to function with the result that the menstrual cycle diminishes and eventually stops. It usually occurs between the 45th and 50th years of life. There may be depression, night sweats, hot flushes, extreme lethargy and diminished libido due to hormone imbalance.

Menorrhagia is an excessive amount of menstrual discharge.

Obstetric Cholestasis (OC) is a form of recurrent jaundice during pregnancy. The mother complains of outbreaks of generalized pruritus (itching) in the third trimester, or occasionally earlier. Symptoms are noticeable on the extremities, especially the palms of the hand and soles of the feet, the trunk, face, breasts, legs and back. No rash is present, with pruritus worse at night, possibly causing insomnia and depression. There may be secondary symptoms of reduced appetite, malaise and gastric discomfort. The condition may become more acute as pregnancy progresses, with relief after the birth. If OC is diagnosed, liver function tests are carried out about six weeks after the birth and repeated until normal. It is not thought that OC causes permanent damage to either the mother or the baby's liver. Recurrence in future pregnancies is possible because of the possibility of genetic links. A programme of healthy eating is recommended during pregnancy with cutting out fatty foods and products high in refined sugar and additives. OC is the most common disorder of liver function during pregnancy, second only to acute viral hepatitis as a cause of jaundice in the third trimester of pregnancy. Increased antenatal surveillance is recommended if symptoms presented are diagnosed as OC.

Orchitis is an inflammation of the testicles.

Ovarian cyst is a tumour of the ovary containing fluid.

Pelvic inflammatory disease (PID) usually begins with vaginitis and may spread to the cervix, uterus, Fallopian tubes and ovaries.

Polycystic ovarian syndrome is due to multiple ovarian cysts and by excess androgen production from the ovaries and adrenal glands, although whether the basic condition begins from the ovaries, adrenal or pituitary glands is unknown. Cysts represent arrested development of the follicles.

Pre-eclampsia is due to high blood pressure, oedema and the presence of albumin in the urine.

Pre-menstrual syndrome (PMS) features physical and/or emotional changes in some women before menstruation. Symptoms include swelling and tenderness in the breasts, temporary weight gain, irritability, loss of concentration, migraine and headaches, constipation, excessive tiredness and sugar craving, depression and uncontrollable outbursts of anger and crying; it can last from three to fourteen days and may begin during the menstrual cycle. It is due to hormonal changes in the body.

Prostatic enlargement (benign) is where the prostate has become enlarged and put pressure on the bladder, causing obstruction to the outflow of urine. In malignancy, changes in the androgen balance may be significant or viruses may be involved.

Prostatitis is an infection of the prostate gland, spread from the urethra or bladder.

Salpingitis is an infection that spreads from the uterus to the Fallopian tubes. It can manifest in acute and chronic inflammation, and leads to fibrous obstruction in the Fallopian tubes and subfertility.

Simmond's disease occurs mostly in women following a difficult labour due to the fall in systemic blood pressure. The pituitary gland becomes wasted and the immediate effect may be failure of milk production (lactation).

Subfertility, a kinder term than infertility, is defined as the inability of a couple to conceive after one year of unprotected intercourse. Causes can be: a major identifiable male factor; female tubal problems and ovulatory disorders; hostile cervical mucus and inadequate intercourse with vaginal factors are uncommon; idiopathic, where there is no apparent explanation; a significant proportion have both male and female problems.

Testicular tumours are usually malignant. The tumour stays localized for some time before spreading via lymph fluid to pelvic and abdominal lymph nodes before entering the blood circulation.

Venereal diseases (VD) are sexually transmitted diseases. Microbes are unable to live outside the body for long periods and microbes produce lesions in the genital area, which discharge infecting microbes. Gonorrhoea is the most common form and in the male may affect the prostate gland, epididymis and testes; in the female infection may affect the vulval glands, vagina, cervix, Fallopian tubes, ovaries and the peritoneum. Syphilis microbes incubate for several weeks, when a primary sore appears at the vulva, vagina, perineum, penis and round the mouth. After several weeks the sore disappears until, 3–4 months later, skin rashes and raised papules appear on external genitalia and vaginal walls. These subside after several months and are followed by a latent period. Sexual transmission occurs during the primary and secondary stages.

Vulvovaginitis is caused by protozoa and is usually sexually transmitted in gonorrhoea.

NERVOUS SYSTEM

Aphasia and dysarthria involve a loss or defect in language caused by brain damage. Partial disturbance is called dysphasia. Dysarthria is disordered articulation, as in paralysis where slowing or incoordination of the muscles of articulation are affected, for example, weakness or incoordination of the speech musculature prevents clear pronunciation of words and can be found in cerebral palsy, multiple sclerosis, Parkinson's disease and motor neurone disease.

Bell's palsy is facial paralysis due to oedema (fluid) of the facial nerve.

Cerebral palsy is a disorder apparent at birth or in childhood, caused by brain damage. Mental retardation, from severe intellectual to mild learning disorders, is common. Physical disability is not necessarily associated with a severe defect of the higher functions of the brain.

Encephalitis is an inflammation of the brain.

Epilepsy is a nervous disorder, characterized by a fit or sudden loss of consciousness, which can be accompanied by convulsions. There are two types of epileptic seizure: *le grand mal* (epileptic fit) and *le petit mal* (a sudden arrest of consciousness, which is of short duration and may be accompanied by staggering, without convulsion).

Headaches are due to pain receptors in the vessels at the base of the brain and in the meninges becoming stimulated by mechanical and chemical means. Nerve impulses are carried centrally via the fifth and ninth cranial nerves. Pain receptors are also present in the muscles of the scalp, neck and face, the sinuses of the skull, the eyes and teeth. The brain itself is almost devoid of pain receptors. There are five reasons for headaches: pressure, when the meninges are moved thus causing pain; subacute headache, with onset and progression over days or weeks, with or without the features of pressure headache, may be due to encephalitis and viral meningitis; single episode of severe headache, is caused by brain haemorrhage, migraine and possibly meningitis; recurrent headaches, such as migraine and tension headaches, are the commonest causes of recurrent pain. Sinusitis, glaucoma and migrainous neuralgia should also be considered. Excess alcohol intake, causing a hangover, is the most obvious cause; chronic headaches usually have a history going back for several years or more, and are due to muscle tension and/or migraine, depression usually accompanies them; headaches following head injury are suggestive of brain lesion.

Herpes Zoster Neuritis (shingles) is caused by the virus that produces chicken pox in children and shingles in adults.

Meningitis is an inflammation of the meninges. There are two major types: viral, which is less serious than the bacterial form

Migraine is an attack of severe headache, often with nausea, vomiting and visual disturbance.

Motor neurone disease is caused by progressive degeneration of cells in the spinal cord, the motor neurones and the corticospinal tracts. Its cause is unknown.

Multiple sclerosis is a disease of the brain and spinal cord, which may be slow in developing the symptoms of paralysis and tremors. In early stages of the disease the myelin sheath (insulating sheath of nerve fibres) becomes hardened resulting in pin-head to pea-sized patches composed of connective tissue. These patches, which are scattered throughout the brain, break up and are absorbed, leaving nerve fibres bare. Connective tissue is later formed between these. Onset of the disease is rare after the age of forty.

Muscle cramp is a prolonged involuntary contraction of muscle fibres, which is very painful.

Muscular dystrophy is a muscle-wasting disease, either with or without increase in muscle, without the nervous system being affected. The cause of the disease is still obscure but it is thought to be hereditary, beginning weakly in childhood.

Myasthenia gravis is an autoimmune disease resulting in muscular weakness with fatigue present with exertion. The body produces antibodies which interfere with the workings of the nerve endings in muscle, which are acted on by chemical transmitters – it is these transmitters that transmit nerve impulses to muscles. Not only voluntary muscles are affected with a resultant lack of contraction but those affecting breathing and swallowing. The thymus gland is important as it is the source of the chemical transmitters which form the antibodies.

Neuralgia simply means 'nerve pain'. Affecting the sensory nerves, its origin is not clearly traceable. Pain can be connected with pressure or inflammation of a nerve. Hence the word is used to define pain associated with a particular nerve or its branches, whatever the cause.

Neuritis means inflammation affecting nerves or nerves localized to one part of the body, e.g. sciatica. The fibrous sheath of the nerve is faulty with nerve fibres being secondarily affected. Inflammation spreading to the nerve from surrounding tissue, too cold or too long-continued irritation by pressure on the nerve may be the cause. If motor nerves are affected, paralysis of the muscle may be present.

Paralysis involves the loss or impairment of motor function in a part due to a lesion of the neural or muscular mechanism. The terms used to describe different types of paralysis are: hemiplegia, paralysis affecting one side of the face with the corresponding arm and leg as a result of disease on one side of the brain; diplegia, a condition of total paralysis in which both sides of the body are affected; monoplegia refers to paralysis of a single limb; paraplegia refers to paralysis on both sides of the body below a certain point, usually below the waist; and quadriplegia refers to paralysis of all four limbs.

Parkinson's disease is due to degenerative changes in the ganglia at the base of the cerebrum. In most cases, this results in a deficiency of the neurotransmitter called dopamine but other neurotransmitters may be included. Symptoms are rigidity of muscles, resulting in loss of facial expression, an affected voice due to the constriction of the laryngeal muscles and those of the tongue and lips. Later, limbs become rigid giving a running gait, tottering, taking short steps and a rolling movement of fingers (as though a cigarette is being rolled). Tremor is caused by excitement and self-consciousness but stops during sleep.

Poliomyelitis is a disease of the brain and spinal cord, with an infecting organism of a virus by the mouth. The virus attacks the motor cells in the spinal cord, especially around the lumbar area of the spine. Cranial nerves and the brain are involved. The virus is eventually excreted in the stools. Symptoms are aches and pains in the limbs with a slight rise in temperature.

Shingles is caused by the herpes zoster virus, similar to chickenpox and causes a belt of small yellow vesicles around the middle of the body.

Spina bifida is a defect in the posterior wall of the spinal wall, usually in the lumbar area. The most serious form is spina bifida cystica, where the meninges, containing the spinal cord and nerves, protrudes through the defect in the spinal canal.

Stroke is a haemorrhage into the brain by the rupture of a blood vessel.

Tetany occurs when nerves are affected by a lack of calcium, causing painful muscle spasms of the hands and feet.

Trigeminal neuralgia or *tic doloureux* is due to severe paroxysms of knife-like, or electric-shock pain lasting seconds, originating from the fifth cranial nerve. Causes can be washing, shaving, a cold wind, or eating which stimulate and provoke pain. The face may be screwed up in agony, hence 'tic', meaning an involuntary movement. Pain does not occur at night and spontaneous remission can last for years before recurring.

SKELETAL SYSTEM AND JOINTS

Ankylosing spondylitis is a rheumatic disease in young adults, especially men. Pain begins in the lumbar spine with stiffness, which progresses to involve the whole spine. The discs and ligaments are replaced by fibrous tissue, making the spine rigid.

Arthritis has two forms: rheumatoid arthritis (RA), where there is a chronic inflammation of the synovial lining in the joint cavity, and osteoarthritis (OA), which consists of mechanical failure of the cartilage and impaired blood supply, due to previous injury or over-weight. The condition affects weight-bearing joints, such as the knees and hips. In both conditions a diet high in acid-forming foods dries out synovial fluid in the joint cavity and eventually eats away the bone.

Bursitis is an inflammation of the joint lining (bursa) caused by injury, friction or pressure.

Carpal tunnel syndrome. The carpal tunnel is a small channel inside the wrist, formed by a group of bones on the back of the hand and a band of ligaments across the base of the palm. The tunnel contains a major nerve, blood vessels and a number of tendons. Pressure on the carpal tunnel causes the nerve, which runs through the tunnel, to become compressed and pinched, which results in paralysis. Symptoms include weakness, pins and needles, redness and swelling, limited range of movement, pain and discomfort, and numbing and tingling sensations in the hand. Repetitive hand movements, diabetes, pregnancy and body

configuration are thought to be causes of the condition.

Fibromyalgia describes a functional condition of voluntary muscle that gives rise to widespread pain arising from muscles and their insertions and can be caused by psychological origin rather than organic.

Fibrositis involves pain, muscular stiffness and inflammation of the soft tissue of the arms, legs and trunk. The cause is unknown and may involve psychological stress, immunological factors and muscular strain.

Frozen shoulder describes a painful, stiff shoulder and is common in adults of any age. Pain may radiate to the arm and is usually more troublesome at night; it is associated with injury or overuse and sometimes has no obvious cause.

Gout is an abnormality of uric acid metabolism, which results in an excess present in the blood with the deposition of urates around the joint. Symptoms are painful inflammation and swelling of the smaller joints, especially those of the big toe and thumb.

Housemaid's knee (bursitis) is an inflammation of the bursa of the patellar in the knee, which becomes distended with serous fluid.

Injury includes bruising, fractures, strains and sprains to any bone, joint, ligament, muscle or tendon in the skeletal frame.

Kyphosis is curvature of the spine, where the concavity of the spine is directed forwards, thereby creating a backwards curvature and a hump-back. It may be caused by postural imbalances, especially in tall adolescent girls who stoop, the obese, or with the elderly who may have osteoporosis.

Lordosis is a curvature of the spine forwards, occurring from the lumbar area of the spine, where the natural curve is forwards. It can be the result of muscular weakness and spinal disease.

Lumbago is caused by pain in the lower part of the back. It may be caused by muscle strain or by a prolapsed intervertebral disc.

Neck pain may be caused by rheumatoid arthritis, ankylosing spondylitis, rheumatism or fibromyalgia. In chronic conditions it is associated with osteoarthritis, which may occur in the lumbar spine as well as the neck. The three lowest cervical discs are often more affected and there is pain and stiffness of the neck with or without pain radiating to the arm. Chronic cervical disc disease is known as cervical spondylosis.

Osteomalacia is the adult form of rickets and is caused by a deficiency of vitamin D or renal (kidney) disease, malabsorption in the small intestine or an inadequate intake.

Osteomyelitis is an inflammation of the marrow of the bone, which leads to infection.

Osteoporosis is a reduced mass of normal bone, caused by the loss of one per cent of bone per year after the menopause. The quality of bone is unaffected, it is the quantity that is deficient. This disease can also be a feature of Cushing's syndrome (an excessive production of cortisol) and with patients who have been on long-term treatment of corticosteroids.

Paget's disease is a disease of the bone affecting the limbs, spine and skull where bone becomes thick and soft causing it to bend. It is thought to be the commonest bone disease in the world.

Polyarthritis is an inflammation of several joints at the same time as seen in rheumatoid arthritis.

Polymyalgia rheumatica is a form of rheumatism with pain in the shoulders and sometimes round the hips and is characterized by extreme early morning stiffness, which eases off during the day. It affects women more than men. Its cause is still unknown.

Reiter's disease is a form of polyarthritis, involving inflammation of the toes and joints with nail thickening and change in skin colour. It can also be linked with urethritis, an inflammation of the urethra.

Rheumatism is a term given for a number of conditions with similar features. They cause musculoskeletal or joint pain that arises from the surrounding structures, such as tendon sheaths and bursae.

Sacroileitis is an inflammation of one or both of the sacroiliac joints, possibly caused by rheumatoid arthritis, Reiter's syndrome infection, ankylosing spondylitis or arthritis linked to psoriasis.

Scoliosis is a curvature of the spine consisting of a bend to one side and partly of a rotary twist. It may result from a disease of the spine, tuberculosis, chronic pleurisy or from bad posture as a child.

Slipped disc is a prolapsed intervertebral disc, which causes pressure on the spinal nerves.

Spondylosis is degeneration of the vertebral discs and joints in the spine. Osteoarthritis is usually implicated. Pain is felt in the neck and lumbar regions and, in these areas, joints may become unstable. This may put pressure on the nerves leaving the lumbar area of the spine with the result that sciatica may be present.

Sprains are injuries related to specific joints, usually consisting of the tearing of a ligament.

Strain is an overuse or stretching of a part, usually a muscle or tendon.

Systemic lupus erythematosus – *see under* Skin disorders.

Tennis elbow is due to the extensor muscles in the forearm at their attachment at the external epicondyle (a protuberance on a long bone).

Tenosynovitis Two tendons are involved in pulling the thumb out and back from the hand, called the abductor pollicis longus and the extensor pollicis longus. These two tendons run in a tunnel over the side of the wrist, just above the thumb. Ligaments that form an arch over the tendons to keep the tendons in place form the tunnel. The two tendons run through a common tunnel in the forearm and are covered with a slippery covering called the tenosynovium. This covering aids in limiting friction as tendons glide back and forth over the thumb. Inflammation of the tenosynovium and tendon is known as tenosynovitis. Symptoms are soreness on the thumb side of the forearm; pain may spread up the forearm or down into the wrist and thumb. As friction increases, the two tendons may squeak as they attempt to move through the restricted tunnel. Increasing pain limits the grasping action for the hand and thumb

Torticollis is due to a contracted state of the cervical muscles producing twisting of the neck. The cause may be congenital or by pressure on the nerves, inflammation of the glands in the neck or to muscle spasm.

Whiplash injuries occur to the neck, usually as a result of a car injury.

MULTI-FACTORIAL DISORDERS

Agoraphobia is a psychological disorder characterized by a sense of fear experienced in open spaces.

Alopecia is hair loss that becomes abnormally visible. It may or may not be permanent, if hair follicles are left intact. It is also associated with hyper/hypothyroidism, pregnancy, and androgen activity in both males and females. Iron deficiency and rapid weight loss associated with dieting and drugs such as lithium and vitamin A and its derivatives also produce diffuse and treatable hair loss.

Burning feet is a condition characterized by a burning sensation on the soles of the feet caused by malnutrition and lack of vitamin B complex.

Claustrophobia is a psychological disorder characterized by a fear of a confined space.

Dementia is a condition characterized by intellectual impairment resulting in forgetfulness. *Alzheimer* type is the most common resulting in loss of memory orientation, judgement, activity and intellectual functioning; it affects language, visio-spatial skills, memory, abstract thought and judgement, and personality. Initially short-term memory loss occurs two to three years prior to development of the disease.

Diaphragmatic fatigue is due to the diaphragm becoming fatigued if the force of inspiration exceeds 40 per cent developed in a maximum effort.

Down's syndrome, which is present from birth, is characterized by mental subnormality in which the patient has Mongolism-like features and a small, round skull. Infant mortality is high, due to other congenital deformities and a lowered resistance to infection.

Healing crisis occurs when a disorder reaches a climax by seeming to appear worse but which then subsides with continuing improvement.

Hernias result in a protrusion of the internal organs through the structures enclosing them. There are several areas of the body where they are found: cerebral, where a part of the brain protrudes through the skull; femoral, where a loop of the intestine protrudes into the femoral canal; incisional, occurring at the site of an old wound; inguinal, where a part of the intestine protrudes through the inguinal canal; and an umbilical hernia, where the weak point in the umbilicus and blood vessels from the placenta enter the foetus (*see* Hiatus Hernia, page 315).

Herpes Simplex is an infectious disease with blister-like, painful vesicles on the skin and mucous membranes. The infection lasts throughout life and vesicles are found on the lips, mouth and face (cold sores), on the genitalia, in the conjunctiva and cornea of the eye, and in the brain where it causes encephalitis or meningitis.

Hirsuties is an excessive growth of a male-type of hair and distribution in females. In females, there is no recognizable evidence of endocrine disease.

Hypothermia is defined as a fall in the rectal temperature to below 35°C. It can lead to fatality if the temperature falls below 32°C. It may occur in cold climates, or be due to depressant drugs, alcohol or hypothyroidism. It is usually the poor and elderly who are affected, the latter having a diminished ability to feel cold accompanied by a decrease in insulating fat layer. Exposure to extremes of temperature and immersion in cold water below 12°C contribute to the condition.

Motion sickness involves a lack of co-ordination between visual and spatial interpretation by the brain.

Muscular dystrophy is a condition where muscle wasting takes place in certain muscles without any affect on the nervous system. The disease appears to run in families, being transmitted by the mother.

Myalgic encephalomyelitis (ME) is a condition in which tiredness, muscle pain, panic attacks, lack of concentration, memory loss and depression occur. ME often follows viral infections of the upper respiratory tract, or gut.

Psychogenic back pain has psychological origins and is associated with young adult females who suffer from continuous unvarying pain, which is described in vivid terms; there is no relief from rest; there is a long history of treatment failures; associated symptoms are headache and a fruitless investigation of symptoms from other systems of the body and which are sometimes accompanied with depression. Difficult life situations are a predisposing factor.

Repetitive strain injury (RSI) is caused by excessive repetitive use of the hands, such as keyboard users and those who work on assembly lines. Although overuse is the fundamental cause, it occurs in stressful circumstances and when other workers are affected.

Restless legs syndrome expresses unpleasant sensations and sometimes involuntary movements in the limbs, usually at night when resting.

Shock occurs when the metabolic needs of cells are not met because of inadequate blood flow. Blood circulation and blood pressure is reduced

Snoring can be caused by smoking, overwork, fatigue, obesity and general poor health.

Toxaemia is a form of blood poisoning caused by absorption of toxins formed at a local site of infection. In pregnancy, it is known as pre-eclampsia and eclampsia.

Toxic shock syndrome is a condition characterized by fever, rash and diarrhoea; it is associated with use of tampons and caused by staphylococcal toxin.

Ulcers are caused by erosion of tissue on the surface of the skin or the membranous lining of any cavity in the body which is slow to heal. Types of ulcer include those found in the mouth, stomach, bowel and varicose ulcers of the leg.

Vasovagal attack is a temporary loss of consciousness due to an abrupt slowing of the heart rate caused by stress, fear, pain or shock, and may be caused by overstimulation of the vagus nerve.

Virus Infections are caused by infective organisms colonizing healthy cells in the body, thus causing disease.

Glossary

Abduction: movement of a limb away from the centre of the body.

Abreaction: is an emotional release caused by re-experiencing unpleasant memories from the past.

Achilles tendon: is a thick tendon that joins the calf muscles to the heel bone (calcaneum). Contraction of the calf pulls the heel upwards.

Acidosis: a condition that results from a decrease in the pH of body fluids.

Active transport: movement of a substance into or out of a cell in a direction opposite that in which it would normally flow by diffusion.

Acute: refers to a short-lived but severe condition.

Adduction: movement of a limb towards the centre of the body.

Adenosine triphosphate (ATP): energy-storing compound found in all cells.

ADH: antidiuretic hormone.

Adhesion: holding together of two surfaces or parts by bands of connective tissue that are normally separate.

Adipose: a type of connective tissue that stores fat.

Aerobic: requiring oxygen.

Albumin: a blood plasma protein and other body fluids that help maintain osmotic pressure of blood.

Alkalosis: results from an increase in the pH of body fluids.

Allergen: a substance that causes sensitivity.

Allergy: an unfavourable reaction to a certain substance that is normally harmless.

Alveolus: one of millions of tiny air sacs in the lungs through which gaseous exchange takes place between the outside air and the blood.

Amino acid: building-block of protein.

Amniotic: fluid-filled sac that surrounds and protects the foetus.

Anabolism: metabolic building of simple compounds into two complex substances needed by the body.

Anaerobic: not requiring oxygen.

Analgesic: relieving pain; an agent that does not cause loss of consciousness.

Angioplasty: is where an insertion of a balloon into constricted blood vessels or a heart valve reopens the affected part.

ANS: autonomic nervous system.

Anterior: toward the front of the body, or ventral aspect.

Antibodies: specific form of blood protein produced in the lymphoid tissue and able to counteract the effects of bacterial antigen and toxin.

Antigen: a foreign substances that produces an immune response.

Aponeurosis: a broad sheet of fibrous connective tissue that attaches muscle to bone or to other muscle.

Areolar: loose connective tissue.

Articulation: means movement between two or more joints.

Benign: a tumour that does not spread; is not recurrent or becoming worse.

Biopsy: removal of tissue for examination, usually under a microscope.

Bradycardia: heart rate of less than 60 beats per minute.

Bronchiole: a small subdivision of the bronchi that branch throughout the lungs.

Bursa: small, fluid-filled sac found in an area subject to stress round bones and joints.

Cancer: tumour that spreads to other tissues and is malignant.

Carbohydrate: simple sugar or compound made from simple sugars linked together, such as starch or glycogen.

Carcinogen: a cancer-forming substance.

Carcinoma: a form of cancer.

Catabolism: metabolic breakdown of substances into simpler substances; includes the digestion of food and the oxidation of nutrient molecules for energy.

Catalyst: a substance that hastens or brings about a chemical change without itself undergoing alteration.

Catheter: a tube that can be inserted into a vessel or cavity to remove fluid, such as urine or blood.

Chlamydia: a type of small bacteria that can exist only in a living cell, causing sexually transmitted diseases and respiratory diseases.

Cholesterol: an organic fat-like compound found in animal fat, bile, blood, myelin, liver and other parts of the body.

Chronic: disorders that are not severe but are continuous or recurring.

Chyle: a milky-like fluid absorbed into the lymphatic system from the small intestine that consists of lymph fluid and droplets of digested fat.

Chyme: a mixture of partially digested food, digestive juices and water formed in the stomach.

Circumduction: movement of parts of the body in circular movements

CNS: central nervous system.

Collagen: flexible white protein that gives resilience and strength to connective tissue, such as bone and cartilage.

Congenital: present at birth.

Cutaneous: referring to the integumentary system (the skin).

Deoxyribonucleic acid: *see* DNA.

Distal: farthest point from the origin of a structure or reference point.

Diencephalon: the region of the brain between the cerebral hemispheres and the midbrain, which contains the thalamus, hypothalamus and the pituitary gland.

DNA: is the abbreviation for deoxyribonucleic acid, the fundamental genetic material contained in the nucleus of a cell, forming part of the chromosomes and carrying genetic information.

Dorsal: relating to the back or posterior part of an organ.

Dorsiflexion: bending backwards, or upwards, of the fingers or toes.

Duct: a tube or channel for the passage of fluid particularly one conveying the secretion of a gland.

ECG: electrocardiograph; an instrument used to study the electric activity of the heart.

Ectopic: applies to a part of the body or a happening in the body outside of its usual place. For example, gestation occurring in the fallopian tubes.

EEG: Electro-encephalography refers to graphically recorded brain waves, used in diagnosis, such as in epilepsy.

Electroconvulsive therapy (ECT): is a form of treatment sometimes used in severe depression where electric shocks are induced in the brain by placing electrodes onto the skull. Amnesia is often a side effect; this form of treatment is rarely used today.

Electrolyte: a compound that forms ions in solution and which conducts an electric current in solution.

Emulsify: to break up fats into small particles.

Endorphins: one of a group of opiate peptides produced naturally in the body at nerve synapses at various points in the central nervous system, where they control pain perceptions, sedation, rise in the pain threshold and euphoria.

Endoscope: a tube-shaped funnel inserted into a cavity in the body used to investigate and treat disorders. Examples are: cystoscope, for examining the bladder; ectoscope, gastroscope, for examining the stomach; and arthroscope, for looking into joints.

Endotoxins: poisons produced by and retained in a bacterium, which are released after the destruction of the bacterial cell.

Epiglottis: a leaf-shaped cartilage that covers the larynx whilst swallowing.

ESR: erythrocyte sedimentation rate, is a test that measures the rate at which red blood cells settle out of suspension in blood plasma. The test is used to determine whether infection or malignancy are present, as proteins in the plasma increase with the incidence of disease, which results in cells settle out more quickly.

Eversion: the feet point outwards away from the centre of the body

Extension: to straighten a joint or part of the body

Flatulence: is a collection of gas in the stomach or bowels. The gas may be forced out via the mouth or anus. It is caused by either fermentation of bacteria containing sulphur or swallowing air.

Flexion: to bend a joint or part of the body

Flexure: a bend or curve.

Foramen: an opening or passageway into or through a bone.

Gland: an organ composed of cells that secrete fluid prepared from blood, either for use in the body or for excretion as waste material; ductless glands secrete contents directly into the blood stream and are called endocrine glands; secretions discharged through a duct are called exocrine glands.

Grommet: a small bobbin shaped tube, used to keep open the incision made in the ear-drum in the treatment of Glue Ear.

Haematology: is the study of diseases of the blood.

Heart murmur: abnormal heart sound.

Heparin: is a substance found in the liver, muscle and lung; prevents coagulation of the blood.

Histamine: a substance released from tissues during an antigen–antibody reaction.

Homeostasis: a state of internal environmental balance; maintenance of body conditions within set limits.

Hyperventilation: an abnormally rapid respiratory rate, causing light-headedness and then unconsciousness by lowering carbon dioxide levels in the blood; present in heart disease and chest disorders.

Ibuprofen: is an analgesic and anti-inflammatory agent; used in treatment for rheumatoid arthritis and other rheumatic disorders.

ICSH: interstitial cell stimulating hormone, another name for luteinizing hormone, found in the male.

Idiopathic: applies to diseases where the cause is unknown.

Ileum: the last portion of the small intestine; can relate to the lower part of the pelvic cavity.

Immunoglobulins: represent many types of antibodies present in the body.

Infarction: a change in an organ where an artery is suddenly blocked, as in thrombosis or embolism.

Inferior: that which is below an internal structure or part of the body.

Innervation: applies to nerve supply to tissue, organ or part of the body carries motor impulses to a part and sensory impulses away from the part to the brain.

Interstitial: between spaces or structures in an organ; between active tissues.

Intracellular: within a cell.

Inversion: the feet point inwards, towards the centre of the body.

Ischaemia: lack of blood supply to an area.

Isometric: muscle contraction where tension is present but there is no change in muscle length; in the calf muscles when walking or pushing against an immovable object.

Isotonic: muscle contraction where the tone in the muscle is the same but the muscle shortens to produce movement.

Lactation: production of milk after childbirth.

Laparoscopy: an investigation by a small incision into the abdominal cavity with a metal cylinder, eye piece and light source.

Lateral: refers to an internal structure or part of the body, which is furthest from the midline.

Libido: is the desire for sexual activity.

Macrophages: are large phagocytes (specialized cells), which form part of the reticuloendothelial system, a part of the immune system; found in the spleen, liver, connective tissues, lymph nodes, bone marrow and central nervous system; collect at sites of infection where they engulf microbes and foreign substances by crushing, strangling and poisoning.

Malleolus: two bony prominences either side of the ankle.

Medial: near the midline, or middle of the body.

Melanin: dark pigment found in skin, some parts of the brain, hair and eyes.

Mesentery: the membranous peritoneal ligament that attaches the small intestine to the back of the abdominal wall.

Mesocolon: peritoneal ligament that attaches the colon to the back of the abdominal wall.

Metabolic rate: the rate at which energy is released from nutrients in the cell.

Metabolism: the physical and chemical processes by which the human body, or other living organism, is maintained.

Metastasis: growth and spread of tumour cells.

Micturition: release of urine from the bladder.

Mitosis: cell division that replicates two daughter cells exactly like the parent.

MRI: magnetic resonance imaging; a method of studying tissue based on nuclear movement following exposure to radio waves in a powerful magnetic field.

Necrosis: tissue death.

Neurolemma: a thin sheath that covers certain peripheral nerve axons and aids in their regeneration.

Neuron: nerve cell.

Oedema: an accumulation of fluid beneath the skin in cavities of the body or the limbs.

Oncology: the study of tumours.

Organ: two or more tissues which function together for a specific purpose.

Os Trigonum: a small bone behind the ankle joint; present in a small percentage of the population; damage caused by springing from the toes or jumping.

Oxidation: chemical breakdown of nutrients for energy.

Pacemaker: sinoatrial (SA) node of the heart, group of cells or artificial device that sets the rate of heart contractions.

Palliative: aims to lessen suffering in the presence of terminal illness.

Palpation: is a method of examining the size, shape and movements related to the surface of the body or internal organs by laying the palm of the hand upon the skin.

Palpitation: is when the heart beats irregularly and with force so that the person is aware of its action.

Pathology: the study of disease.

Pathophysiology: the study of the physiologic basis of disease.

Peristalsis: wave-like contraction preceded by a wave of dilation that travels along the walls of a tubular organ.

pH: acid and alkaline balance present in blood represented from 0 to 14, with acid content from 0 to 7 and alkaline content from 7 to 14. The body is predominately alkaline at 7.4.

Phagocytosis: is where bacteria are engulfed by specialized white cells (*see* macrophages).

Phrenic nerve: supplies the diaphragm beginning at the third, fourth and fifth cervical spinal nerves, extending down the neck through the thoracic cavity to the diaphragm.

Physiology: the study of the function of living organisms.

PID: Pelvic Inflammatory Disease.

Plantarflexion: bending the fingers or toes towards the ground.

Pneumothorax: an accumulation of air in the pleural space.

PNS: peripheral nervous system.

Posterior: the back, or behind the body.

Prolapse: means a part of the body which slips downwards, especially the uterus or rectum.

Pronation: turning the palm of the hand downwards; lying face downwards.

Prophylaxis: the prevention of disease.

Proprioceptor: sensory receptor that aids in judging body position and changes in position, located in muscles, tendons and joints.

Prostaglandins: a group of hormones, formed by fatty acids, produced by many cells, which have a variety of effects including on the brain, lungs, uterus and semen; activity includes cardiac, respiratory and digestive process and cause uterine contractions.

Protein: organic compound made of amino acids, containing nitrogen, hydrogen, carbon, and oxygen; sometimes sulphur and phosphorus.

Prosthesis: a prosthesis is an artificial replacement for a part of the body such as an eye, limb or denture.

Proximal: point nearest to a point of origin, or reference point.

Psychosomatic: means unexpressed and repressed emotions; results in structural or physiological changes in the body.

Psychosis: any major mental disorder of organic or emotional origin marked by a derangement of the personality.

Pulse: wave of increased blood pressure in the vessels produced by contraction of the heart.

Referred pain: is pain felt in a part of the body which has its origin in another part.

Reflex: an involuntary response to a stimulus.

Ribonucleic acid (RNA): a substance required for protein manufacture in the cell.

Serotonin: a substance widely distributed in body tissue, especially in the platelets, lining of the gastrointestinal tract, where it inhibits gastric secretion and stimulates smooth muscle in the walls of the small intestine; in the brain it participates in the transmission of nerve impulses and is thought to be involved in controlling states of consciousness and moods; also believed to have a similar function as histamine in inflammation.

Somatic: relating to the body as opposed to the mind.

Sphincter: a muscular ring that controls the size of an opening.

Stasis: inhibition of the normal flow of body fluids, such as blood, lymph, urine or the contents of the digestive tract.

STD: sexually transmitted diseases.

Stenosis: a narrowing of a duct or canal.

Steroid: certain lipids that include the hormones of the adrenal cortex and the sex glands.

Subcutaneous: under the skin.

Subluxation: means a sprain or partial dislocation.

Sudoriferous: producing sweat or referring to the sweat glands.

Superior: that which is above an internal structure or part of the body.

Supine: turning of the palm of the hand upwards; lying on the back with face upwards.

Suspension: a mixture that will separate unless shaken.

Synapse: a junction between two nerves or between a nerve and an effector.

Syndrome: a group of symptoms characteristic of a disorder.

Systemic: referring to a generalized infection or condition.

Tissue: a group of similar cells that perform a specialized function.

Torsion: applies to twisting of organs or tumours attached to the body, which narrow blood vessels and structures.

Toxin: any poisonous compound, usually referring to that produced by bacteria.

Viscera: is the medical term for organs and glands within the body.

Warfarin: is a drug that acts as an anticoagulant of the blood.

Water on the brain: is another term for hydrocephalus and meningitis.

Withdrawal symptoms: are unpleasant side effects, physical or mental, when withdrawing from a drug; symptoms include sweating, tremors and vomiting.

Organizations

For details of professional, accredited training in reflexology, contact The Chiron Training in Reflexology, P.O. Box, 3544, Christchurch, Dorset BH23 5XE, tel: 01425 271257.

PROFESSIONAL ORGANIZATIONS WHO WILL SUPPLY ACCREDITED TRAINING SCHOOLS AND PRACTITIONERS

Where the therapy is not so widely known, an explanation of benefits is given with the organization concerned.

Affiliation of Crystal Healing Organizations
Crystals are placed on specific parts of the body where the energy field needs rebalancing.
72 Pasture Road, Goole
East Yorks
tel: 01405 769 119

Alcoholics Anonymous
General Service Office
London WC1X 8QF
tel: 0171 352 3001 (London)

Stonebrow House
Stonebrow
York YO1 2NJ

Alcohol Concern
275 Gray's Inn Road
London WC1X 8QF
tel: 0171 833 3471

Aromatherapy Organizations Council
(Umbrella Organization)
The Secretary
3 Latymer Close, Braybrooke
Market Harborough
Leicester LE16 8LN
tel: 01858 434242

Association of Reflexologists
For a free copy of the practitioner register, send an A4 sae to:
27 Old Gloucester Street
London WC1N 3XX
tel: 0990 673320

Ayurvedic Medical Association UK
Asian Indian system based on balancing the three elements, or doshas, in the body. Usually involves herbal medicine, massage, sauna, pulse diagnosis and dietary advice.
The Hale Clinic
7 Park Crescent
London W1N 3HE
tel: 0171 631 0156

Bach Flower Therapy
The Bach Centre
Mount Vernon, Sotwell
Wallingford
Oxfordshire OX10 0PZ
tel: 01491 834678

Birmingham Obstetric Cholestasis Support Group
4 Shenstone Close, Four Oaks
Sutton Coldfield
Birmingham B74 4XB
tel: 0121 353 0699

Bowen Association
Non-invasive therapy that works the connective tissue of muscle. Used for sports injuries, headaches, asthma and jet lag.
PO Box 182, Witney
Oxon OX8 5YD
tel: 01993 705769

British Acupuncture Council
Park House, 206–208 Latimer Road
London W10 6RE
tel: 0181 964 0222

British Association for Counselling (BAC)
1 Regent Place, Rugby
Warwickshire CV21 2PJ
tel: 01788 550899

British Chiropractic Association
Equity House
29 Whitley Street, Reading
Berks RG2 0EG
tel: 0118 975 7557

British Massage Council
Greenbank House
65a Adelphi Street
Preston
Lancs PR1 7BH
tel: 01772 881063

Colonic International Association
Cleanses the colon using purified water to flush away toxic waste, faeces, gas and mucus deposits.
16 Englands Lane
London NW3 4TG
tel: 0171 483 1595

Craniosacral Therapy
Body treatment, using subtle
manipulative techniques to aid in
rebalancing the body.
27 Old Gloucester Street
London WC1N 3XX
tel: 01886 884121

Feldenkrais Guild UK
Gentle therapy that encourages
awareness of movement and relieves
emotional, muscular and joint problems by increasing flexibility.
PO Box 370
London N10 3XA

**General Council and Register of
Naturopaths**
Uses diet, osteopathy and
hydrotherapy to treat illness and
rebalance.
Goswell House, 2 Goswell Road
Street, Somerset BA16 OJG
tel: 01458 840072

**Guild of Naturopathic
Iridologists**
The whole body is based on the
appearance of the eyes, since the
nervous system comes to the surface
of the body at this point. Examination of the iris pinpoints weakness.
94 Grosvenor Road
London SW1V 3LF
tel: 0171 834 3579

Homeopathic Trust
Hahnemann House
2 Powis Place, Great Ormond Street
London WC1N 3HT
tel: 0171 837 9469

**International Association for
Colour Therapy**
Treats mental, emotional and physi-
cal problems.
PO Box 3, Potter's Bar
Hertfordshire EN6 3ET

**ISDD (The Institute for the
Study of Drug Dependence)**
Waterbridge House, 32–36 Loman
Street, London SE1 0EE

Kinesiology Federation
Based on the principle that muscle
groups are related to body parts.
Muscle testing is used to detect
energy imbalances and blockages
through light touch, deep massage
and dietary advice.
PO Box 83, Sheffield S7 2YN
tel: 0114 281 4064

**Manual Lymphatic Drainage
(MLD)**
Gently stimulates the lymphatic sys-
tem, which supports the immune
system and helps to clear waste.
Aids lymphoedema, wounds, frac-
tures and chronic conditions.
PO Box 149, Wallingford
Oxfordshire OX10 7LD

**McTimoney Chiropractic
Association**
21 High Street, Eynsham
Oxfordshire OX8 1HE
tel: 01865 880974

Narcotics Anonymous
UK Service Office
PO Box 1980, London N19 3LS
tel: 0171 730 0009 or Freephone:
0800 214274

National Drugs Helpline
tel: 0800 77 66 00

**National Federation of Spiritual
Healers (NFSH)**
Old Manor Farm Studio
Church Street, Sunbury-on-Thames
Middlesex TW16 6RG
tel: 0891 616080

**National Institute of Medical
Herbalists**
56 Longbrook Street, Exeter
Devon EX4 6AH
tel: 01392 426022

Osteopathic Information Service
(Umbrella Organization)
PO Box 2974, Reading
Berks RG1 4YR
tel: 0118 951 2051

**Register of Chinese Herbal
Medicine**
PO Box 400, Middlesex HA9 9NZ
tel: 0171 224 0883

Rolfing – Bodywork
Deep manipulation of muscular
connective tissue to rebalance the
body by improving posture, relieving injuries and releasing trapped
emotions.
For further details call 0171 834
1493.

Shiatsu Society
Shiatsu means 'finger pressure' as
practitioners work with fingers and
thumbs to rebalance energy. An
ancient Japanese pressure point
technique, worked on the body's
pressure points.
Interchange Studios, Dalby Street
London NW5 3NQ
tel: 0171 813 7772

**Society for the Promotion of
Nutritional Therapy**
PO Box 47, Heathfield
East Sussex TN21 8ZX
tel: 01825 872921

**UK Council for
Psychotherapy (UKCP)**
167–169 Great Portland Street
London W1N 5FB
tel: 0171 436 3002

UK Polarity Therapy Association
Uses bodywork, awareness skills,
diet and stretching to heal.
Monomark House
27 Old Gloucester Street
London WC1N 3XX
tel: 01483 417714

Bibliography

MEDICAL BOOKS

Anon., *The First Aid Manual. 1997,* Dorling Kindersley, London.
A comprehensive manual, used and recommended by the St John Ambulance, the Red Cross and other organizations.

Gosling, J. & Harris P., *The Human Anatomy Colouring Book*, 1996, Mosby, USA.
A good learning aid, providing the medium of colour which helps students learn the systems of the body.

Pearce, Evelyn, *Anatomy & Physiology for Nurses*, Faber, 1995, London.
A good, basic training manual on anatomy and physiology.

Riddle, J., *Anatomy & Physiology Applied to Nursing*, Churchill Livingstone, 1985, New York.
A good, basic clinical training manual on anatomy and physiology.

Ross, Janet S. & Wilson, Kathleen J., *Anatomy & Physiology in Health and Illness*, Churchill Livingstone, 1989, London.
An English clinical training manual that expects readers to have a comprehensive understanding of anatomy and physiology. Good for nurses training in reflexology who wish to revise.

Rowntree, D., *Learn How to Study,* Warner Books, 1993, London.
A comprehensive guide for the student to study with many methods of learning to suit the individual.

Wood, Memmler Cohen, *The Human Body in Health and Disease*, Lippincott & Williams, 1992, New York.
An American clinical training manual in anatomy and physiology, comprehensive with a good page layout and written in simple language. Recommended for students in training.

POCKET DICTIONARIES

Good reference dictionaries are essential for a practising reflexologist and the following are recommended.

Dorland, William Alexander Newman, *Dorland's Pocket Medical Dictionary*, W.B. Saunders, 1995, New York.

Macpherson, G. (ed.) by *Black's Medical Dictionary*, A & C Black, 1992, London.

Weller, Barbara F. & Wells, Richard J., *Baillière's Medical Dictionary*, Baillière Tindall, 1990, London.

MISCELLANEOUS

Appleton, Nancy, *Lick The Sugar Habit*, Avery, 1997, USA.
An informative book on the effects of sugar on the body.

Becker, Robert and Selden, Gary, *Body Electric*, Aquarius, 1997, USA.
An informative book of the body as an energy field.

Bohm, David, *The Implicate Order*, Routledge & Kegan Paul, 1981, London.
An in-depth book suitable for serious students interested in new physics.

Brennan, Barbara Ann, *Hands of Light*, Bantam New Age Books, 1988, USA.
A must for all students in training in complementary medicine. Detailed drawings and text on understanding the human energy field.

Byers, D., *Better Health with Foot Reflexology*, Ingham Publishing, Inc., 1983.
A follow-up book on reflexology written by Eunice Ingham's nephew.

Capra, Fritjof, *The Tao of Physics,* Flamingo, 1991, London.
An exciting work by a renowned physicist on the nature of new physics. Suitable for the very serious student who wishes to understand energy from innovative concepts.

Capra, Fritjof, *The Turning Point*, Bantam New Age Books, 1988, New York.
An in-depth book written by a leading physicist in his field. Suitable for the very serious student who wishes to understand and develop understanding of energy concepts.

Everly, Jr., G.S., *A Clinical Guide to the Treatment of the Human Stress Response,* Plenum, 1989, New York.
A clinically written book for specialists in the field. Suitable for those wishing to develop an in-depth understanding of the stress response.

Furlong, M., *Flight of the Kingfisher,* Flamingo, 1997, London.
A beautifully detailed book on the Aboriginal culture.

Ingham, Eunice D., *Stories the Feet Have Told and Stories the Feet Can Tell,* Ingham Publishing, Inc., 1984.
The original work of Eunice Ingham who developed the 'Ingham Method' of working with reflexology in the 1930s. A must for every student training in reflexology or for those interested in learning more about the therapy.

Ostrom, J., *Understanding Auras,* Aqaurius, 1993, London.
A good introduction to the aura. Suitable for all students and the lay reader.

Pierrakos, John C., *The Core Energetic Process,* Monograph, 1977, New York.
An in-depth book suitable for the serious student interested in learning more about the human energy field and health problems.

Reich, Wilhelm, *Character Analysis,* Vision Press, 1950, London.
The theory and development of how the development of the physical body depends on the infant's emotional life from birth. Suitable for the very serious student who wishes to develop understanding of physical energy, or train in body psychotherapy.

Rinpoche, S., *The Tibetan Book of Living and Dying,* Rider, 1992, London.
The Eastern perspective of living and dying. A must for the serious student in complementary therapy training.

Sheldrake, R., *A New Science of Life,* Paladin, 1987, London.
An overview of new concepts of life and new physics. Suitable for the very serious student who wishes to understand concept of energy and manifestation of life forms.

Sheldrake, R., *The Rebirth of Nature,* Rider, 1990, London.
A metaphysical book, written by a well-known physicist. Suitable for the serious student who wishes to understand new physics and life forms.

Sills, F., *The Polarity Process,* Element Books, 1991, UK.
Based on the development of Ayurvedic medicine, this book is a mine of information for the serious student in understanding energy concepts, based on polarity therapy.

Walker, Kristine, *Hand Reflexology,* Key Books, 1996.
A text book for students.

REFERENCES

Dagogo-Jack, Samuel, et.al., *Robust Leptin Responses to Dexamethasone In Obese Subjects,* Journal of Clinical Endocrinology and Metabolism, Vol. 82 (10), pp. 3230–222, October 1997.

Fitzgerald, William H. and Bowers, Edwin F., *Zone Therapy,* Mokelumne Hill CA, Health Research, 1917.

Ghalioungui, Paul, *Health and Healing in Ancient Egypt,* Cairo, Dar Al-Maaref, 1965.

Head, Henry, *On Disturbance of Sensation with Especial reference To The Pain of Visceral Disease Parts I and II,* Brain, 1883.

Head, Henry, W., Rivers, H.R. and James, Sherren, *The Afferent Nervous System from a New Aspect,* Brain, 1905.

Ingham, Eunice, *Zone Therapy,* Ingham Publishing, Rochester, New York, 1945.

Kumar, Parveen and Clark, Michael, *Clinical Medicine,* Saunders, 1994, London.

Mookerjee, Ajit, *Tantra Asana,* Basilius Presse, Basel Switzerland, 1971.

Raine-Fenning, N. and Kilby, M. Division of Foetal Medicine, Birmingham Women's Hospital, *Foetal and Maternal Medicine Review,* 1997: 9:1-17, Cambridge University Press.

Riley, Elizabeth Ann, *Class Lessons in Zone Therapy, Reflex Technique and Hook Work, Correspondence Course in Zone Therapy, Reflex Technique and Hook Work,* Mokelumne Hill CA, Health and research, 1959.

Riley, Joe Shelby, *Zone Reflex,* Mokelumne Hill, CA, Health research, 1942.

Tay, Geraldine and Khaw, Eu Hooi, *The Rwo Shur Health Method,* Trans. Gerdine Co., 1988.

Index

333